Parenting and Child/Adolescent Development: Current Updates and Global Perspectives

Parenting and Child/Adolescent Development: Current Updates and Global Perspectives

Guest Editors

Elitsa Dimitrova
Apolinaras Zaborskis

MDPI

Basel • Beijing • Wuhan • Barcelona • Belgrade • Novi Sad • Cluj • Manchester

Guest Editors

Elitsa Dimitrova
Department of Demography
Institute for Population and
Human Studies – Bulgarian
Academy of Sciences
Sofia
Bulgaria

Apolinaras Zaborskis
Department of Preventive
Medicine & Health Research
Institute
Lithuanian University of
Health Sciences
Kaunas
Lithuania

Editorial Office
MDPI AG
Grosspeteranlage 5
4052 Basel, Switzerland

This is a reprint of the Special Issue, published open access by the journal *Children* (ISSN 2227-9067), freely accessible at: https://www.mdpi.com/journal/children/special_issues/7839X9JHQQ.

For citation purposes, cite each article independently as indicated on the article page online and as indicated below:

Lastname, A.A.; Lastname, B.B. Article Title. *Journal Name* **Year**, *Volume Number*, Page Range.

ISBN 978-3-7258-6161-3 (Hbk)
ISBN 978-3-7258-6162-0 (PDF)
https://doi.org/10.3390/books978-3-7258-6162-0

Contents

About the Editors

Elitsa Dimitrova

Elitsa Dimitrova is an Associate Professor in Sociology and Social Demography at the Institute for Population and Human Studies, Bulgarian Academy of Sciences and Plovdiv University Paisii Hilendarski. She works in the field of fertility and family studies, young people's health and well-being, early child education and care, child poverty and social exclusion, demographic and family policies, work-life balance, parental leave arrangements and social sustainability.

Apolinaras Zaborskis

Apolinaras Zaborskis Professor Habilated Doctor graduated from the Faculty of Biophysics of Kaunas Institute of Medicine (Lithuania). He is currently a Professor Emeritus at the Faculty of Public Health of the Lithuanian University of Health Sciences. His areas of research include the lifestyle of children and adolescents, health and quality of life, health inequalities, and biostatistics. He has published more than 200 scientific articles.

children

MDPI

Editorial

Parenting and Child/Adolescent Development: Current Updates and Global Perspectives

Elitsa Dimitrova [1,*] and Apolinaras Zaborskis [2]

1 Institute for Population and Human Studies, Bulgarian Academy of Sciences & Plovdiv University Paisii Hilendarski, 1000 Sofia, Bulgaria

2 Department of Preventive Medicine & Health Research Institute, Faculty of Public Health, Medical Academy, Lithuanian University of Health Sciences, A.Mickevičiaus 9, LT-44307 Kaunas, Lithuania; apolinaras.zaborskis@lsmu.lt

* Correspondence: e.dimitrova@iphs.eu

This Special Issue, titled "Parenting and Child/Adolescent Development: Current Updates and Global Perspectives", brings together a diverse collection of ten articles that examine the complex challenges and opportunities shaping children's and adolescents' lives today. Despite addressing varied topics and contexts, the articles converge on several cross-cutting themes: the central role of the family in development, the dynamic balance between risk and protective factors, the necessity of cultural sensitivity, the value of interventions that strengthen families, and the importance of broader systemic supports. Expanding on these themes in light of both the contributions in this issue and the wider scholarly literature offers a more nuanced understanding of how children's lives unfold within their developmental contexts.

1. Introduction

Family dynamics, parenting practices, and parent/caregiver–child relationships have a formative influence on children's health, well-being, and socioemotional, cognitive, and neurobiological development, with effects that extend into later life [1,2]. Family connectedness, communication, and relationships with parents and relatives not only provide important role models but also shape identity formation and the adoption of skills and behaviors during adolescence [3,4]. For adolescents in particular, connections with family, peers, and community play a critical role in their development, as argued by Robert Blum and colleagues [5]. Supportive networks of parents, peers, and teachers have been shown to improve adolescent mental and behavioral health, with lasting benefits across the life course [6,7]. By contrast, youth development programs that frame adolescents as problems to be fixed tend to be ineffective, yet governments and non-governmental organizations continue to invest in them [8].

The evidence reviewed above demonstrates that family dynamics and relationships are central to child and adolescent development across multiple domains—including health, well-being, socioemotional functioning, cognition, and neurobiological processes. Importantly, their influence extends across diverse cultural, social, and economic contexts and is not confined to Western, high-income settings. Alongside this recognition, scholarship increasingly emphasizes the interconnectedness of ecological systems—families, peers, schools, and communities—and the ways in which these overlapping spheres interact to collectively shape developmental trajectories.

At the same time, a substantial body of research continues to document the limited effectiveness of punitive or deficit-oriented interventions that frame young people primarily as problems to be managed [8]. These findings have fueled momentum toward evidence-based approaches that promote positive youth development, emphasizing strengths, agency, and supportive environments. This global reorientation reflects not only a rejection of narrow, problem-focused models but also a paradigm shift toward holistic, contextually grounded strategies. Such approaches acknowledge the diversity of adolescent experiences, highlight the critical role of relational and ecological supports, and position adolescents as active partners in shaping their own health, well-being, and future prospects [5,9,10].

The articles published in this Special Issue respond directly to current challenges in the field facing children, adolescents, and families today. Accordingly, this editorial article seeks to organize them around several cross-cutting themes that address both enduring concerns and emerging opportunities. Together, these contributions are expected not only to deepen our understanding of how development unfolds across diverse contexts but also to illuminate innovative pathways for advancing research, informing practice, and shaping policy.

2. The Family as a Central Developmental Context

Family processes are consistently shown to be pivotal in shaping developmental trajectories. Jeong and Bang (contribution 1) highlight how adolescents in immigrant marriage families often provide "unavoidable family assistance, even under pressure." Their experiences reveal both empathy toward immigrant mothers and stress when paternal involvement is diminished. Similarly, Chan et al. (contribution 2) emphasize that parental "emotion talk" significantly shapes preschoolers' expression of anger, sadness, and positive emotions, supporting the notion that parental practices are central to children's socioemotional development.

The literature broadly confirms that families constitute the primary ecological system in Bronfenbrenner's (1979) Ecological Systems Theory [11]. Parenting behaviors, family communication, and emotional climates all affect how children regulate emotions, develop social skills, and manage stress [12]. Positive co-parenting, as Seijo et al. (contribution 3) argue, is associated with "healthy development of children," reinforcing that family harmony is a cornerstone of resilience. Conversely, conflict, neglect, or imbalanced role expectations, as seen in both immigrant families and foster care transitions, may create stressors with long-term consequences.

3. The Interplay of Risk and Protective Factors

A second unifying theme is the constant interplay between vulnerabilities and buffers. Nesmith (contribution 4) shows that foster youth aging out of care are at risk of "homelessness and social disconnection," yet the Bridges Transitions Framework fostered moderate to high levels of social support and higher school enrollment compared with state averages. Similarly, Valentic et al. (contribution 5) reveal that "maternal monitoring" strongly protects Croatian adolescents against substance use and bullying, while Dimitrova and Alexandrova-Karamanova (contribution 6) demonstrate that parental unemployment and economic stress increased Bulgarian adolescents' health risk behaviors during the pandemic.

This duality is echoed in developmental criminology. Zúñiga et al. (contribution 7) identify biological, socioemotional, and contextual risk factors that elevate the likelihood of transgressive behavior, while protective factors include "cognitive, socioemotional, and personality development aspects." Together, these findings confirm Masten's (2001) seminal argument that resilience is "ordinary magic," emerging when protective processes such as supportive relationships, self-regulation, and positive identity buffer the effects of adversity [13].

Protective factors often work relationally: Hadar (contribution 8) demonstrates how music therapy empowered displaced families to rediscover a "sense of agency… through controlling the musical environment." This aligns with Bowlby's (1969) Attachment Theory, which emphasizes the role of secure caregiver–child bonds in mitigating trauma [14]. Risk and protection, therefore, must be viewed not as static traits but as dynamic processes embedded in everyday interactions.

4. Cultural and Contextual Sensitivity

Across contexts, the studies demonstrate that children's development is inseparable from cultural expectations and structural realities. Chan et al. (contribution 2) found cultural differences between Chinese American and Mexican American preschoolers: Mexican American children expressed more anger and sadness, reflecting cultural norms around emotional expression. Jeong and Bang (contribution 1) emphasize that Korean adolescents in immigrant families felt a "natural" obligation to support their mothers, shaped by Confucian traditions of filial duty and gender role expectations.

Correia et al. (contribution 9) in Cape Verde show how a family education program enhanced parental competence, but the degree of benefit varied across clusters, suggesting that cultural beliefs and parenting profiles mediate outcomes. Likewise, Seijo et al. (contribution 3) adapted the Coparenting Relationship Scale for Spanish parents, demonstrating the necessity of ensuring psychometric tools are culturally valid.

The literature reinforces this need for cultural grounding. Harkness and Super's (1994) developmental niche framework argues that cultural settings shape parental ethnotheories, daily routines, and physical environments, which in turn shape child development [15]. Without attending to these cultural lenses, interventions risk being ineffective or even harmful [16].

5. The Importance of Interventions That Strengthen Families

Another shared theme is the promise of interventions that empower families rather than targeting children in isolation. Hadar (contribution 8) illustrates how dyadic music therapy "restored the children's freedom of play" and parents' sense of competence. Correia et al. (contribution 9) show that the Family Education and Support Program promoted positive parenting practices and increased parental efficacy. Nesmith (contribution 4) demonstrates that integrating a structured transition framework into foster care supports internal coping and social support among youth leaving care.

These interventions reflect a paradigm shift toward systemic and relational approaches. Child–Parent Psychotherapy [17,18] has long emphasized the dyad as the unit of intervention, while Triple P [19,20] and other evidence-based parenting programs highlight the role of parental self-efficacy in promoting child well-being. The findings across the ten studies support the view that strengthening parental skills, fostering supportive co-parenting, and providing structured guidance during transitions yield protective ripple effects for children.

6. The Role of Broader Systems

Finally, the studies highlight how families are embedded in larger systems—schools, communities, and governments—that profoundly affect child outcomes. Groff et al. (contribution 10) found that "live online classes protected parents and children" during homeschooling, while a lack of adequate support compounded stress. Dimitrova and Alexandrova-Karamanova (contribution 6) show how macroeconomic shocks such as "income reduction and temporary lay-offs" cascaded into adolescent substance use. Zúñiga et al. (contribution 7) emphasize that risk and protective factors extend to "family, school, peers, socioeconomic situation and governance," requiring multi-level interventions.

This resonates with Bronfenbrenner's ecological model [11], which situates the child within interconnected systems from the microsystem of family to the macrosystem of policy and culture. Public health crises like COVID-19 and structural conditions like unemployment demonstrate that no family operates in isolation. Research on social determinants of health [21] further underscores how inequities in income, housing, and education shape child outcomes long before individual-level interventions take place.

7. Conclusions

In synthesizing these ten studies, five cross-cutting themes stand out. Families remain the central developmental context, but their ability to nurture is shaped by the interplay of risk and protective factors, the cultural milieu in which they operate, the strength of interventions that empower them, and the broader systems within which they are embedded. Together, the evidence paints a picture of child and adolescent development as a dynamic process—shaped by both vulnerability and resilience, grounded in culture, and profoundly relational.

To move forward, research and practice must adopt an integrated perspective: one that not only identifies risks but also strengthens protective mechanisms across levels, from parent–child relationships to community supports and public policy. Doing so honors the complexity of children's lived experiences while advancing the goal shared across all these studies: enabling every child to grow in environments that promote health, competence, and well-being.

Author Contributions: Conceptualization, E.D. and A.Z.; methodology, E.D. and A.Z.; writing—original draft preparation, A.Z.; writing—review and editing, E.D.; visualization, A.Z.; supervision, E.D.; project administration, E.D. All authors have read and agreed to the published version of the manuscript.

Funding: This research received no external funding.

Conflicts of Interest: The authors declare no conflicts of interest.

List of Contributions:

1. Jeong, Y.; Bang, K.-S. Family Assistance Experiences of Adolescents in Marriage Immigrant Families. *Children* **2025**, *12*, 862. https://doi.org/10.3390/children12070862.
2. Chan, M.; Taw, M.; Eisenberg, N.; Zhou, Q. Relations Between Parental Emotion Talk and Preschoolers' Emotion Expressions in Low-Income Chinese American and Mexican American Families. *Children* **2025**, *12*, 52. https://doi.org/10.3390/children12010052.
3. Seijo, D.; Fariña, F.; Fernández, M.P.; Arce, R. Adaptation of the Coparenting Relationship Scale Questionnaire to Spanish Parents with Offspring. *Children* **2024**, *11*, 535. https://doi.org/10.3390/children11050535.
4. Nesmith, A.A. Managing Major Life Changes: An Exploratory Study Using the Bridges Transitions Framework to Help Foster Youth Prepare for Discharge. *Children* **2025**, *12*, 22. https://doi.org/10.3390/children12010022.
5. Valentic, M.; Simetin, L.; Mayer, D.; Simetin, F.; Pavic, I. The Impact of Parental Monitoring on Exposure to Multiple Substances and Bullying in Croatian Students. *Children* **2024**, *11*, 1292. https://doi.org/10.3390/children11111292.
6. Dimitrova, E.; Alexandrova-Karamanova, A. Family Dynamics, Socioeconomic Hardships, and Health Risk Behaviours of Bulgarian Adolescents during the COVID-19 Pandemic. *Children* **2024**, *11*, 1016. https://doi.org/10.3390/children11081016.
7. Zúñiga, D.; Carretta, F.; Contreras, M.; Cornejo, E.; Gallardo, C.; Guichapani, I.; Muñoz, C. Systematic Review of Psychosocial Risk and Protective Factors in Children Reported from Developmental Criminology. *Children* **2024**, *11*, 974. https://doi.org/10.3390/children11080974.

8. Hadar, T. Parenting in the Face of Trauma: Music Therapy to Support Parent–Child Dyads Affected by War and Displacement. *Children* **2024**, *11*, 1269. https://doi.org/10.3390/children11101269.
9. Correia, A.; Martins, C.; Santos, R.d.; Hidalgo, V.; Jesus, S.N.d.; Nunes, C. Who Benefits Most from the Family Education and Support Program in Cape Verde? A Cluster Analysis. *Children* **2024**, *11*, 782. https://doi.org/10.3390/children11070782.
10. Groff, L.V.M.; Elgendi, M.M.; Stewart, S.H.; Deacon, S.H. Long-Term Mandatory Homeschooling during COVID-19 Had Compounding Mental Health Effects on Parents and Children. *Children* **2024**, *11*, 1072. https://doi.org/10.3390/children11091072.

References

1. Bornstein, M.H. (Ed.) *Handbook of Parenting*, 3rd ed.; Routledge: New York, NY, USA, 2015.
2. Britto, P.R.; Lye, S.J.; Proulx, K.; Yousafzai, A.K.; Matthews, S.G.; Vaivada, T.; Perez-Escamilla, R.; Rao, N.; Ip, P.; Fernald, L.C.H.; et al. Nurturing care: Promoting early childhood development. *Lancet* **2017**, *389*, 91–102. [CrossRef] [PubMed]
3. Merlo, G.; Snellman, L.; Sugden, S.G. Connectedness: The Updated and Expanded Pillar of Lifestyle Psychiatry and Lifestyle Medicine. *Am. J. Lifestyle Med.* **2025**, 15598276251345455. [CrossRef] [PubMed]
4. Too, E.K.; Chongwo, E.; Mabrouk, A.; Abubakar, A. Adolescent Connectedness: A Scoping Review of Available Measures and Their Psychometric Properties. *Front. Psychol.* **2022**, *13*, 856621. [CrossRef] [PubMed]
5. Blum, R.W.; Lai, J.; Martinez, M.; Jessee, C. Adolescent connectedness: Cornerstone for health and wellbeing. *BMJ* **2022**, *379*, e069213. [CrossRef] [PubMed]
6. Hoferichter, F.; Kulakow, S.; Hufenbach, M.C. Support From Parents, Peers, and Teachers Is Differently Associated with Middle School Students' Well-Being. *Front. Psychol.* **2021**, *12*, 758226. [CrossRef] [PubMed]
7. Ehsan, A.; Klaas, H.S.; Bastianen, A.; Spini, D. Social capital and health: A systematic review of systematic reviews. *SSM Popul. Health* **2019**, *8*, 100425. [CrossRef] [PubMed]
8. Petrosino, A.; Turpin-Petrosino, C.; Hollis-Peel, M.E.; Lavenberg, J.G. 'Scared Straight' and other juvenile awareness programs for preventing juvenile delinquency. *Cochrane Database Syst. Rev.* **2013**, *4*, CD002796. [CrossRef] [PubMed]
9. Patton, G.C.; Sawyer, S.M.; Santelli, J.S.; Ross, D.A.; Afifi, R.; Allen, N.B.; Arora, M.; Azzopardi, P.; Baldwin, W.; Bonell, C.; et al. Our future: A Lancet commission on adolescent health and wellbeing. *Lancet* **2016**, *387*, 2423–2478. [CrossRef] [PubMed]
10. World Health Organization. *Working for a Brighter, Healthier Future: How WHO Improves Health and Promotes Well-Being for the World's Adolescents*; World Health Organization: Geneva, Switzerland, 2020.
11. Guy-Evans, O. Bronfenbrenner's Ecological System Theory. *Simply Psychol.* **2025**. Available online: https://www.simplypsychology.org/bronfenbrenner.html (accessed on 19 September 2025).
12. Starrs, B. *Adolescent Configuration Styles, Parenting and Psychotherapy: A Relational Perspective*, 1st ed.; Routledge: London, UK, 2023.
13. Masten, A.S.; Narayan, A.J.; Wright, M.O. Resilience Processes in Development: Multisystem Integration Emerging from Four Waves of Research. In *Handbook of Resilience in Children*; Goldstein, S., Brooks, R.B., Eds.; Springer Nature: Cham, Switzerland, 2023. [CrossRef]
14. Jones, S.M. Attachment Theory. In *The International Encyclopedia of Interpersonal Communication*; Berger, C.R., Roloff, M.E., Wilson, S.R., Dillard, J.P., Caughlin, J., Solomon, D., Eds.; John Wiley & Sons, Inc.: Hoboken, NJ, USA, 2015. [CrossRef]
15. Harkness, S.; Super, C.M. The developmental niche: A theoretical framework for analyzing the household production of health. *Soc. Sci. Med.* **1994**, *38*, 217–226. [CrossRef] [PubMed]
16. Rogoff, B. *The Cultural Nature of Human Development*; Oxford University Press: New York, NY, USA, 2003.
17. Lieberman, A.F.; Van Horn, P.; Ghosh Ippen, C. Toward evidence-based treatment: Child–Parent Psychotherapy with preschoolers exposed to marital violence. *J. Am. Acad. Child Adolesc. Psychiatry* **2005**, *44*, 1241–1248. [CrossRef] [PubMed]
18. Shafi, R.M.A.; Bieber, E.D.; Shekunov, J.; Croarkin, P.E.; Romanowicz, M. Evidence Based Dyadic Therapies for 0- to 5-Year-Old Children with Emotional and Behavioral Difficulties. *Front. Psychiatry* **2019**, *10*, 677. [CrossRef] [PubMed]
19. Sanders, M.R. Triple P-Positive Parenting Program: Towards an empirically validated multilevel parenting and family support strategy for the prevention of behavior and emotional problems in children. *Clin. Child Fam. Psychol. Rev.* **1999**, *2*, 71–90. [CrossRef] [PubMed]
20. Sanders, M.R.; Kirby, J.N.; Tellegen, C.L.; Day, J.J. The Triple P-Positive Parenting Program: A systematic review and meta-analysis of a multi-level system of parenting support. *Clin. Psychol. Rev.* **2014**, *4*, 337–357. [CrossRef] [PubMed]
21. Marmot, M. Social determinants of health inequalities. *Lancet* **2005**, *365*, 1099–1104. [CrossRef] [PubMed]

children

MDPI

Article

Family Assistance Experiences of Adolescents in Marriage Immigrant Families

Yeseul Jeong [1,2] and Kyung-Sook Bang [3,*]

1 College of Nursing, Keimyung University, Daegu 42601, Republic of Korea; yeseuljeong@kmu.ac.kr
2 Research Institute of Nursing Science, Keimyung University, Daegu 42601, Republic of Korea
3 College of Nursing, The Research Institute of Nursing Science, Seoul National University, Seoul 03080, Republic of Korea
* Correspondence: ksbang@snu.ac.kr; Tel.: +82-2-740-8819

Abstract

Background/Objectives: Family assistance by adolescents (e.g., cooking, cleaning, listening to family members) is a common phenomenon. However, the impact of such assistance on adolescent development remains a topic of debate. Increasingly, the importance of adolescents' own perceptions and interpretations is being emphasized in understanding how family assistance influences their development. Adolescents in marriage immigrant families may face unique psychosocial challenges as they support their immigrant parents. This study explores the family assistance experiences of adolescents in marriage immigrant families. **Methods**: Data were collected through one-on-one in-depth interviews with 10 adolescents aged 13–18 years from currently married marriage immigrant families, all of whom were born in Korea. The interviews were conducted between October and November 2022. The data were analyzed using interpretative phenomenological analysis. **Results**: The family assistance experiences were categorized into three main themes, namely, "Old enough to help—naturally, and rightly so", "Foreign mother whom I naturally come to help", and "Unavoidable family assistance, even under pressure", and 10 subordinate themes. The adolescents provided support naturally, grounded in familial obligation and empathy toward their immigrant mothers. When the native Korean father shared the responsibilities, the assistance was not perceived as burdensome. However, diminished paternal involvement, traditional gender role expectations, and unmet emotional or academic needs led to more negative perceptions and psychological stress. **Conclusions**: Support systems are needed to ensure that adolescents do not assume sole responsibility for both the native father's and the immigrant mother's roles within marriage immigrant families.

Keywords: adolescent; immigrant family; family assistance; parentification; qualitative research; phenomenology

1. Introduction

In South Korea, international marriages have rapidly increased from 3.7% of all marriages in 2000 to 10.1% in 2023 [1]. Accordingly, the number of children from multicultural families has increased approximately fivefold, from 58,007 in 2008 to 299,440 in 2022 [2]. In particular, the number of adolescent children aged 13 to 18 surged from 6176 in 2008 to 80,840 in 2022 [2].

Adolescence is a developmental period marked by extensive physical, psychosocial, and cognitive growth, during which individuals prepare for a healthy transition into adulthood. During this time, various factors can influence adolescents' growth and development, and family support is one such factor. Family assistance refers to activities such as helping with household chores or caring for younger siblings, as well as providing moderate emotional support, including listening to and empathizing with family members [3]. This concept is distinct from not only parentification, whereby developmentally inappropriate adult roles or responsibilities are expected from children [4,5], but also young caregiving, whereby children provide intensive and time-consuming care such as assisting with meals, dressing, or toileting for ill, disabled, or aging family members [3]. During adolescence, individuals experience significant physical growth, social interactions, skill acquisition, and enhanced cognitive and social awareness, all of which can improve their capacity to assist others [6]. Consequently, adolescents may become more capable of supporting their families, and parents may, in turn, come to expect more assistance from them. Performing newly assigned roles and meeting these expectations can, in turn, influence adolescents' development and well-being.

Family assistance has both positive and negative effects on adolescents' health and development [3,7]. For example, positive health outcomes, such as improved sleep quality, fewer physical symptoms, and reduced physiological stress responses, have been reported [8–10]. Conversely, other studies have found associations between family assistance and negative outcomes, such as increased substance use or elevated levels of C-reactive protein (CRP), a biomarker of inflammation [11,12]. While the fragmented nature of the existing studies presents a limitation, the inconsistency in the findings highlights the complexity of the effects that family assistance may have on individuals, suggesting that its impact is not straightforward.

For adolescents from immigrant families, the types and levels of family assistance expected may differ due to their family's migration background; nonetheless, both positive and negative outcomes have been reported in this group as well. Immigrant adolescents may act as cultural and linguistic brokers for their parents—who typically adapt to the host society more slowly—and may take on responsibilities uncommon among their non-immigrant peers, such as translating official documents or assisting with family financial issues [13]. While such roles may expose these adolescents to experiences of discrimination or psychological stress due to excessive responsibilities [14,15], they may also foster family adaptation and the development of adolescents' social skills, self-efficacy, and self-esteem [13].

These divergent findings in the existing literature suggest that the impact of family assistance is shaped not only by the task itself but also by contextual factors and adolescents' own perceptions of their roles. One study reported that family assistance in high-conflict households is linked to increased substance use [11]. Additionally, Lam et al. [16] found that family assistance has been associated with depressive symptoms and declining academic performance only in contexts of high parental conflict or low family values [16]. Similarly, Lazarevic [15] found that among immigrant adolescents, negative family dynamics can exacerbate the burdens of discrimination and lead to role reversals, indicating the importance of context in shaping these experiences. These findings highlight the need to explore adolescents' subjective experiences of family assistance.

Despite this need, the extant literature has focused on parentification or young caregiving [14,17], and comprehensive research on adolescents' everyday family assistance and their own perceptions and meanings of such experiences is lacking.

Particularly, examining the family assistance experiences of adolescents from marriage immigrant families—who are likely to face compounded difficulties owing to their background—from their own perspectives is essential as a foundational step in supporting their healthy development and adjustment. Therefore, this study seeks to comprehensively explore the lived experiences and meanings of family assistance among adolescents from marriage immigrant families through interpretative phenomenological analysis (IPA).

2. Materials and Methods

2.1. Research Design

This study employed a qualitative research design using IPA to deeply examine the family assistance experiences of adolescents from marriage immigrant families.

2.2. Data Collection

2.2.1. Participant Selection

This study recruited participants through purposive sampling. Participants were adolescents, aged 13–18 years (mean age: 14 years), who were born in Korea and from marriage immigrant families, in which the parents were currently married. All the participants could communicate in Korean, were legally minors, living in households, and without intellectual or physical disabilities. All the immigrant parents were mothers, and their countries of origin were the Philippines, Vietnam, Pakistan, and Indonesia.

2.2.2. Participant Recruitment

Participants were recruited by posting study announcements at two multicultural centers, one community children's center, and one online community for marriage immigrants. Adolescents who saw the announcement and expressed interest contacted the researcher directly, received a detailed explanation of this study, and subsequently decided to participate.

2.2.3. Data Collection Procedure

Data were collected through one-on-one in-depth interviews conducted from November to December 2022. The interview method, location, and time were decided based on participant preferences. Nine interviews were conducted at cafes or a private room in the center, and one was conducted using a real-time video-conferencing platform. As the data collection occurred during the COVID-19 pandemic, the participant chose to participate online. The mode of interview did not pose any limitations.

To create a comfortable atmosphere, the researcher offered refreshments and engaged in icebreaking activities before the interviews. Participants also completed a general demographic questionnaire. Special care was taken to build a rapport with participants, particularly by the adult female researcher, who explicitly expressed appreciation and respect for the adolescents as experts on their own experiences, thereby minimizing the discomfort stemming from adult–adolescent hierarchies.

The interviews were guided by a semi-structured protocol developed through a pilot study. The interview guide consisted of approximately ten open-ended questions. Examples of these questions included the following: "Can you describe a typical day at home?", "How is household labor shared in your family?", "How do you usually help your family?", "How do your family members respond when you help?", and "What is your relationship like with your parents?" Follow-up and probing questions were used when necessary to further clarify or explore participants' responses.

Each interview lasted for an average of 1 h and 35 min, and all the interviews were conducted once per participant. The interviews were audio-recorded, the researcher took field notes during the interviews, and all the recordings were transcribed verbatim by the researcher. Two participants reviewed their transcripts to verify the accuracy of the transcriptions and ensure that their statements were accurately reflected. The data collection was concluded when saturation was reached, that is, when no new themes or information emerged and the interview content became repetitive with no additional insights.

2.3. Data Analysis

The data were analyzed following the IPA approach outlined by Smith and Nizza [18] and Smith, Flowers, and Larkin [19]. IPA is a qualitative research methodology that inductively explores how individuals perceive and make sense of their lived experiences. Rooted in phenomenology, hermeneutics, and idiography, IPA involves interpreting data collected from participants through the processes of phenomenological reduction and the hermeneutic circle. This approach emphasizes an in-depth, rigorous, and detailed examination of specific cases, aiming to illuminate participants' experiences through rich descriptions and analyses that capture both individual and shared meanings.

The data collection and analysis were conducted concurrently. We maintained a reflexive stance throughout the process to prevent the fore-conception from distorting participants' lived experiences. The transcripts and field notes were repeatedly examined to not only become immersed in the data but also identify the distinctive and structural elements of each participant's experience. Exploratory notes were developed and synthesized into experiential statements. These statements were then physically arranged and clustered to develop a table of personal experiential themes for each participant. After conducting the individual case analyses, a cross-case analysis was performed to derive group experiential themes and subthemes, which were subsequently labeled as themes and subthemes, respectively.

2.4. Ethical Considerations

This study was reviewed and approved by the Institutional Review Board (IRB) of Seoul National University to ensure the ethical protection of research participants (IRB No. 2209/003-012), and the ethical procedures were strictly followed.

Before the data collection, an online pre-meeting was conducted with potential participants to explain this study using a shared screen displaying the consent form and study explanation. Participants were informed of this study's objectives, procedures, use of audio recordings, data anonymization, and data storage and usage. Participation was entirely voluntary, and it was explained that participants could withdraw at any time without any disadvantage; if withdrawn, all the data would be immediately discarded. Written informed consent was obtained from both the participants and their legal guardians, and consent was reconfirmed on the day of the interview before proceeding.

2.5. Rigor

The researchers were trained in qualitative research methods and had hands-on experience of conducting and analyzing qualitative studies. Prior to the data collection, the relevant literature and media were critically reviewed, and one researcher (YJ) reflected on the personal experiences of having immigrant relatives. A pilot study was conducted to develop the interview guide, which was further refined during this study based on the emerging themes. Purposeful sampling ensured the selection of appropriate participants, and the data collection continued until saturation was reached. Efforts were made to create a comfortable interview environment, empathize with participants' experiences, and affirm them as experts on their own lived realities. The researcher (YJ) collected data directly from participants and transcribed it verbatim. To enhance the analytical rigor, the analysis was thoroughly interpretative and focused on individual cases before synthesizing across cases, following Smith and Nizza's [18] approach. Bracketing was applied throughout the process to reduce the bias from the researchers' fore-conceptions. Additionally, feedback was obtained from a third party experienced in qualitative research, and the results were member-checked with two participants.

To enhance transparency and rigor, this study followed the COREQ checklist [20], detailing the participant recruitment, data collection, analysis, and findings. Efforts were made to ensure a logical writing structure and clarity, with detailed descriptions and appropriate quotations.

3. Results

3.1. General Characteristics of the Participants

The study participants were 10 adolescents from marriage immigrant families. The majority were female (n = 7, 70.0%) and high school students (n = 6, 60.0%) (Table 1). The average age of the participants was 15 years (range: 13–18), and the average ages of their fathers and mothers were 53.6 years (range: 45–63) and 39.1 years (range: 34–55), respectively. The mothers' countries of origin were the Philippines (n = 4, 40.0%), Vietnam (n = 4, 40.0%), Pakistan (n = 1, 10.0%), and Indonesia (n = 1, 10.0%). According to the adolescent participants, their immigrant mothers' Korean language proficiency was rated as "high" in the following areas: speaking by eight participants (80.0%), listening by six participants (60.0%), reading by two participants (20.0%), and writing by two participants (20.0%).

Table 1. Characteristics of the participants.

Participant No.		1	2	3	4	5	6	7	8	9	10
Age		13	17	17	18	13	14	14	14	13	17
Sex		Female	Male	Female	Male	Female	Female	Female	Male	Female	Female
Age of Father		45	50	51	61	63	56	54	57	47	52
Age of Mother		34	42	41	40	40	34	35	35	35	55
Father's Educational Level		High school	Under-graduate	Middle school	Under-graduate	High school	High school	High school	High school	High school	High school
Mother's Educational Level		Middle school	Under-graduate	Under-graduate	Graduate	Under-graduate	Primary school	Under-graduate	High school	High school	Under-graduate
Mother's Country of Origin		Pakistan	Philippines	Philippines	Philippines	Philippines	Vietnam	Vietnam	Vietnam	Vietnam	Indonesia
Mother's Korean Profi-ciency	Speaking	High	High	High	Low	High	Middle	High	High	High	High
	Listening	High	Middle	High	Middle	High	Middle	High	High	Middle	High
	Reading	Middle	Middle	Middle	Middle	High	Low	High	Middle	Middle	Middle
	Writing	Middle	Middle	Middle	Low	Low	Low	High	High	Low	Middle
Age of Sibling(s)		11, 5				32, 29	13	12	3		18

3.2. Experiences of Family Assistance Among Adolescents from Marriage Immigrant Families

The family assistance experiences of adolescents from marriage immigrant families were categorized into three main themes, namely, "Old enough to help—naturally, and rightly so", "Foreign mother whom I naturally come to help", and "Unavoidable family assistance, even under pressure", with a total of ten subthemes being identified (Table 2).

Table 2. List of themes and subthemes of the family assistance experiences of adolescents in marriage immigrant families.

Theme 1. Old enough to help—naturally, and rightly so
(1) Things that an adolescent—not a child—can take on
(2) Learning and preparing for the tasks I will face when I grow up
(3) Family means helping one another.

Table 2. *Cont.*

Theme 2. Foreign mother whom I naturally come to help
(1) Being told to help my immigrant mother (2) Driven by empathy for my immigrant mom (3) Assisting with mom's small but constant language struggles
Theme 3. Unavoidable family assistance, even under pressure
(1) Carrying the weight of the father's role too soon (2) Forced into traditional but outdated roles (3) Unassisted academic struggles (4) A language barrier too thick to truly touch the heart

3.2.1. Old Enough to Help—Naturally, and Rightly So

This theme describes the participants' internal standards and perceptions that led them to accept family assistance as a natural and rightful responsibility.

Things That an Adolescent—Not a Child—Can Take on

All the participants engaged in various household chores, such as laundry and cleaning, to help their families. While some assistance was voluntary, most occurred in response to direct requests from parents. The adolescents recognized that the type and degree of assistance expected by their parents changed as they matured. Tasks that were once difficult owing to physical limitations or immaturity were now manageable thanks to their growth and development. They understood the new expectations as something feasible due to their physical and emotional maturity, which helped them accept these roles regardless of whether the tasks were voluntary.

> *"The food waste bin is kind of big. So, my parents started asking me to take it out once I got tall enough". (Participant 7)*

> *"Now that I'm 14, I guess they trust me more. When I was younger, they didn't really believe in me". (Participant 1)*

The participants expressed satisfaction and a sense of achievement when completing difficult or higher-responsibility tasks. When their parents acknowledged or praised their efforts, they perceived themselves as capable and competent, thus contributing to a positive self-image.

> *"My mom and dad say I have a knack for taking care of my little sibling. When the baby sleeps well, it feels nice and fulfilling". (Participant 1)*

Learning and Preparing for the Tasks I Will Face When I Grow up

Most participants helped their mothers, who primarily managed the household duties. They learned chores step-by-step from their parents and assisted them accordingly. The responsibilities were not overly burdensome in terms of the difficulty, quantity, frequency, or responsibility, so the participants viewed the tasks as somewhat annoying but manageable. Moreover, they regarded the experience as a form of learning and preparation for adulthood—a way of acquiring skills they would eventually need.

> *"When I vacuumed the wrong way, my dad said, 'This is how you should do it', and demonstrated it to me". (Participant 8)*

> *"I think of it as practice for when I grow up. I'll have to clean like this then, too". (Participant 3)*

Family Means Helping One Another

The participants frequently heard from both family and society that children should help their parents and that family members were supposed to support each other. This message helped internalize family assistance as a natural responsibility. Additionally, their own experiences of receiving help from relatives purely because of familial ties further reinforced the value of mutual support. To them, helping their family was a way to not only uphold family values but also repay the support they had received. The participants evaluated themselves as "good" people by duly embracing these family values, showing that family support can help form positive self-evaluation.

> *"When I was sick, my mom and I went to the university hospital with my aunt. She helped with the diagnosis and explained everything to my mom". (Participant 6)*

> *"I might not be the best at everything, but I think I'm decent. I listen to my parents and try to do what they ask, even if I'm not good at it". (Participant 1)*

3.2.2. Foreign Mother Whom I Naturally Come to Help

This theme captures how the participants perceived their immigrant mothers as individuals in need of help and how assisting their mothers became a familiar, normalized part of their lives from a young age.

Being Told to Help My Immigrant Mother

The participants repeatedly reported hearing throughout their upbringing that they should help their immigrant mothers. Their Korean fathers would often explain that their mothers came to Korea alone, without family, and may feel lonely, encouraging the children to understand and support them. Moreover, their immigrant mothers often requested help because of physical or emotional fatigue resulting from working. These messages naturally shaped the perception that helping their lonely and exhausted mothers was expected and necessary, leading the participants to accept family assistance with little resistance. However, in situations where their own emotional struggles conflicted with their mothers' needs, the participants sometimes felt compelled to suppress or relinquish their own needs. This reveals that the acceptance of family assistance is not always solely grounded in positive motivation.

> *"(When I tell my dad I'm upset with mom) he says I should help her because she came from Vietnam all alone without her family and must be really lonely... When I hear that, I feel like I have to understand and help her, not that I want to". (Participant 9)*

Driven by Empathy for My Immigrant Mom

By living closely with their immigrant mothers, the participants came to understand that their mothers had different backgrounds and experiences from those of themselves or native Koreans. Through everyday observations, they recognized the chronic difficulties and isolation that their mothers faced in Korean society. Sometimes, they tried to put themselves in their mothers' shoes and empathized with the hardship of living in a foreign country. In particular, hearing about the discrimination their mothers faced simply for being immigrants reinforced their motivation to support them.

> *"If I went to another country where I didn't speak the language and went to the hospital with a friend, and people were speaking in words I didn't understand... I'd ask my friend what was going on". (Participant 5)*

> *"When my mom talks about being discriminated against, I feel like it must be really tough for her. It makes me think, 'I should be on her side at least.'" (Participant 10)*

Assisting with Mom's Small but Constant Language Struggles

Language brokering for their immigrant mothers was an inevitable part of family assistance for all the participants. While their mothers could communicate reasonably well through speaking and listening in Korean, they still needed help with reading and writing. Although the whole family shared in supporting the mother's language needs, the Korean father often played the primary role—handling official communications with schools, banking, and interpreting text messages. The participants also contributed to the language brokering, especially when their fathers were unavailable. While this task felt burdensome when they were younger, as their Korean language and problem-solving skills improved, the participants began to view it as a minor, manageable responsibility—"annoying, but not difficult". Regardless of its difficulty, language brokering was a recurring duty for all the participants with immigrant mothers.

> *"Mom isn't great at figuring out Korean words on her own, so she always asks dad. If he's not home, she asks me". (Participant 9)*

> *"For things like writing a report in Korean, I think I started doing that in first grade. It used to be hard, sitting there going over it and fixing it... But these days, I can just run it through a grammar checker quickly, so it's okay". (Participant 7)*

3.2.3. Unavoidable Family Assistance, Even Under Pressure

This theme explores the experiences of adolescents from marriage immigrant families who provide assistance to their families while under psychological pressure.

Carrying the Weight of the Father's Role Too Soon

In most participants' households, the father was seen as the primary economic provider and symbolic head of the family. This perception persisted even after the father's retirement, and he continued to be regarded as the pillar of the family. For the participants, helping their fathers was not limited to everyday support; it implied sharing major responsibilities, such as earning income and maintaining the family. Under normal circumstances, they were not expected to assume or share these roles. However, due to structural changes such as their father's retirement in his 60s, deteriorating health, or the birth of a much younger sibling, the participants began to gradually take on some of their fathers' responsibilities. In this context, they were expected to prepare for financial independence and internalize a sense of responsibility to eventually step into the father's role in the near future.

> *"When I was told we were having a new baby, my dad said, 'I'm getting old, and if something happens to me, you—my eldest son—must lead the family. You can't act like a child anymore. I'm sorry, but I want you to mature earlier than other kids.'" (Participant 8)*

In Korea's college-entrance-focused society, it is atypical for children to immediately support themselves financially upon becoming adults. The participants also believed that studying hard was their main duty as adolescents. Thus, being asked to shoulder part of the father's burden caused them to feel overwhelmed and confused. However, they understood that such requests reflected the family's difficult circumstances and felt unable to reject them. The belief that they must share the weight of being the family's pillar caused considerable psychological pressure, often leading to feelings of helplessness and depression.

> *"The thought of having to earn money as soon as I become an adult is kind of stressful. So I try not to think about it... a sort of helplessness?" (Participant 4)*

> *"Getting the role of the next family head at such a young age made me feel mentally overwhelmed and stressed. I didn't believe in depression before, but now... I realize it's real". (Participant 8)*

Forced into Traditional but Outdated Roles

Some traditional values were used to justify forcing the participants to help their families, even when they did not agree with such values. The participants wished to reject outdated beliefs and obligations, but, as minors, they could not easily oppose adult authority within the household and were sometimes coerced into undesired family assistance. In particular, patriarchal gender role stereotypes had negative effects on all the adolescents, regardless of their gender. On the one hand, female participants were scolded if they were not good at cooking or cleaning, causing them to feel unjustly and unfairly treated. Male participants, on the other hand, internalized traditional norms that labeled them as "the next family head", leading them to feel immense responsibility and pressure. These outdated gender role expectations contributed to feelings of inequality, negative emotion, and psychological burden among the participants.

> *"Times have changed a lot, right? But I just think to myself, 'It's not like that anymore...' When grandma says things like, 'You have to eat what you're given if you want to be liked by your future in-laws, and you must be good at housework if you want to get married.' I hate that". (Participant 7)*

> *"If you're the eldest son, the family's pillar, you must be able to take responsibility, bear the burden, endure hardship... and I think you're expected to have a strong sense of sacrifice too". (Participant 8)*

Unassisted Academic Struggles

The participants viewed "studying hard" and "obeying their parents" as forms of helping their parents. Focusing on academics reduced the parents' worries and was therefore considered a form of emotional support. Likewise, obeying parental instructions without causing stress was seen as a way to support the parents psychologically.

> *"I think it's good to be respectful to the parents who went through so much to have me. I try not to speak rudely, and I try to listen when they ask me to do something. I just want to keep them from being stressed". (Participant 1)*

Despite their strong sense of duty toward pursuing academic success, many participants struggled due to a lack of parental support. According to the participants, immigrant mothers often did not attend school meetings or access academic information because of language and experiential limitations. Unlike typical households where the mothers actively support their children's education, the immigrant mothers in these families are unable to provide substantial help with academics or career planning. Although the participants sometimes sought help from their fathers, they often could not provide effective support due to a lack of knowledge, limited availability, or lower educational attainment. While academic support is generally considered a parental responsibility, the participants had to accept and assist themselves in this role, leading to feelings of disappointment and burden. Some even had to take responsibility for younger siblings' studies in place of their parents, which they found unfair and stressful.

> *"Most people talk to their parents about GPA and the college entrance exam. But my mom and dad don't really know much about that, so we don't talk about it. I wish I could talk to them—even just to get some advice". (Participant 10)*

> *"It's hard to ask my dad to help my younger brother with homework... Honestly, no one in our house is good at studying. My dad only finished high school, and my mom doesn't speak Korean well. So if not me, then who?" (Participant 6)*

A Language Barrier Too Thick to Truly Touch the Heart

With the exception of a few participants who primarily communicated with their mothers in English (Participants 2, 3, and 4), most did not speak their mothers' native language, and communication with their mothers occurred primarily in Korean. While the participants generally rated their mothers' Korean language proficiency as "high", this was found to be limited to basic, everyday communication. The participants experienced language barriers with their immigrant mothers particularly in situations requiring detailed explanations or emotional communication. Due to limitations in their Korean proficiency, some mothers employed a closed and directive communication style when asking for help, or gave vague instructions without sufficient explanation. These interactions were often perceived as authoritarian, leading to misunderstandings and negative emotions. Emotional and supportive conversations that might have resolved such issues could not take place effectively because of the language barrier. Consequently, the participants felt frustration and resentment toward their mothers, and repeated communication failures sometimes led them to develop negative perceptions vis-à-vis their mothers' foreign identities.

> *"Since she's Vietnamese, she often talks in a very shortened way. It made me wish mom spoke better Korean... or even that she were just Korean. Then we could communicate better". (Participant 9)*

> *"Mom tends to just say, 'Do what I say, I'm tired', and things like that... Since she's a foreigner, I think it's hard for her to express things properly in Korean". (Participant 7)*

4. Discussion

This study is a qualitative investigation conducted to explore the experiences and meanings of family assistance among adolescents from marriage immigrant families. In-depth interviews were conducted with 10 Korean-born adolescents from marriage immigrant families, and the data were analyzed using IPA.

The first theme, "*Old enough to help—naturally, and rightly so*", revealed that adolescents from marriage immigrant families naturally engaged in helping their families as part of their development, grounded in strong family values. They perceived these responsibilities as part of growing up and a preparatory process for adulthood. This finding aligns with prior studies that emphasize the significance of family values in collectivist Asian cultures [14], where family values have been shown to predict adolescents' family assistance behaviors [21]. Asian adolescents often grow up in environments that emphasize loyalty to family, obedience to parents, and expectations to contribute to family welfare. Even when faced with difficulties, such cultural contexts can foster the acceptance of assigned roles [14]. The participants in this study unreservedly accepting routine requests for family assistance as natural can be interpreted as being influenced by this cultural background.

The natural acceptance of family support roles observed among the participants in this study may stem not only from their cultural backgrounds but also from the adolescents' positive evaluations of helping their families—such as feelings of pride, a sense of self-efficacy, and fulfillment of their roles as family members. Aumann and Titzmann [22] reported that adolescents from German immigrant families in Switzerland engaged in more technology mediation activities than their native peers. This finding is particularly noteworthy given that the study focused on European immigrant families, rather than Asian or Latin American families, who are typically more associated with strong familism values. Such results suggest that family assistance behaviors among immigrant adolescents may not solely be the result of internalized cultural values.

Previous studies have also found that immigrant adolescents' support for their families is related to both the social adaptation of immigrant parents [23] and adolescents' positive emotional states [10]. These findings imply that family support can be perceived not merely as a duty or cultural expectation but as a subjective and positive experience. The increase in positive affect observed during family assistance in Shen and colleague's [10] study may be associated with adolescents' sense of contributing to the family, fostering agency and a sense of positivity. Similarly, the participants in the present study expressed feelings of pride or evaluated themselves as "good" individuals through their family assistance experiences, suggesting that helping one's family can be understood as a self-affirming and agentic act rather than a mere obligation. This aligns closely with the findings from previous research.

In cultural groups that emphasize family values, family assistance has been linked to positive developmental outcomes, including increased positive affect [10] and prosocial behaviors [9,21]. Thus, helping one's family may serve not only as role fulfillment but also as a contributor to adolescents' psychological and social development. However, when the expectations for adolescents to support their families become excessive, negative outcomes may arise. For instance, Mejia and colleagues [24] found that while fulfilling familial expectations was associated with a positive self-image among early Asian adults, failure to meet such expectations correlated with a negative self-image and symptoms of depression. Therefore, for family assistance to promote adolescent development, identifying and addressing value mismatches within the family, such as traditional gender roles, is necessary. Additionally, the level of expectations held by both adolescents and their families must be assessed. Moreover, where discrepancies exist, adjustments should be made accordingly.

The participants' experiences of family assistance were twofold: a positive preparation for adulthood and a source of perceived unfairness. These experiences could vary depending on the degree of parental involvement. While household labor can function as a process of socialization that fosters responsibility and the internalization of family norms, it can also serve as a means of compensating for labor shortages caused by demographic or economic limitations [25]. When parents share household tasks with their children, this can promote family closeness, instill values around labor, and foster responsibility and patience [26]. Conversely, when children are left to perform such tasks alone, they may interpret their contributions as a form of forced labor, especially when seen as a substitute for adult responsibilities [27]. This perception of unfairness can lead to negative outcomes, such as depression, substance use, and diminished self-efficacy or self-esteem, and may be indicative of parentification [5].

These results particularly highlight the psychological vulnerabilities of female adolescents in relation to family assistance. Several studies have shown that daughters are more likely to take on family responsibilities compared with sons [7,28,29]. Moreover, some findings indicate that the amount of housework that daughters perform is comparable to that of their fathers [28]. However, few studies have directly examined the relationship between fathers' participation in housework and daughters' experiences of parentification or perceived unfairness. Therefore, future research should explore how fathers' involvement in household labor affects female adolescents' perceptions and mental health more specifically.

The second theme, *"Foreign mother whom I naturally come to help"*, illustrates how the participants form their perceptions of helping their immigrant mothers based on their upbringing and everyday experiences. Messages about their mothers' hardships and isolation, conveyed over time, fostered empathy and a sense of moral obligation. The participants consistently acted as language brokers for their immigrant mothers, perceiving the role as a familial responsibility rather than a major burden. Difficult tasks were typically handled by the Korean—non-immigrant—fathers; thus, the adolescents did not bear the full burden. This contrasts sharply with previous research that suggests language brokering can lead to a reversal of parent–child roles and an intense psychological burden [14,30]. For example, Cho and colleagues [14] studied early adult children in Asian immigrant families in the U.S. who took on vital administrative tasks for survival, such as handling health insurance, housing applications, and utility bills, instead of their parents. These tasks were often accompanied with the fear of making costly errors and added significant stress. Conversely, the participants in this study grew up in South Korea and had native-born Korean fathers, who belonged to the majority of the population. These fathers handled official documents and public communications, reducing the children's burden and creating a different language-brokering experience. Furthermore, considering previous research emphasizing the importance of language acquisition through formal schooling [31], it is likely that adolescents in multicultural families in South Korea—having been born and raised in the country and having learned Korean as a first language through the national curriculum—experienced little difficulty communicating in Korean on behalf of their mothers.

Furthermore, Crafter and Iqbal [32] emphasized that the context in which language brokering occurs is important, especially in hostile environments. Immigrant children acting as intermediaries with native adults may face discrimination and microaggression, reinforcing their marginalized identity and negatively affecting their well-being. They may also feel anxious about making mistakes because of their limited proficiency in either language [30]. However, the participants in this study were fluent in Korean and did not bear the sole responsibility for complex tasks, thereby significantly lowering their exposure to such risks. The supportive involvement of their Korean fathers allowed them to share the burden of brokering in a less stressful manner.

The theme "*Unavoidable family assistance, even under pressure*" revealed that the adolescents in marriage immigrant families often found themselves in inescapable roles, leading to psychological strain. The participants were burdened by having to assume their fathers' responsibilities, forced to adhere to outdated traditional values, and left to manage their academic and emotional needs without adequate parental support, often leading to disappointment or even disillusionment with their marriage immigrant family background.

Despite the presence of socially vulnerable immigrant mothers, the family assistance provided by the adolescents in marriage immigrant families did not amount to full-scale parentification, such as the reversal of parent–child roles. A key reason for this was the presence and involvement of Korean, native-born, fathers. As members of the dominant cultural group, these fathers were capable of addressing the challenges faced by the immigrant mothers because of their familiarity with Korean society and its systems. Although the children were also born and raised in Korea, their limited experience and capabilities meant that they could not assume such responsibilities to the same extent as their fathers. When difficulties arose in helping their mothers, the adolescents were able to rely on their fathers to take over, which significantly reduced their psychological burden and limited the scope of their responsibilities. However, the heavy role of Korean fathers in these households also meant that any absence or loss of function—due to illness, aging, or retirement—posed a significant risk to the family. Some participants reported experiencing psychological and economic stress because of their fathers' older age or deteriorating health. The average age of the participants' fathers was 53.6 years, compared to 39.1 years for the mothers. This reflects national data from 2004 to 2008, when immigrant women commonly matched with significantly older Korean husbands [33]. For example, between 2004 and 2009, the age gaps between immigrant wives and their Korean husbands were as follows: 0–9 years (24.7–33.3%), 10–19 years (46.9–54.8%), and 20+ years (16.5–18.4%). This contrasts with Korean couples from the same period, where only 4.0–5.9% had an age gap of 10 years or more [34]. These differences suggest that marriage immigrant families with adolescent children today often have fathers who are significantly older than their peers in non-multicultural households. In this study, the participants with fathers near to or over 60 years of age reported changes in their households due to the father's physical or economic limitations, resulting in psychological distress, such as pressure to become financially independent (Participant 4), anxiety about their father's health (Participant 5), and a burden related to becoming the next family head (Participant 8). These findings highlight the socioeconomic and emotional vulnerabilities of children in marriage immigrant families with older fathers. There is a clear need for future research and policy development to assess and support the psychological well-being of these adolescents.

The participants in this study perceived "studying hard" and listening to their parents as forms of emotional support for their parents. This perception aligns with previous findings that report a positive association between adolescents' family caregiving behaviors and their academic engagement, suggesting that in family-centered cultures, a sense of familial responsibility can be internalized as academic motivation [9]. However, emphasizing academic immersion in the absence of substantial emotional and academic support from parents may lead to heightened stress among adolescents.

In cultures influenced by Confucian values, children's academic achievement is regarded as a crucial familial duty. Consequently, children are not expected to contribute much to household chores [35]. Furthermore, supporting their academic pursuits is greatly emphasized. Nevertheless, the participants in this study were often expected to assist both their mothers, who were raising children alone in unfamiliar environments, and their fathers, who supported them, placing them in dual caregiving roles.

Notably, children in marriage immigrant families may experience psychological vulnerability, as they are exposed to a dual burden: being expected to achieve academic success while simultaneously assisting their families, often without sufficient academic support from their mothers because of language barriers. To mitigate these challenges, it is essential to not only enhance marriage immigrant mothers' understanding of the host country's educational system but also establish structural and ongoing support for career exploration and academic development among adolescents from marriage immigrant families. Such interventions may help reduce the risk of mental health issues caused by academic stress [36], alleviate feelings of guilt experienced by mothers who are unable to provide adequate academic support to their children [37], and ease the burden on native fathers who assume additional familial roles [38].

Finally, the participants expressed emotional distress stemming from communication failures with their immigrant mothers. Repeated breakdowns in communication—due to language barriers and emotionally closed interactions—led some participants to give up trying to communicate their emotions and even to develop negative perceptions of their mothers' foreign identities. Immigrant mothers often have difficulty expressing subtle emotions in Korean [39] and tend to engage in surface-level conversations with their spouses, lacking emotional depth [40]. Furthermore, the cultural norms of emotional restraint in Asian families [14,41] discourage adolescents from openly expressing negative emotions to their parents. However, the quality of parent–child communication is a critical factor affecting adolescent mental health, including depression, anxiety, and suicidal ideation [42]. Therefore, family-based programs that promote open communication and enhance immigrant mothers' open and emotional communication skills are urgently needed to support the well-being of adolescents in marriage immigrant families.

5. Conclusions

This study employed IPA to explore and deeply understand the family caregiving experiences and their significance among adolescents from marriage immigrant families. Through this analysis, three superordinate themes were identified namely, "Old enough to help—naturally, and rightly so", "Foreign mother whom I naturally come to help", and "Unavoidable family assistance, even under pressure". Additionally, 10 subordinate themes were identified.

Although this study was initially designed to investigate experiences of parentification among adolescents in marriage immigrant families, the research question being partially revised during the course of the in-depth interviews and data analysis has presented a limitation. The original design anticipated that adolescents in marriage immigrant families would take on additional responsibilities due to their immigrant parent's background and that these roles might involve a certain level of burden. However, the findings revealed that such roles were predominantly undertaken by the native Korean fathers, who were adults and citizens of Korea, rather than by the minor children who were born and raised in the country. Consequently, the typical indicators of parent–child role reversal or high levels of responsibility assumed by the child were not clearly observed. This necessitated iterative revisions to the research question, which may be considered a limitation of this study.

Additionally, some of this study's participants were recruited through an online community primarily composed of Filipino marriage immigrant women working as English teachers in Korea. This recruitment channel implies that the participants' mothers generally had a relatively high level of education, which may pose certain limitations to the generalizability of the findings.

Lastly, all the participants in this study were adolescents from families with immigrant mothers and native Korean fathers, despite the absence of such restrictions in the recruitment process. This may reflect broader demographic patterns in South Korea, where the majority of marriage-based immigration involves immigrant women marrying Korean men; in fact, such unions account for 81.8% of all international marriages in the country [43]. While this limits the applicability of the findings to families with immigrant fathers, the results nonetheless offer valuable insights into the dominant family structure among multicultural families in Korean society.

Based on the findings and limitations of this study, the following directions for future research are proposed. First, further qualitative studies should explore the nature and psychological impact of family assistance among adolescents in families in which the native Korean parent is absent or plays a minimal role. Second, quantitative research is needed to assess the psychological distress experienced by immigrant spouses and adolescent children in contexts where the role of the native parent is diminished. Finally, intervention programs should be developed and empirically tested to address the communication challenges and lack of open dialogue between marriage immigrant mothers and their children, as identified in this study.

Author Contributions: Conceptualization, Y.J. and K.-S.B.; data curation, Y.J.; formal analysis, Y.J. and K.-S.B.; investigation, Y.J.; methodology, Y.J. and K.-S.B.; supervision, K.-S.B.; validation, Y.J. and K.-S.B.; writing—original draft, Y.J.; writing—review and editing, Y.J. and K.-S.B. All authors have read and agreed to the published version of the manuscript.

Funding: This research received no external funding.

Institutional Review Board Statement: Informed consent was obtained from all subjects involved in this study.

Informed Consent Statement: This study was conducted in accordance with the Declaration of Helsinki, and approved by the Institutional Review Board of Seoul National University (IRB No. 2209/003-012, approved on 6 September 2022).

Data Availability Statement: The data generated and analyzed in this study are not publicly accessible due to the sensitive and personal nature of the information shared by vulnerable participants.

Acknowledgments: The authors gratefully acknowledge the participants for their meaningful contributions and willingness to share their lived experiences, which were essential to conducting this study.

Conflicts of Interest: The authors declare no conflicts of interest.

Author Contributions: This article is based on the first author's doctoral dissertation submitted to Seoul National University in 2023, with revisions and enhancements made for publication.

References

1. Statistics Korea. Status of International Marriages. 2024. Available online: https://www.index.go.kr/unity/potal/main/EachDtlPageDetail.do?idx_cd=2430 (accessed on 19 March 2025).
2. Ministry of Gender Equality and Family. Yearly Statistics on Multicultural Families. 2023. Available online: https://www.mogef.go.kr/mp/pcd/mp_pcd_s001d.do?mid=plc503&bbtSn=704964 (accessed on 17 May 2025).
3. Armstrong-Carter, E.; Olson, E.; Telzer, E. A unifying approach for investigating and understanding youth's help and care for the family. *Child Dev. Perspect.* **2019**, *13*, 186–192. [CrossRef]
4. Boszormenyi-Nagy, I.; Spark, G.M. Parentification. In *Invisible Loyalties: Reciprocity in Intergenerational Family Therapy*; Routledge: New York, NY, USA, 1973; pp. 151–165.
5. Dariotis, J.K.; Chen, F.R.; Park, Y.R.; Nowak, M.K.; French, K.M.; Codamon, A.M. Parentification Vulnerability, reactivity, resilience, and thriving: A mixed methods systematic literature review. *Int. J. Environ. Res. Public Health* **2023**, *20*, 6197. [CrossRef] [PubMed]
6. Telzer, E.H.; Fuligni, A.J. A longitudinal daily diary study of family assistance and academic achievement among adolescents from Mexican, Chinese, and European backgrounds. *J. Youth Adolesc.* **2009**, *38*, 560–571. [CrossRef]
7. East, P.L. Children's provision of family caregiving: Benefit or burden? *Child Dev. Perspect.* **2010**, *4*, 55–61. [CrossRef] [PubMed]
8. Armstrong-Carter, E.; Ivory, S.; Lin, L.C.; Muscatell, K.A.; Telzer, E.H. Role fulfillment mediates the association between daily family assistance and cortisol awakening response in adolescents. *Child Dev.* **2020**, *91*, 754–768. [CrossRef]
9. Armstrong-Carter, E.; Telzer, E.H. Bidirectional spillover across days between family assistance and physical health experiences during adolescence. *J. Fam. Psychol.* **2021**, *35*, 875–885. [CrossRef]
10. Shen, Y.; Zheng, Y.; Garza, A.R.; Reisz, S. Latinx adolescents' daily family assistance and emotional well-being before and amid the COVID-19 pandemic: A pilot measurement burst study. *J. Res. Adolesc.* **2024**, *34*, 1107–1114. [CrossRef]
11. Telzer, E.H.; Gonzales, N.; Fuligni, A.J. Family obligation values and family assistance behaviors: Protective and risk factors for Mexican–American adolescents' substance use. *J. Youth Adolesc.* **2014**, *43*, 270–283. [CrossRef]
12. Fuligni, A.J.; Telzer, E.H.; Bower, J.; Irwin, M.R.; Kiang, L.; Cole, S.W. Daily family assistance and inflammation among adolescents from Latin American and European backgrounds. *Brain Behav. Immun.* **2009**, *23*, 803–809. [CrossRef]
13. Jugert, P.; Titzmann, P.F. Developmental tasks and immigrant adolescent's adaptation. In *Contextualizing Immigrant and Refugee Resilience: Cultural and Acculturation Perspectives*; Güngör, D., Strohmeier, D., Eds.; Springer International Publishing: Cham, Switzerland, 2020; pp. 33–50.
14. Cho, S.; Glebova, T.; Seshadri, G.; Hsieh, A. A phenomenological study of parentification experiences of Asian American young adults. *Contemp. Fam. Ther.* **2025**, *47*, 275–287. [CrossRef]
15. Lazarevic, V.; Guan, S.-S.A.; Weisskirch, R.S. Experiences of discrimination and language brokering: Exploring risks and protective factors. *Cult. Divers. Ethn. Minor. Psychol.* **2024**, *30*, 130–142. [CrossRef] [PubMed]
16. Lam, C.B.; Greene, K.M.; McHale, S.M. Housework time from middle childhood through adolescence: Links to parental work hours and youth adjustment. *Dev. Psychol.* **2016**, *52*, 2071–2084. [CrossRef] [PubMed]
17. Saragosa, M.; Frew, M.; Hahn-Goldberg, S.; Orchanian-Cheff, A.; Abrams, H.; Okrainec, K. The young carers' journey: A systematic review and meta ethnography. *Int. J. Environ. Res. Public Health* **2022**, *19*, 5826. [CrossRef] [PubMed]
18. Smith, J.A.; Nizza, I.E. *Essentials of Interpretative Phenomenological Analysis*; American Psychological Association: Washington, DC, USA, 2022.

19. Smith, J.A.; Flowers, P.; Larkin, M. *Interpretative Phenomenological Analysis: Theory, Method and Research*, 2nd ed.; SAGE Publisher Ltd.: London, UK, 2022.
20. Tong, A.; Sainsbury, P.; Craig, J. Consolidated criteria for reporting qualitative research (COREQ): A 32-item checklist for interviews and focus groups. *Int. J. Qual. Health Care* **2007**, *19*, 349–357. [CrossRef]
21. Zhao, C.; White, R.M.B.; Roche, K.M. Familism values, family assistance, and prosocial behaviors among U.S. Latinx adolescents. *J. Early Adolesc.* **2022**, *42*, 914–936. [CrossRef]
22. Aumann, L.; Titzmann, P.F. Technical brokering of immigrant adolescents in Switzerland: A developmental-acculturative perspective. *J. Child Fam. Stud.* **2022**, *31*, 185–196. [CrossRef]
23. Titzmann, P.F.; Gniewosz, B. With a little help from my child: A dyad approach to immigrant mothers' and adolescents' socio-cultural adaptation. *J. Adolesc.* **2018**, *62*, 198–206. [CrossRef]
24. Mejia, Y.; Supple, A.J.; Plunkett, S.W.; Kulish, A.L.; Stein, G.L. The role of perceived familial expectations on depressive symptoms and self-esteem in emerging adulthood: A cultural analysis. *Emerg. Adulthood* **2021**, *10*, 971–977. [CrossRef]
25. Blair, S.L. Children's participation in household labor: Child socialization versus the need for household labor. *J. Youth Adolesc.* **1992**, *21*, 241–258. [CrossRef]
26. Glen, H.; Elder, R.D.C., Jr. Ties to family and land. In *Children of the Land: Adversity and Success in Rural America*; University of Chicago Press: Chicago, IL, USA, 2000; pp. 61–85.
27. Kim, K.-J.; Lee, Y.-S. Household tasks that children do with or without parents. *Surv. Res.* **2020**, *21*, 141–167. [CrossRef]
28. Kim, K.-J.; Lee, Y.-S. Parents' and children's housework: Modeling by children's gender and age. *Korea J. Popul. Stud.* **2019**, *42*, 1–25. [CrossRef]
29. Schulz, F. Mothers', fathers' and siblings' housework time within family households. *J. Marriage Fam.* **2021**, *83*, 803–819. [CrossRef]
30. Gustafsson, K.; Norström, E.; Höglund, P. Language interpreting and brokering in Swedish public service institutions: The use of children for multilingual communication. *J. Lang. Law.* **2019**, *71*, 13–26.
31. Figueiredo, S. Comparison of cognitive performance between two generations of immigrant school-aged children: Child development change over time. *J. Cogn. Educ. Psychol.* **2020**, *19*, 121–140. [CrossRef]
32. Crafter, S.; Iqbal, H. Child language brokering as a family care practice: Reframing the 'parentified child' debate. *Child. Soc.* **2022**, *36*, 400–414. [CrossRef]
33. Lee, H.-K. Characteristics of internationally married couples and their families. In *Korean Social Trends 2010*; Statistics Korea: Daejeon, Republic of Korea, 2010; pp. 47–53.
34. Statistics Korea. Marriages by Age Difference Between First-Time Couples by Region (2004–2009). Available online: https://kosis.kr/statHtml/statHtml.do?orgId=101&tblId=DT_1B83A08&conn_path=I2 (accessed on 20 March 2025).
35. Lee, C.F.; Tang, S.M. Young children's housework participation in Taiwan: Serial multiple mediations. *Int. J. Environ. Res. Public Health* **2022**, *19*, 15448. [CrossRef]
36. Steare, T.; Gutiérrez Muñoz, C.; Sullivan, A.; Lewis, G. The association between academic pressure and adolescent mental health problems: A systematic review. *J. Affect. Disord.* **2023**, *339*, 302–317. [CrossRef]
37. Lee, E.-A. Urban marriage migrant women's role of a mother and their identities: Focusing on the experience of child education. *J. Korean Women Stud.* **2013**, *29*, 115–146.
38. Cheon, J.-H.; You, Y.-L. Understanding the lives of multi-cultural family husbands in their biographical contexts. *J. Community Welf.* **2018**, *64*, 115–156. [CrossRef]
39. Oh, H. A qualitative study on communication difficulty mothers of multicultural families experience in rearing child. *J. Spec. Child. Educ.* **2015**, *17*, 215–237.
40. Jang, E.-K.; Ryu, J.-A. A qualitative study on husbands' experience in marital conflict in multicultural families. *J. Agric. Ext. Community Dev.* **2015**, *22*, 117–133.
41. Bi, X.; Wang, S. Parent-adolescent communication quality and life satisfaction: The mediating roles of autonomy and future orientation. *Psychol. Res. Behav. Manag.* **2021**, *14*, 1091–1099. [CrossRef] [PubMed]
42. Zapf, H.; Boettcher, J.; Haukeland, Y.; Orm, S.; Coslar, S.; Fjermestad, K. A systematic review of the association between parent-child communication and adolescent mental health. *JCPP Adv.* **2024**, *4*, e12205. [CrossRef] [PubMed]
43. Statistics Korea. Index Nuri e-National Index. *Statistics Korea*. 2024. Available online: https://www.index.go.kr/unity/potal/main/EachDtlPageDetail.do?idx_cd=2819 (accessed on 17 May 2025).

children

MDPI

Article

Relations Between Parental Emotion Talk and Preschoolers' Emotion Expressions in Low-Income Chinese American and Mexican American Families

Megan Chan [1], Michelle Taw [1], Nancy Eisenberg [2] and Qing Zhou [1,*]

[1] Department of Psychology, University of California Berkeley, Berkeley, CA 94720, USA
[2] Department of Psychology, Arizona State University, Tempe, AZ 85281, USA; nancy.eisenberg@asu.edu
* Correspondence: qingzhou@berkeley.edu

Abstract: Background/Objectives: Preschool children learn to express emotions in accordance with sociocultural norms. Parental emotion talk (ET) has been theorized to shape these processes. Limited research has examined preschoolers' observed emotion expressions and emotion-related behaviors in culturally diverse samples. We sought to explore the following: (1) cultural group differences and similarities in observed emotion expressions (anger, sadness, and positive emotions) and emotion-related behaviors between Chinese American and Mexican American preschoolers, and (2) the concurrent links between parental ET and children's emotion expressions. **Methods**: In a sample of 86 children (age range = 38 to 70 months, 62% girls) from low-income immigrant families (Mexican Americans/MA = 43 and Chinese Americans/CA = 43), the observed children's emotion expressions and emotion-related behaviors were coded based on a frustration-eliciting task. Parental ET quality and quantity were coded from transcripts of a parent–child shared reading task. **Results:** MA children expressed more anger and sadness, but the two groups did not differ on positive emotions or emotion-related behaviors. Multiple regressions showed that children whose parents engaged in more ET expressed higher levels of anger and sadness and used more non-feeling state languages than children whose parents engaged in less ET. **Conclusions**: The results revealed cultural variations in preschool-age children's emotion expressions and provided support for associations between parental ET and children's emotion expressions.

Keywords: parental emotion talk; preschoolers' emotion expressions; culture

1. Introduction

Parental emotion talk (ET), a common emotion socialization practice during early childhood, plays a critical role in shaping children's socioemotional competence [1]. Despite the acknowledgement that how parents socialize children's emotions depend on sociocultural norms and values [1], there is a dearth of research on parental ET in non-Western families and its links to children's emotion expressions. As the number of immigrant families continues to rise in the United States and elsewhere, it is crucial to understand parental use of emotion talk and its roles in children's socioemotional development in immigrant families. Such knowledge can inform the development and dissemination of culturally competent parent education and family engagement programs in culturally diverse and immigrant communities. To fill these gaps, the present study sought to explore the following (1) cultural group differences and similarities in emotion expressions (anger, sadness, and positive emotions) and emotion-related behaviors (attention to target, gaze

 https://doi.org/10.3390/children12010052

aversion, and verbalization) between Chinese American and Mexican American children using an observational approach, and (2) the concurrent links between parental ET and children's emotion expressions.

1.1. Preschool-Age Children's Emotion-Related Behaviors and Emotion Expressions

The ability to express emotions in a regulated and appropriate manner is a crucial component of emotional competence in Western cultures [2]. With the development of cognitive, language, and motor skills, preschool-age children learn to regulate their emotions and adapt emotion expressions in alignment with social and cultural norms and expectations [2]. Researchers have identified several types of emotion-related behaviors in young children during emotion-evoking situations. For example, attention control refers to the ability to focus or shift one's attention voluntarily to facilitate emotion management [3]. Gaze aversion (averting one's gaze or looking away) is a basic form of self-distraction or attention control [4]. As children develop more sophisticated verbal skills, they increasingly utilize language as a tool for regulating emotions [5]. As such, self-verbalization (including labeling emotions) is commonly observed among preschoolers in emotion-evoking situations [6]. In sum, preschoolers' emotion-related behaviors reflect their developing emotion regulation skills.

Children's emotion-related behaviors often co-occur with and are thus related to their expressions of positive and negative emotions, although the direction of such associations varies by valence and situational contexts. For example, in predominantly White samples, positive relations were observed between preschoolers' expressions of positive emotions (e.g., smiling) and fidgeting [7,8]. Using behavioral data from the same sample of preschoolers as the present paper but assessed with a different paradigm (unfair sharing), we found that children's gaze aversion was positively associated with negative emotion expressions, whereas fidgeting was positively associated with positive emotion expressions and negatively associated with negative emotion expressions [9]. Because the relations between emotion expressions and emotion-related behaviors vary by situations [4], it is important to investigate these associations in different situations to get a better understanding of young children's emotion regulatory processes.

1.2. Parental Emotion Talk and Its Links to Children's Emotion Expressions

Emotion talk (ET) refers to conversations involving the labeling of emotions, references to the cause or elicitors of emotions, and the appropriateness or consequences of emotions and emotion-related behaviors [10]. Parental ET is theorized to shape children's emotion expressions through multiple pathways (e.g., emotion arousal, emotion understanding, and emotion control values). First, by engaging in ET, parents teach, coach, and model constructive emotion regulatory strategies (e.g., labeling, validating, and cognitive restructuring) and culturally appropriate emotion expressions. Second, parental ET or other mental state talk can promote children's emotion understanding, theory of mind, perspective taking, and emotion vocabulary [11], which in turn facilitate emotion regulation and expression [12]. Third, parents' use of emotion language and modeling of emotion regulation strategies can shape children's emotion control values [13]. Research conducted with adults showed that individuals' emotion control values (e.g., the beliefs that one should or can control one's emotions) are associated with their emotion regulation strategies and emotion-related behavioral and physiological responses [14,15].

Consistent with these theories, the quality and elaborateness of parental ET has been linked to children's higher effortful control (a temperament-based self-regulatory process related to emotion regulation), better emotion understanding, and more prosocial behaviors. For example, a latent factor reflecting both the quantity and elaborateness of parental

ET predicted school-age children's higher effortful control in a longitudinal study of Chinese American immigrant families [16]. In a sample of upper to middle-class, predominantly White families, the mothers' emotion explanations were associated with preschoolers' greater emotion situation knowledge and greater prosocial behaviors [17].

It is important to note that the relation between parental ET and children's emotion expressions is bidirectional, such that children with dispositional tendencies to experience or express intense emotions might elicit certain types of parenting behaviors, including ET. In a longitudinal study of parental ET with toddlers in a predominantly Latino sample, Lorenzo et al. (2023) found that toddlers' externalizing problems prospectively and positively predicted maternal ET, whereas maternal ET did not predict a child's externalizing behaviors [18]. One interpretation is that the mothers whose children had high levels of externalizing behavior increased the use of ET to teach or scaffold their children's emotion regulation in frustrating situations. However, Vu et al. (2022) found some support for bidirectional relations between mothers' emotion socialization strategies (e.g., emotion dismissing and emotion coaching) and children's (4–8 years of age) anger and sadness reactions to disappointment in Chinese immigrant families [19].

1.3. Cultural Variations in Parental ET and Children's Emotion Expressions

Emotion models are mental representations of expected, valued, appropriate, and desirable emotional patterns within a cultural context, which serve to shape individual emotional experiences and expressions [20]. Although both Chinese and Mexican cultures are considered collective cultures, they differ in specific emotion values. In Chinese/Asian cultures, open expression of emotions in public is discouraged due to its potential threat to interpersonal harmony [21]. Moreover, the experience of low-arousal positive emotions (e.g., calm) is preferred over high-arousal positive emotions (e.g., excitement) in Chinese/Asian individuals [22]. Influenced by these cultural values, Chinese/Asian families might discourage children from experiencing and expressing high-arousal positive emotions, dampen children's high-intensity positive emotion, or model emotion suppression [23]. In contrast, related to the Latino cultural values of *respeto* (i.e., obedience/conformity to authority, deference, decorum, and socially appropriate public behaviors [24], and *simpatía* (i.e., the preference for social interactions characterized by warmth and emotional positivity and avoidance of conflict/overt negativity [25], Latino cultures value open expressions of positive emotions while discouraging expressions of negative emotions. In line with these cultural values, compared to Latino-heritage (and European-heritage) young adults, Asian-heritage young adults rated positive emotions as the least desirable to experience and the least appropriate to express, whereas Latino-heritage young adults rated negative emotions as less desirable compared to Asian-heritage young adults [20]. Influenced by these cultural values, Latinx families might encourage and model open expressions of positive emotions and create opportunities to savor or enhance children's positive emotions.

In line with theorized cultural influences on emotion socialization, past studies have found some evidence of cultural variations in parental ET. For example, Luo and colleagues (2014) [26] found that during parent–child shared book reading, Chinese mothers were most likely to emphasize negative consequences of inappropriate behaviors and referred to emotions less frequently than mothers from other U.S. ethnic groups (African American, Mexican, and Dominican families). In a previous study using data from the same sample as the present paper, we found that MA parents used more negative emotion words and emotion reasoning and engaged in more elaborate ET than did CA parents during shared picture book reading [9]. However, this study did not examine the link between parental ET and children's emotion expressions.

Cultural variations in emotion values are also expected to shape children's emotion expressions and emotion-related behaviors through emotion socialization. However, few studies have examined cultural group variations in children's emotion expressions using observational methods, and the findings are mixed. For example, European American girls smiled more than Mainland Chinese and Chinese American girls and displayed higher disgust-related expressions and greater overall expressivity than Mainland Chinese girls [27]. Using two emotion situations (resistance to temptation and a "mishap" paradigm), Wang and Barrett (2015) [28] found that American preschoolers expressed more happiness and sadness than Chinese preschoolers. Although the two groups did not differ on overall expressiveness in anger, the Chinese children's anger showed a cumulative pattern across contexts. The findings suggest that cultural group differences in emotional expressiveness may be "dimension-specific, emotion-specific, and context-specific" ([28] p. 420). On the other hand, Mexican American toddlers expressed more positive affect than negative affect during parent–child free play [29], consistent with Latino value of *simpatía* [30].

To our knowledge, few studies have sampled Mexican- and Chinese-heritage children in the same study and examined the similarities and differences in emotion expressions and emotion-related behaviors by cultural group. As an exception, using data from the same sample as the present study, we previously found that MA preschoolers displayed a higher intensity of positive (but not negative) emotions than CA preschoolers when treated unfairly (in an unfair sharing task), although the two groups did not differ in the expression of negative emotions [9]. Moreover, MA preschoolers displayed more frequent emotion-related behaviors than CA children, which may have been driven by the overall higher intensity or duration of emotion expressions [9]. However, the question remains whether the cultural group variations in children's emotion expressions generalize to other situations (e.g., a frustration-eliciting task). Moreover, the study did not examine the links between parental ET and children's emotion expressions and emotion-related behaviors.

When studying parental ET and children's emotion expressions, it is important to consider other sociocultural and individual factors, such as gender/sex, parental education, and family income, which have been linked to emotion socialization. For example, a cumulative risk index capturing multiple family risks (e.g., low income, single-parent status, larger household size, and lower parental education) was associated with the mothers' less frequent use of expressive encouragement and problem-focused responses in response to children's negative emotions [31]. Moreover, the mothers' education levels have been negatively related to their displays of unsupportive emotion reactions [31] and positively related to their use of positive emotion words, emotion questions, and emotion explanations [32]. Parents' emotion socialization differed according to the child's sex: parents of preschoolers engaged in more elaborate emotion conversations with their daughters than with their sons [33]. Moreover, parental education and child's age were associated positively with parental emotion talk [9].

1.4. The Present Study

The present study has two aims. First, we used an observational approach to assess children's emotion expressions (anger, sadness, and positive emotions) and emotion-related behaviors (attention to target, gaze aversion, and verbalization) during a frustration paradigm in two cultural groups: Chinese American and Mexican American preschoolers. We compared cultural group differences and similarities in the frequency of children's emotion-related behaviors and intensity of emotion expressions. Based on prior findings [20,30,34], we hypothesized that MA children would express more positive affect than CA children. Due to past mixed findings on cultural differences in anger expression [28,34] and negative expressions [9], we tested cultural group differences in anger and sadness expression as an exploratory aim. This hypothesis will be tested using independent-sample t-tests. Because no prior studies have compared children from the two cultural groups on emotion-related behaviors, we tested this as an exploratory hypothesis.

Second, we examined the unique relations of parental ET to children's emotion-related behaviors and emotion expression, controlling for other demographic factors (family SES, child's age, sex, and generation status). This hypothesis will be tested using multiple regression analyses. Based on prior findings showing that parental ET is associated positively with child's emotion regulation [16,32] and emotion understanding [35] in older children, we hypothesized that parental ET would be associated positively with children's emotion-related behaviors. Due to lack of prior research on parental ET and children's emotion expressions, we tested the relations between parental ET and children's emotion expression as an exploratory hypothesis.

2. Materials and Methods

2.1. Participants

The study utilized data from a cross-sectional study on language and socioemotional development of dual language learners in immigrant families (data were collected between March 2013 and March 2016). The sample consisted of a total of 86 children (age range = 38 to 70 months, M = 54.4 months, SD = 7.11, 62% girls) and their parents, with 43 children from Mexican American (MA) families and 43 children from Chinese American (CA) families in a metropolitan area in Northern California. Three MA children and one CA child were excluded from the analysis because their video data were not captured due to equipment malfunctions during assessment. The average length of parental education was 9.6 years (equivalent to some high school, range = 2.5–16.0 years, SD = 3.84). Eighteen percent of children were first generation (born outside of the US), 78% were second generation (born in the U.S. with at least one foreign-born parent), and 6% were third generation (born in the U.S. with two U.S.-born parents). The average family per capita income in the past year was $5166.8 (range = $1000 to $24,166.7, SD = $5166.8).

We conducted independent sample t-tests (for continuous variables) and chi-square tests of independence (for categorical variables) to compare the MA and CA groups on demographic variables (child's age, sex, generation status, parental education, and family income). The two groups differed on child's generation status: the CA group had more first-generation children, and the MA group had more third-generation children, $\chi^2(df = 2) = 23.4$, $p < 0.001$. No group difference was found with parental education or family income. Furthermore, prior analyses conducted using data from the present sample found no significant cultural group differences in children's English receptive and expressive vocabulary [9].

2.2. Procedures

Participants were recruited from 15 Head Start preschool centers in Northern California serving high concentrations of either Chinese-speaking or Spanish-speaking families. To be eligible, the child had to meet the following criteria: (1) be between 36–71 months of age, (2) be enrolled at a Head Start program for at least 3 days per week, (3) able understand and speak some English and either Chinese (Cantonese or Mandarin) or Spanish, (4) have both parents self-identifying as ethnically Chinese or Mexican. Children who were diagnosed with a speech or language disorder or who were receiving speech or language services were excluded from the study.

The parent–child dyad participated in a 2.5 h assessment, either at the university laboratory or at their homes, based on the parents' preference. The assessment included parent questionnaires, one-on-one child emotion and behavioral tasks, and parent–child interaction tasks. Child participants were interviewed in their preferred language (18% in English and 82% in Cantonese/Mandarin or Spanish), during which they played games with bilingual research assistants and were tested on their linguistic and socioemotional development. Parents also completed parent questionnaires administered in their preferred language (10% in English, 90% in Cantonese/Mandarin or Spanish) by bilingual research assistants. Children were given a small prize, and parents received $70 for participation.

2.3. Measures

2.3.1. Demographic Variables (Parent Report)

Parents were administered the adapted version of the Family and Demographics and Migration History Questionnaire [36] by a bilingual interviewer. Items included the child's sex, the child's age, the parent's age, the parent's length of stay in the US, maternal education, paternal education, annual per capita income, and child's generation.

2.3.2. Parental Emotion Talk (Observed)

Shared picture book reading task. We recorded parent–child book-sharing interactions using a picture book "Frog, where are you" [37] with no words. The book contains 29 black and white illustrations depicting a little boy's journey to find his lost frog. Parents were given 5 min to read the story with their child in their preferred language, which could be English, Cantonese, Mandarin, or Spanish. The visual images in the book evoke various emotions, such as happiness, anger, fear, and sadness, prompting parents and children to engage in emotion talk during the storytelling process. Shared book reading tasks are commonly used in research on parent–child interactions as they can elicit rich and complex language from parents, including emotion talk [17]. For example, Huang and Kan (2021) [38] used three picture book storytelling tasks to examine parental emotion talk in Cantonese-speaking Chinese American immigrant families with preschool-age children and found that Chinese American parents' use of emotion words and emotion reasoning did not differ across the books.

Emotion talk coding scheme. The Frog Storytelling Task recordings were transcribed and scored using a coding manual adapted from Spinrad and Eisenberg (2010) [39], which had been previously validated in a sample of Chinese American families with school-age children [6,32]. Two bilingual coders proficient in both Chinese and English coded the Chinese American sample, whereas two bilingual coders proficient in Spanish and English coded the Mexican American sample. The coders worked independently on each sample and resolved discrepancies through post-discussions. The measurement of emotion talk (ET) included three components: the number of emotion words, the number of ET comments and questions, and the overall elaborateness of ET. Interrater reliabilities, assessed using intra-class correlations (ICCs), were 0.93 for parental emotion words, 0.71 for parental emotion questions, 0.74 for parental emotion reasoning, and 0.62 for overall ET elaborateness. According to Koo and Li (2016) [40], ICCs between 0.50 and 0.75 are considered to indicate moderate reliability, and those between 0.75 and 0.90 are considered to indicate good reliability. Therefore, the ET codes demonstrated moderate-to-good interrater reliabilities in the present sample. Only parental ET variables were used in the analysis because child ET variables had low frequencies and little variability in the present sample.

Emotion words. The coders counted the number of emotion words uttered by the parent during the book-reading task. Emotion words included words that express affective states (e.g., "mad" 生氣/enojada, "unhappy" 不開心/infeliz, "afraid" 害怕/temerosa, ...)

and words that are related to emotional states without naming the specific emotion (e.g., "laugh", "naughty", "tired" ...) The counted emotion words were categorized as having a positive or negative valance.

Emotion talk comments and questions. Three types of parental emotion comments or questions were categorized, and the frequencies of utterance were counted: linking, emotion questions, and emotion reasoning. Linking refers to parental linking of the story to personal experiences (e.g., "I told you; bees sting you because they get mad since the beehive is their home"). Emotion questions refer to a parent's raising of questions regarding the character or the child's emotional state (e.g., "Why is the boy mad?"). Emotion reasoning refers to a parent providing explanations for a character's feeling (e.g., "The little boy is happy because he saw that the little frog is with its family").

Global quality (elaborateness) of emotion talk. The coders rated each parent on a global code of ET quality based on the parent's storytelling behaviors throughout the whole task, using a 3-point scale (1 = no ET present, 2 = low quality of ET, 3 = high quality of ET). Coders evaluated the quality of ET based on the elaborateness of ET (the levels of detail and sophistication, the amount of information conveyed regarding emotions, and the degree to which parents engaged children in the discussion of emotions). Low quality of ET (a rating of 2) was represented by use of short statements and simple questions, such as "The boy is sad" and "Is the boy unhappy?" High quality of ET (a rating of 3) was represented by the use of detailed explanations of emotions (e.g., "The boy got angry because the jar is broken, right?"), questions that elicits the child's own thoughts (e.g., "What do you think he is feeling?"), and sentences that take the perspective of the character (e.g., "The boy named Luis scolded the dog and told him that he needed to behave").

Data reduction of ET variables. To reduce the number of parental ET variables, we conducted an exploratory factor analysis with the seven ET variables using Principal Axis Factoring. Based on the scree plot, one factor was extracted, which accounted for 59% of total variance. Two ET variables (linking and self-reporting of emotion) did not load onto the factor and were dropped from subsequent analyses. The other five ET variables had factor loadings larger than 0.30: positive emotion words (0.33), emotion questions (0.47), overall quality of ET (0.67), emotional reasoning (0.74), and negative emotion words (0.80). Based on these results, we computed a composite score of parental ET by averaging the standardized scores of the above five ET variables, with a higher score on the ET composite indicating more frequent ET behaviors and more elaborate ET.

2.3.3. Children's Emotion Expressions and Emotion-Related Behaviors (Observed)

Attractive toy in a transparent box task. The LAB–TAB Preschool Battery's Attractive Toy in a Transparent Box Task [41] was utilized to evaluate children's emotion expression and regulation. During this task, children were asked to select a toy they liked, which was then locked in a transparent box by the experimenter. The child was given a set of incorrect keys and instructed to use them to open the box and access the toy. After a 4 min interval, the experimenter returned, apologized, and provided the child with the correct key, allowing them to finally play with the toy.

Coding scheme. The task was recorded on video and analyzed using a coding scheme that included codes for affect and behavior. Emotion expression was measured by the intensity and duration of the observed affect, and emotion-related behaviors were measured by the frequency of observed behaviors. The videos, which were approximately 6–7 min in length, were segmented into 5 s epochs using ELAN (Version 5.9), a psycholinguistic software [42]. An average of 74.8 epochs and 77.5 epochs were coded for each video in the MA and CA samples, respectively. Two trained coders who were proficient in Spanish coded the MA sample, while two trained coders who were proficient in Cantonese and

Mandarin coded the CA sample. The coders scored the videos independently and resolved any differences in coding through consensus meetings.

Emotion expression codes. The coders assessed children's expression of anger, sadness, and positive affect in each 5 s epoch, taking into consideration facial, vocal, and bodily displays. Emotion expression was rated on a 4-point scale, where 1 indicated the absence of emotion, 2 indicated low-intensity expression, 3 denoted moderate-intensity expression or prolonged low-intensity expression, and 4 indicated intense expression or prolonged moderate-intensity expression. For each emotion expression, the ratings were averaged across all epochs. Interrater reliabilities (computed as intraclass correlations/ICCs) between the two coders were 0.93 for expressed positive affect, 0.82 for expressed anger, and 0.52 for expressed sadness.

Emotion-related behavioral codes. Twelve behavioral codes were employed to capture children's emotion-related behaviors during the task. In the current study, four of these behavioral variables were selected and coded in 5 s epochs, namely attention to target objects, gaze aversion, feeling–state language, and non-feeling–state language. Codes of 0 were used to indicate the absence of a behavior, whereas codes of 1 represented the presence of a behavior. The average of codes across all epochs was used for each emotion-related behavior variable in the data analyses. ICCs between coders were acceptable: 0.92 for attention to target, 0.88 for gaze aversion, 0.69 for feeling–state language, and 0.97 for non-feeling–state language. The feeling–state language variable was dropped due to extremely low frequency.

2.4. *Data Analytic Plan*

First, after data screening and descriptive analyses, independent-sample t-tests were performed to test for cultural group differences in the means of parental ET and children's emotion variables. Second, zero-order correlations were computed to examine the associations between socio-demographic variables and parental ET and children's emotion expressions. Socio-demographic variables that were significantly correlated with both parental ET and children's emotion expressions were included as covariates in subsequent analyses testing the relations between parental ET and child's emotion variables. Third, multiple regressions were computed to test the unique relations between parental ET and children's emotion expressions/behaviors, controlling for socio-demographic covariates. All analyses were conducted in IBM SPSS (Version 27).

3. Results

3.1. *Descriptive Statistics and Cultural Group Comparisons*

Descriptive statistics for parental emotion talk (ET), children's emotion expression variables, and demographic variables are reported in Table 1. Based on the cutoffs of 2 and 7 for skewness and kurtosis respectively [43], all the study variables were normally distributed. There were significant differences between the MA and CA groups: (a) in parental ET, MA parents scored higher, t(df = 78) = 3.75, $p < 0.001$, Cohen's d = 0.65; (b) in children's expressed anger, MA children displayed more anger, t(df = 84) = 9.99, $p < 0.001$, Cohen's d = 0.26; and (c) in children's expression of sadness, MA children scored higher, t(df = 84) = 3.01, $p = 0.003$, Cohen's d = 0.23.

Table 1. Descriptive statistics of study variables by cultural groups.

Variables	Mexican American Sample (n = 43)		Chinese American Sample (n = 43)	
	Mean	SD	Mean	SD
Parental emotion talk [1]	0.26_a	0.65	-0.29_b	0.65
Child's positive emotions [2]	1.55	0.31	1.44	0.38
Child's anger [2]	1.70_a	0.34	1.16_b	0.11
Child's sadness [2]	1.37_a	0.25	1.22_b	0.22
Child's attention to target [3]	0.85	0.10	0.85	0.13
Child's gaze aversion [3]	0.17	0.11	0.19	0.15
Child's non-feeling state language [3]	0.12	0.11	0.08	0.12
Child's age	55.22	6.96	53.48	7.23
Average parent education	10.28	3.29	8.90	4.26
Per capita income	$4664	$3875	$5646.9	$3406.8
Family SES composite [4]	0.04	0.65	−0.04	0.77

Notes. [1] Parental emotion talk is a composite computed as the mean of standardized scores of the five ET variables (positive and negative emotion words, emotion questions and reasoning, and overall elaborateness of ET). [2] Child's positive emotions, anger, and sadness are the mean ratings across epochs coded on a 4-point scale (from 1 = absence of emotion expression to 4 = intense expression or prolonged moderate intensity expression). [3] Child's attention to target, gaze aversion, and non-feeling state language are computed as the average presence (0 = not present, 1 = present) of such behavior across all epochs. [4] Family SES composite was computed as the mean of standardized parental education and family income variables. Means with different subscripts differ at $p = 0.05$ level across the two cultural groups (MA vs. CA) by independent-sample t-tests.

3.2. Correlations Among Demographic and Study Variables

Zero-order correlations among parental ET and children's emotion expression and emotion-related behaviors, as well as demographic variables (child's sex, age, generation status, and family SES), are presented in Table 2. Significant positive correlations were found between the quality and elaborateness of parental ET and children's expressions of anger (r = 0.32) and sadness (r = 0.28), and use of non-feeling state language (r = 0.27) during the frustration task. It is worth noting that children's emotion expression variables were mostly unrelated to each other, except for a positive correlation between expressed anger and expressed sadness (r = 0.32) and a negative correlation between gaze aversion and attention to target (r = −0.96).

Table 2. Zero-order correlations among demographic and study variables.

Variables	1	2	3	4	5	6	7	8	9	10
1. Child's sex [1]	–									
2. Child's age	0.02	–								
3. Child's generation status [2]	−0.02	0.19	–							
4. Family's SES	−0.09	0.07	0.14	–						
5. Parental emotion talk	−0.05	0.03	0.12	0.16	–					
6. Child's expressed positive emotions	−0.07	0.12	0.13	−0.05	−0.07	–				
7. Child's expressed anger	−0.14	0.27 **	0.33 **	0.12	0.32 **	0.04	–			
8. Child's expressed sadness	−0.05	0.04	0.19	0.03	0.28 *	−0.10	0.32 **	–		
9. Child's attention to target	0.07	0.20	−0.09	0.16	0.06	−0.04	0.17	−0.10	–	
10. Child's gaze aversion	−0.13	−0.18	0.04	−0.15	−0.12	0.02	−0.21	0.03	−0.95 ***	–
11. Child's non-feeling state language	−0.12	0.23 *	0.03	−0.10	0.27 *	0.14	0.10	0.07	0.03	−0.03

Notes. [1] Child's sex is coded as follows: 0 = girls, 1 = boys; [2] Child's generation is coded as: 1 = 1st generation, 2 = 2nd generation, 3 = 3rd generation. *** $p < 0.001$, ** $p < 0.01$, * $p < 0.05$.

Regarding the demographic variables, child's age was positively correlated with children's expressions of anger (r = 0.27) and use of non-feeling state language (r = 0.23). Children's generational status was positively correlated with their use of anger, such that second- or third-generation children expressed more anger than first-generation children (r = 0.32). Child's sex or family's SES was unrelated to any parental ET or child's emotion expression or regulation variables. Based on the correlation results, we included child's age and generation status as covariates in subsequent analyses, testing the relations between parental ET and child emotion variables.

3.3. Multiple Regressions Testing the Relations of Parental ET to Children's Emotion Expressions

Six multiple regressions were computed to test the relation of the parental ET composite to each of the six children's emotion expression variables, controlling for child's age and generation status. As shown in Table 3, parental ET, child's age, and generation status were entered as simultaneous predictors. The regression equation accounted for significance variances in three dependent variables: child's expressed anger ($R^2 = 0.23$, $p < 0.001$), expressed sadness ($R^2 = 0.12$, $p < 0.05$), and non-feeling state language ($R^2 = 0.21$, $p < 0.001$). Specifically, child's generation status (ß = 0.28) and parental ET (ß = 0.28) were positively associated with child's expressed anger. Parental ET was positively associated with child's expressed sadness (ß = 0.25). Moreover, child's age (ß = 0.38) and parental ET (ß = 0.27) were positively associated with child's use of non-feeling state language. For the six regression models tested in Table 3, we further tested whether culture group moderated the relation between parental ET and child outcomes by adding the culture group (0 = MA, 1 = CA) and the multiplicative term of culture group × parental ET as predictors. None of the interaction terms was significant. Thus, no evidence of moderation by cultural group was found.

Table 3. Multiple regressions predicting children's emotion expressions from parental emotion talk.

Predictors	Regression 1: Predicting Child's Expressed Positive Affect		Regression 2: Predicting Child's Expressed Anger		Regression 3: Predicting Child's Expressed Sadness	
	ß	B (SE)	ß	B (SE)	ß	B (SE)
Child's age	0.13	0.01 (0.01)	0.18	0.01 (0.01)	−0.07	−0.02 (0.004)
Child's generation status	0.13	0.09 (0.09)	0.28	0.22 * (0.08)	0.21	0.10 (0.05)
Parental emotion talk	−0.09	−0.05 (0.06)	0.28	0.15 ** (0.05)	0.25	0.08 * (0.04)
	$R^2 = 0.05$		$R^2 = 0.23$ ***		$R^2 = 0.12$ *	
Predictors	**Regression 4: Predicting Child's Attention to Target**		**Regression 5: Predicting Child's Gaze Aversion**		**Regression 6: Predicting Child's Non-feeling State Language**	
	ß	B (SE)	ß	B (SE)	ß	B (SE)
Child's age	0.20	0.003 (0.002)	−0.16	−0.003 (0.002)	0.38	0.01 *** (0.002)
Child's generation status	−0.10	−0.02 (0.03)	0.05	0.12 (0.03)	−0.10	−0.02 (0.02)
Parental emotion talk	0.07	0.01 (0.02)	−0.12	−0.02 (0.02)	0.27	0.04 * (0.02)
	$R^2 = 0.04$		$R^2 = 0.04$		$R^2 = 0.21$ ***	

Notes. ß = standardized regression coefficient; B = unstandardized regression coefficient; SE = standard error of regression coefficient. * $p < 0.05$, ** $p < 0.01$, *** $p < 0.001$.

4. Discussion

This is one of the first observational studies that examined the link between parental ET and children's emotion expressions and emotion-related behaviors among low-income Mexican American and Chinese American families. Using independent-sample t-tests, we found that MA children expressed more anger and sadness during the frustration task compared to CA children, although the two groups did not differ in expressed positive emotions or emotion-related behaviors. Moreover, MA parents used more ET during shared book reading than did CA parents. Using multiple regressions and controlling for sociodemographic covariates, we found that the children whose parents used more ET in shared reading expressed more anger and sadness and used more non-feeling states languages during the frustration paradigm.

Tested as an exploratory hypothesis, we found that MA children displayed more anger and sadness during the frustration task than CA children. Because no prior studies have directly compared MA and CA children from similar socioeconomic background on emotion expressions using observational measures, we can only compare the study results with the finding of Kim et al. (2023) [9], which used observational data from the same sample but with a different emotion paradigm (unfair treatment). Contrary to our results, Kim et al. (2023) [9] did not find cultural group differences in children's expressions of anger during the unfair sharing paradigm. It is important to note that the frustration task (attractive toy in a transparent box) examined in the present paper differs from the unfair sharing task examined in Kim et al. (2023) [9]: the unfair sharing task involves social interactions with an adult (the interviewer shares a bag of candies with the child), whereas the frustration task involves minimum interactions with the social partner (the child was asked to open the transparent box on their own without the interviewer present). Thus, the two situations differ in the emotion display rules. Although it might seem impolite or inappropriate for children to express negative emotions when interacting with an adult in both Latino and East Asian cultures, displaying negative emotions while trying to solve a frustrating problem on one's own is not necessarily viewed as inappropriate in either Latino or East Asian cultures. Therefore, culturally based emotion models are situation specific. While there are general cultural variations in the desirability and appropriateness of expressing different types of emotions, the emotion display rules depend on the interpersonal and personal goals of specific situations. It is interesting that preschool-age children in U.S. immigrant families living in the same geographic region are displaying divergent patterns of situation-specific emotion expressions that are consistent with the emotion models of their heritage cultures.

On the other hand, contrary to our hypothesis that MA children would display more positive emotions than CA children, we did not find significant culture group difference in positive emotion expressions. This is different from Kim et al. (2023) [9], which found that MA children displayed more positive emotions and emotion-related behaviors (gaze aversion, self-soothing, and fidgeting) than CA children during the unfair sharing paradigm. However, an examination of group means (in Table 1) suggested that the result is in the expected direction: MA children (M = 1.55) had a higher mean in expressed positive emotions than CA children (M = 1.44) in the frustration paradigm, although it did not reach statistical significance. Perhaps the frustration paradigm offered limited opportunity for observing children's positive emotions. Therefore, the situational context of the frustration paradigm, coupled with the small sample size, might have limited our ability to detect cultural group differences in expressed positive emotions.

Our second exploratory aim was to examine the unique relations between parental emotion talk and children's emotion expression and emotion-related behaviors. Using a series of multiple regressions, we found that after controlling for child's age and generation status, parental ET positively predicted children's expressed anger and sadness and their use of non-feeling state languages. Thus, the children whose parents used more ET during shared book reading expressed more anger and sadness and used more non-feeling state language during the frustration task than the children whose parents used less emotion talk. These results are generally in line with prior studies showing that parental ET was associated with child's emotion regulation [16,32] and emotion understanding [35], although no prior studies have examined the specific links between ET and preschool-age children's emotion expressions. Overall, our results indicate a general pattern that parents who used more ET tended to have children who are more emotionally expressive. Although we did not examine the mechanisms that might underly this association, we can speculate on a few possibilities. First, parents who use more ET might convey to children that it is okay to express and talk about emotions (via shaping children's emotion control values), which in turn can shape children's emotion expressions and emotion-related behaviors [14,15]. Second, it is also possible that children who are temperamentally more expressive elicit more ET in parents (e.g., by creating more opportunities for parents to respond to and talk about children's emotions or by making parents more attuned to children's emotions and more motivated to provide scaffolding for children's emotion regulation [18]. Future studies should replicate these relations in other samples and investigate the mechanisms using longitudinal data.

5. Limitations and Conclusions

The study has several limitations. First, the cross-sectional design did not allow us to test the directionality of the relations between parental ET and child's emotions, which is of theoretical importance given the transactional nature of parent–child interactions. Second, the small sample size offered limited statistical power for testing cultural group variations in strengths of relations between ET and emotion expressions. Third, the interrater reliability for children's expressed sadness was low, partly because children were allowed to move freely during the tasks, and their facial expressions were often obstructed by the box or shadow, making it difficult to code expressed sadness (which involves more subtle facial expressions and behaviors than anger or positive emotions). Also, we did not code other types of negative emotions (e.g., fear, anxiety). Fourth, the brief frustration task did not provide sufficient opportunity to observe a full range of emotion-related behaviors during this age period, such as self-soothing, self-talk, and problem-solving behaviors. Future research should use multiple methods and tools to assess children's emotion expressions and emotion-related behaviors across different situations to obtain a better understanding of cultural variations in emotion models. Fifth, the shared picture book reading task might not capture the full range of parent–child ET in daily life. Moreover, because the ET coding theme was originally developed in English based on conversations in European American families and only includes explicit verbal references to emotions, it might not capture subtle or indirect references to emotions in Spanish or Chinese languages. Future research can use qualitative or mixed methods to capture unique aspects of parent–child discourse related to emotions in Mexican and Chinese families.

In sum, this study revealed culture group similarities and differences in preschool-age children's emotion expressions and emotion-related behaviors in low-income immigrant families. Regardless of culture, children whose parents used more emotion talk during shared book reading expressed more anger and sadness and used more non-feeling states languages in the frustration-eliciting situation. The findings highlighted emotion talk as a potential mechanism through which culturally based values and norms in emotion expressions are transmitted. The findings have implications for school-based socioemotional learning and parent psycho-education programs for promoting socioemotional development in early childhood. Specifically, these programs need to be sensitive to cultural variations in how parents and children express and communicate emotionally, and cultural adaptations might be necessary to enhance the programs' fit with and potential to engage immigrant families from diverse backgrounds.

Author Contributions: Conceptualization, Q.Z., M.C., M.T. and N.E.; methodology, Q.Z., M.C., M.T. and N.E.; software, Q.Z.; validation, M.C., M.T. and Q.Z.; formal analysis, Q.Z., M.C. and M.T.; investigation, Q.Z.; resources, Q.Z.; data curation, Q.Z.; writing—original draft preparation, M.C., M.T. and Q.Z.; writing—review and editing, N.E.; visualization, Q.Z.; supervision, Q.Z.; project administration, Q.Z.; funding acquisition, Q.Z. All authors have read and agreed to the published version of the manuscript.

Funding: This research was funded by a seed grant from the Institute for the Study of Societal Issues, University of California Berkeley (to Qing Zhou). Work on this manuscript was also supported by a grant from the National Institute of Health (R01HD091154) to Qing Zhou and Yuuko Uchikoshi and a National Science Foundation Graduate Research Fellowship to Megan Chan.

Institutional Review Board Statement: This study was conducted in accordance with the Declaration of Helsinki and was approved by the Institutional Review Board of the corresponding author's institution on 12 November 2012.(Protocol No. #2012-06-4454).

Informed Consent Statement: Informed consent was obtained from all subjects involved in the study.

Data Availability Statement: The data is available upon request due to privacy and ethical reasons.

Acknowledgments: The authors would like to thank all families, preschool teachers, staff, and directors who have participated in or assisted with the study, as well as the graduate and undergraduate students who have assisted with the study.

Conflicts of Interest: The authors declare no conflicts of interest. The funders had no role in the design of the study; in the collection, analyses, or interpretation of data; in the writing of the manuscript; or in the decision to publish the results.

References

1. Eisenberg, N.; Cumberland, A.; Spinrad, T.L. Parental socialization of emotion. *Psychol. Inq.* **1998**, *9*, 241–273. [CrossRef] [PubMed]
2. Chaplin, T.M.; Klein, M.R.; Cole, P.M.; Turpyn, C.C. Developmental change in emotion expression in frustrating situations: The roles of context and gender. *Infant Child Dev.* **2017**, *26*, e2028. [CrossRef] [PubMed]
3. Thompson, R.A. Emotion dysregulation: A theme in search of definition. *Dev. Psychopathol.* **2019**, *31*, 805–815. [CrossRef]
4. Grolnick, W.S.; Bridges, L.J.; Connell, J.P. Emotion regulation in two-year-olds: Strategies and emotional expression in four contexts. *Child Dev.* **1996**, *67*, 928–941. [CrossRef] [PubMed]
5. Cole, P.M.; Armstrong, L.M.; Pemberton, C.K. The role of language in the development of emotion regulation. In *Child Development at the Intersection of Emotion and Cognition*; Calkins, S.D., Bell, M.A., Eds.; American Psychological Association: Washington, DC, USA, 2010; pp. 59–77. [CrossRef]
6. Chan, M.; Williams, A.I.; Teng, Y.P.T.; Zhou, Q. Links between parent-child emotion talk and preschoolers' socioemotional behaviors in Chinese-heritage families. *Early Educ. Dev.* **2023**, *34*, 366–386. [CrossRef]
7. Garrett-Peters, P.T.; Fox, N.A. Cross-cultural differences in children's emotional reactions to a disappointing situation. *Int. J. Behav. Dev.* **2007**, *31*, 161–169. [CrossRef]
8. Liew, J.; Eisenberg, N.; Reiser, M. Preschoolers' effortful control and negative emotionality, immediate reactions to disappointment, and quality of social functioning. *J. Exp. Child Psychol.* **2004**, *89*, 298–319. [CrossRef] [PubMed]
9. Kim, Y.; Williams, A.I.; Liu, C.; Zhou, Q. Dynamic associations between emotion expressions and strategy use in Chinese American and Mexican American preschoolers. *Emotion* **2023**, *23*, 460–472. [CrossRef]
10. Camras, L.A. *Emotional Development Across the Lifespan*; Guilford Publications: New York, NY, USA, 2022.
11. Fivush, R.; Haden, C.A.; Reese, E. Elaborating on elaborations: Role of maternal reminiscing style in cognitive and socioemotional development. *Child Dev.* **2006**, *77*, 1568–1588. [CrossRef] [PubMed]
12. Streubel, B.; Gunzenhauser, C.; Grosse, G.; Saalbach, H. Emotion-specific vocabulary and its contribution to emotion understanding in 4- to 9-year-old children. *J. Exp. Child Psychol.* **2020**, *193*, 104790. [CrossRef] [PubMed]
13. Denham, S.A.; Bassett, H.H.; Zinsser, K.; Wyatt, T.M. How preschoolers' social–emotional learning predicts their early school success: Developing theory-promoting, competency-based assessments. *Infant Child Dev.* **2014**, *23*, 426–454. [CrossRef]
14. Mauss, I.B.; Butler, E.A. Cultural context moderates the relationship between emotion control values and cardiovascular challenge versus threat responses. *Biol. Psychol.* **2010**, *84*, 521–530. [CrossRef] [PubMed]
15. Zerwas, F.K.; Tharp, J.A.; Chen, S.; Mauss, I.B. Individual differences in social power: Links with beliefs about emotion and emotion regulation. *J. Personal.* **2023**, *91*, 314–331. [CrossRef]
16. Curtis, K.; Zhou, Q.; Tao, A. Emotion talk in Chinese American immigrant families and longitudinal links to children's socioemotional competence. *Dev. Psychol.* **2020**, *56*, 475–488. [CrossRef] [PubMed]
17. Garner, P.W.; Dunsmore, J.C.; Southam-Gerrow, M. Mother–child conversations about emotions: Linkages to child aggression and prosocial behavior. *Soc. Dev.* **2008**, *17*, 259–277. [CrossRef]
18. Lorenzo, N.E.; Bahrick, L.E.; Bagner, D.M. Examining the trajectory of parent emotion talk in mothers of toddlers: A predominantly Latine sample. *Infant Behav. Dev.* **2023**, *70*, 101801. [CrossRef] [PubMed]
19. Vu, K.T.T.; Cheah, C.S.L.; Halberstadt, A.G. Chinese immigrant child and maternal reactions to disappointment: Cultural fit impacts the bidirectional associations. *Soc. Dev.* **2023**, *32*, 445–462. [CrossRef]
20. Senft, N.; Campos, B.; Shiota, M.N.; Chentsova-Dutton, Y.E. Who emphasizes positivity? An exploration of emotion values in people of Latino, Asian, and European heritage living in the United States. *Emotion* **2021**, *21*, 707–719. [CrossRef] [PubMed]

21. Matsumoto, D.; Yoo, S.H.; Fontaine, J. Mapping expressive differences around the world: The relationship between emotional display rules and individualism versus collectivism. *J. Cross-Cult. Psychol.* **2008**, *39*, 55–74. [CrossRef]
22. Tsai, J.L.; Knutson, B.; Fung, H.H. Cultural variation in affect valuation. *J. Personal. Soc. Psychol.* **2006**, *90*, 288–307. [CrossRef]
23. Song, Q.; Yang, Y.; Doan, S.N.; Wang, Q. Savoring or dampening? Maternal reactions to children's positive emotions in cultural contexts. *Cult. Brain* **2019**, *7*, 172–189. [CrossRef]
24. Calzada, E.J.; Fernandez, Y.; Cortes, D.E. Incorporating the cultural value of *respeto* into a framework of Latino parenting. *Cult. Divers. Ethn. Minor. Psychol.* **2010**, *16*, 77–86. [CrossRef] [PubMed]
25. Acevedo, A.M.; Herrera, C.; Shenhav, S.; Yim, I.S.; Campos, B. Measurement of a Latino cultural value: The Simpatía scale. *Cult. Divers. Ethn. Minor. Psychol.* **2020**, *26*, 419. [CrossRef]
26. Luo, R.; Tamis-LeMonda, C.S.; Kuchirko, Y.F.; Ng, F.; Liang, E. Mother–child book-sharing and children's storytelling skills in ethnically diverse, low-income families. *Infant Child Dev.* **2014**, *23*, 402–425. [CrossRef]
27. Camras, L.; Bakeman, R.; Chen, Y.; Norris, K.; Cain, T. Culture, ethnicity, and children's facial expressions: A study of European American, Mainland Chinese, Chinese American, and adopted Chinese girls. *Emotion* **2006**, *6*, 103–114. [CrossRef] [PubMed]
28. Wang, J.; Barrett, K.C. Differences between American and Chinese preschoolers in emotional responses to resistance to temptation and mishap contexts. *Motiv. Emot.* **2015**, *39*, 420–433. [CrossRef]
29. Lindsey, E.W.; Caldera, Y.M.; Rivera, M. Mother–child and father–child emotional expressiveness in Mexican-American families and toddlers' peer interactions. *Early Child Dev. Care* **2023**, *183*, 378–393. [CrossRef]
30. Ruby, M.B.; Falk, C.F.; Heine, S.J.; Villa, C.; Silberstein, O. Not all collectivisms are equal: Opposing preferences for ideal affect between East Asians and Mexicans. *Emotion* **2021**, *12*, 1206–1209. [CrossRef] [PubMed]
31. Shaffer, A.; Suveg, C.; Thomassin, K.; Bradbury, L.L. Emotion socialization in the context of family risks: Links to child emotion regulation. *J. Child Fam. Stud.* **2012**, *21*, 917–924. [CrossRef]
32. Tao, A.; Zhou, Q.; Lau, N.; Liu, H. Chinese American immigrant mothers' discussion of emotion with children: Relations to cultural orientations. *J. Cross-Cult. Psychol.* **2013**, *44*, 478–501. [CrossRef]
33. Adams, C.; Kuebli, J.; Boyle, P.A.; Fivush, R. Gender differences in parent-child conversations about past emotions: A longitudinal investigation. *Sex Roles* **1995**, *33*, 309–323. [CrossRef]
34. Chung, S.; Zhou, Q.; Anicama, C.; Rivera, C.; Uchikoshi, Y. Language proficiency, parenting styles, and socioemotional adjustment of young dual language learners. *J. Cross-Cult. Psychol.* **2019**, *50*, 896–914. [CrossRef] [PubMed]
35. Tompkins, V.; Benigno, J.P.; Kiger Lee, B.; Wright, B.M. The relation between parents' mental state talk and children's social understanding: A meta-analysis. *Soc. Dev.* **2018**, *27*, 223–246. [CrossRef]
36. Roosa, M.W.; Liu, F.F.; Torres, M.; Gonzales, N.A.; Knight, G.P.; Saenz, D. Sampling and recruitment in studies of cultural influences on adjustment: A case study with Mexican Americans. *J. Fam. Psychol.* **2008**, *22*, 293–302. [CrossRef]
37. Mayer, M. *Frog, Where Are You?* Dial Press: New York, NY, USA, 1969.
38. Huang, S.; Kan, P.F. Cross-linguistic transfer between aspect in Cantonese and past tense in English in Cantonese- English bilingual preschool children. *Int. J. Speech-Lang. Pathol.* **2021**, *24*, 385–394. [CrossRef] [PubMed]
39. Spinrad, T.; Eisenberg, N. *Codebook: Toddler Emotion Development Project*; Unpublished manual; T. Denny Sanford School of Social and Family Dynamics and Department of Psychology, Arizona State University: Tempe, AZ, USA, 2010.
40. Koo, T.K.; Li, M.Y. A guideline of selecting and reporting intraclass correlation coefficients for reliability research. *J. Chiropr. Med.* **2016**, *15*, 155–163. [CrossRef] [PubMed]
41. Goldsmith, H.H.; Rothbart, M.K. *Coding Gestural Behavior with the NEUROGES-ELAN System*, Version 3.0.; Technical Manual, Department of Psychology, University of Wisconsin: Madison, WI, USA, 1996.
42. Lausberg, H.; Sloetjes, H. Coding gestural behavior with the NEUROGES¬ELAN system. *Behav. Res. Methods Instrum. Comput.* **2009**, *41*, 841–849. [CrossRef]
43. West, S.G.; Finch, J.F.; Curran, P.J. Structural equation models with nonnormal variables: Problems and remedies. In *Structural Equation Modeling: Concepts, Issues, and Applications*; Hoyle, R.H., Ed.; Sage Publications, Inc.: New York, NY, USA, 1995; pp. 56–75.

children

MDPI

Article

Adaptation of the Coparenting Relationship Scale Questionnaire to Spanish Parents with Offspring

Dolores Seijo [1], Francisca Fariña [2], María Paula Fernández [3,*] and Ramón Arce [1]

[1] Forensic Psychology Unit, Department of Political Science and Sociology, Faculty of Psychology, University of Santiago de Compostela, 15782 Santiago de Compostela, Spain; mariadolores.seijo@usc.es (D.S.); ramon.arce@usc.es (R.A.)
[2] Department AIPSE, University of Vigo, 36310 Vigo, Spain; francisca@uvigo.gal
[3] Department of Psychology, Oviedo University, Plaza Feijoo, 33003 Oviedo, Spain
* Correspondence: paula@uniovi.es

Abstract: The scientific literature supports that practicing positive coparenting leads to the healthy development of children. Consequently, professional interest in parenting and coparenting has experienced significant growth, and evaluating coparenting is crucial in family psychology for establishing action protocols in clinical practice. An instrument highly regarded within the scientific community for evaluating coparenting dynamics is *The Coparenting Relationship Scale* (CRS). This research aims to achieve two objectives: first, to adapt the CRS for the Spanish population of both engaged and separated/divorced parents and to ascertain its reliability, validity, and factorial invariance psychometric properties; second, to assess the effectiveness of the total coparenting measure in categorizing sample participants. A cross-sectional non-experimental investigation was conducted to address these objectives. The first objective was answered by conducting an instrumental study, and the second by an exploratory study using classification techniques and a causal-comparative study using multivariate inferential methods. It was concluded that the model comprising 20 items across two factors, *Positive Coparenting* and *Negative Perception of Coparenting*, is the simplest and best fit for the Spanish parent sample; it is invariant regarding gender and marital status, and the measures derived from each factor demonstrate reliability and convergent and discriminant validity. The resulting questionnaire for Spanish parents is named CRS-$S_{Eg\text{-}S\&D}$. The *Coparental Vitality* measure calculated using the total weighted measure of CRS-$S_{Eg\text{-}S\&D}$ allows the sample of participants to be divided into three differentiated clusters called *Coparental Robustness*, *Moderate Coparenting*, and *Coparenting Rickets*.

Keywords: coparenting; coparenting relationship scale/CRS; engaged and separated/divorced parents; construct; convergent validity; discriminate validity; factorial invariance; coparental vitality

1. Introduction

The scientific literature strongly supports the importance of coparenting in the proper development of children [1–4]. The exercise of parenting refers to the set of activities related to the care and education of children that each parent carries out, regardless of their legal or biological relationship [1,3,5,6]. Coparenting refers to how parents or caregivers relate to each other as such [7], irrespective of their sex. Today, the construct of coparenting has been decoupled from the gender role and is applied to all types of intact families [2].

When parents or parental figures agree to meet the needs of their children, they share the responsibilities of their upbringing by distributing the tasks related to their care, protection, and education, and they support each other in the parental role by facilitating and promoting positive interactions with their children (i.e., children must perceive that their parents agree on the rules they must follow; children must perceive that their parents address issues related to them together, support each other as parents, and avoid contradictions or competition between them in front of them). If the above description is true, they are exercising positive coparenting [1,4,8–12]. The coparenting relationship, although different from the couple relationship since it includes a romantic relationship between adults [9], is closely connected to it [7] and is of capital importance. Not in vain, the study of coparenting began by examining how the quality of the relationship that parents maintain when they have divorced influences their children [13–16]. It has been shown that when parents maintain a good relationship, their parental behaviors are positive, and the coparenting is harmonious; in addition to having advantages for themselves, it has clear advantages for their children, directly affecting their physical and psycho-emotional well-being [4,17–22], demonstrating that it is a powerful protective factor [2], for example, against addictions [4]. Often, when parents are separated or divorced, the consequences on their children are negative and contrary to these [2,4,13–16].

Thus, scientific and professional interest in parenting and coparenting has grown exponentially, and the evaluation of coparenting has become an essential issue in family psychology, both for research protocols and intervention in clinical practice [14]. This growing interest has led to the development of numerous self-report instruments aimed at capturing some of the multiple aspects that the construct entails [7,18], among them the *Parenting Alliance Inventory* [23], the *Coparenting Questionnaire* [24], and the *Coparenting Inventory for Parents and Adolescents* [25].

One of the instruments that has had the most significant impact and is best received by the scientific community is the Coparenting Relationship Scale (CRS) [26]. This scale can be used for families with children from infancy to adolescence. Based on family systems theory, Feinberg [9] proposes an ecological theoretical model of coparenting. (This model establishes the distribution between parents of the duties and responsibilities related to childcare. The parents agree on parenting between themselves and establish the roles of each one for joint management of the family, forming a coalition between the co-parental figures in front of the child. Each parent reinforces the other in their role as parents without any questioning or criticism between them). Thus, it places the coparenting relationship or the coparenting subsystem within the context of a broader family system where other social systems (e.g., economic context, religious context, and employment situation) are identified between which connections exist, where different family processes develop (it is considered that families are not static, but instead constantly changing due to the development processes of each family member), and where the main facets of the coparenting relationship are exercised [7,27,28]. New partners and children must be incorporated into the family naturally without posing an obstacle to the parental relationship.

The CRS questionnaire developed by Feinberg et al. [26] has been translated into multiple languages. The adequacy of its dimensional structure (long and short, 35 and 14 items, respectively) has been analyzed in different countries (Portugal, Sweden, France, Romania, and Spain/Spanish-speaking countries), and for samples with very *diverse particularities*, such as divorced parents (Portugal: [29]), father's prenatal (Portugal: [30]), primiparous and multiparous fathers (Sweden: [31]), mothers (Portugal: [32]), minority and heterosexual people (Portugal: [33]), and parents of both sexes and all marital statuses in Portugal [34], France [35], Romania [36], and Spain/Spanish speakers [37].

Plá [37] translated and adapted the CRS questionnaire into Spanish in its two versions, long and short. However, it manifests important deficiencies in its approach and in the validation process, which we can summarize in five points. First, the sample consisted of 489 parents with at least one adolescent child between 11 and 18 years old. A total of 51.1% of the participants lived in Uruguay, and 48.9% lived in Spain. Furthermore, the Spanish participants were of 18 different nationalities. Assuming that the translation of the items had content that Spanish speakers of the 18 nationalities equally understood, it is very risky to believe that the dimensional structure found is valid for all of them because the different origins contain cultural differences, a widely documented aspect. In this sense, Bornstein [38] and Sun [4] have shown that the interaction between parents and children and cultural context may impact family functions, and Ronaghan et al. [7]

insist that the country of the people can mediate the quality of parenting. Second, Feinberg et al. [26] found in the dimensional structure that the *Division of Labor* factor comprises only two items. Plá [37] added three more items, with common sense but without proven empirical support for this factor to be better represented. Third, Plá [37] tests the 7-factor model found by Feinberg et al. [26] in an exploratory way; however, they perform this task using Principal Component Analysis (PCA) instead of using Exploratory Factor Analysis (EFA). This aspect has been highly criticized by experts who unanimously conclude that PCA is not valid to study the dimensional structure of a questionnaire [39–42]. Fourth, Pla [37] does not show the descriptive statistics of the items referring to the central tendency, variability, and distribution, and this aspect is essential to evaluate the adequacy of the items. However, it does display the homogeneity index (HIc, the corrected correlation of each item with the test) and Cronbach's alpha if the item is eliminated. It can be seen that item 5 has a value of 0.267, 0.221, and 0.297 in the long and short versions and in the belonging factor, respectively (the experts consider HIc < 0.30 [42–44] inadequate). It is also noted that the reliability of the questionnaire would increase significantly if this item were eliminated. This aspect has been observed in the adaptation of the questionnaire to other languages [29,32–34,36], and in all cases, it has been taken into account, and the item has been eliminated. However, it was not taken into account by Plá [37]. Fifth, in the request for seven factors (the same model found by Feinberg et al. [26]), two were underrepresented (appeared with two and three items, respectively), and one factor was overrepresented (appeared with eleven items). Consequently, since the seven factors of the CRS represented four theoretical domains (see Feinberg [9]), Plá confused domains with factors and requested four factors. Plá [37] finally concludes that the factors that make up the dimensional structure of the CRS-r are four, and demonized *Support received* or *Coparenting strength* (items 2, 3, 6, 10, 17, 19, 24, 25, 26, 27, 28, and 30 that correspond to the original scales *Coparenting Closeness*, *Coparenting Support* and *Coparenting Agreement*), *Exposure to Conflict* (for items 24–28, this factor remains fully equivalent to the factor of the original scale of the same name), *Agreement-non-sabotage* (items 8, 9, 11, 12, 13, 15, 16, 21, and 22, which correspond to the original scales *Coparenting Agreement* and *Coparenting Undermining*), and *Support given or solidarity* (items 1, 4, 5, 7, 14, 18, 20, 23, 31, 32, 33 that correspond to the original scales *Endorse Partner Parenting* and *Division of Labor*—it is necessary to remember that three more items were added to this factor). Item 29 of the original scale appeared unloaded and was the only item that was decided to be eliminated. However, in the final solution found by Plá [33], items 6 and 18 show a loading of <0.40, and items 18 and 33 are complex. Although both characteristics invalidate the relevance of the items [42,45,46], Plá [37] does not give importance to this aspect.

In this way, assuming that the items that make up the CRS include all the content of the coparenting construct that Feinberg et al. [26] identified, considering that "The advantages of this measure will also facilitate the assessment of the domains of coparenting in clinical practice, allowing intervention to capitalize on areas of strength and focus on improving areas of difficulty" [26] (p. 12), and considering that the adaptation and validation of the CRS scale to the Spanish population sample carried out by Plá [37] was not made appropriately, in this research, we propose two objectives. The first is to adapt *The Coparenting Relationship Scale* (CRS) [26] to the Spanish population of engaged parents (Eg) and separated or divorced parents (S&D) and to study its psychometric properties, that is, to determine its dimensionality, to test the hypothesis of factorial invariance as a function of sex and marital status, to study the reliability of the measure, and to examine evidence of validity. The second is to evaluate the strength of the total coparenting measure to classify the sample participants into different categories and thus deepen the knowledge of the coparenting construct.

A cross-sectional non-experimental investigation was carried out to respond to the stated objectives. The first objective was answered by conducting an instrumental study that followed the standards required for the construction, adaptation, and development of tests [47,48]. The second was answered by conducting an exploratory study using classification techniques and a causal-comparative study using multivariate inferential methods.

2. Materials and Methods

2.1. Participants

A total of 3155 parents submitted the answer booklet. Initially, the responses of 13 participants who had been widowed were eliminated (and for obvious reasons, their responses were not useful for the instrumental study because they were not coparenting). As a result, a total of 3142 participants were potentially useful to carry out the instrumental research: 2754 (87.65%) engaged parents (Eg, never separated or divorced, regardless of whether they are married or cohabiting together) [84.02% (n = 2314) and 15.97% (n = 440), respectively] and 388 (12.34%) separated or divorced (S&D) parents (188 S and 199 D).

First, a thorough study of the participants' responses to the CRS items was conducted to clean the database [42,46] and preserve the sample of participants with useful responses to carry out the analysis. We began by identifying all *illegitimate cases* [42] (p. 85); these were those whose responses were useless for the intended objective, therefore lack value, and add substantial error variance to the analysis [42] (p. 85). Illegitimate cases were considered, such as those arising from non-responses to all scale items, for obvious reasons, and those arising from random response patterns likely to threaten the quality of the measure when carrying out a factor analysis. Random responses are a set of responses where individuals respond with little thought or reflection [49] due to a lack of preparation, reactivity to observation, lack of motivation to cooperate with the test, disinterest, or fatigue [49–53]. In this sense, it was established to reject the responses of those participants who did not respond to 40% or a greater percentage of the items in the CRS questionnaire. The argument is the following: This behavior could be due to a good intention (to respond later in a more reflective way, but never did so), but it could also be due to a lack of motivation and/or commitment to the research for which they had given their consent. On the other hand, of those participants whose response rate was complete, it was decided to eliminate those participants who maintained the same response level in more than 50% of the items (levels 3 and 6 were the most selected).

Thus, 218 participants did not respond to any item on the scale, 271 left the responses to more than 40% of the items blank, and 102 gave the same response to more than 50% of the items. In total, 591 participants submitted the booklet with little or no commitment to the research. We considered the pattern of their responses to be random; therefore, their responses were useless for the analysis. Thus, the responses of 2551 people are potentially useful for data analysis.

Among these, 124 people left some items empty (between 1 and 5 items), possibly due to random (MAR) or non-random (NMAR) causes. They were also eliminated because they represent a percentage of less than 5% (4.86%), and their elimination does not threaten the validity of the statistical and substantive conclusions of the analysis results [54]. As a result, the sample finally consisted of 2427 parents.

2.2. Sociodemographic Characteristics of the Sample

Regarding marital status, 90.1% (n = 2187) are Eg and 9.9% (n = 240) are D&S (technically, distributed in the same proportion, 4.9%, n = 119, are separated and 5%, n = 121, are divorced). The number of women is four times greater than that of men [women are 80.4% (n = 1951) of the sample, and men are 19.6% (n = 475)], and the mean age is 40.42 years [SD = 5.67; range 1–66 years; bias = −0.291 and kurtosis = 1.27].

On the other hand, 96.4% do not have other children from previous relationships. Only 3.6% (n = 87) have children from previous relationships [2.7% (n = 66) have one more child from earlier relationships, 0.8% (n = 19) report having two children from previous relationships, and only 2 people have 3 children from previous relationships]. Regarding the age of those children they have with previous partners, for people who have a child, the age of these children is between 1–33 years (M = 17.74; SD = 6.39). Of those who have two children, the first is in the range of 10–29 years (M = 19.65; SD = 5.88), and the second is in the range of 1–25 years (M = 15.68; SD = 6.33). Those who have three children (which are only two people) have had children after a long time because the first is in a range of 21–24 years (M = 22.5; SD = 2.12), the second is in a range of 21–23 years (M = 22; SD = 1.40), and the third is in the range of 19–27 years (M = 23; SD = 5.65).

Regarding the current family at the time they participated in this research, 89.4% (n = 2154) is a primary family (both are biological or adoptive parents), 3.3% (n = 80) is a reconstructed family (at home, there is a stepfather/stepmother), 3.7% (n = 89) is a family of single parents, and 3.5% (n = 84) state that they are in a different situation from the previous ones. Regarding the number of children living at home, the most frequent situation is where 2 children live together, 55% (n = 1336), followed by where only one child lives together, 33.8% (n = 820). Far removed from these two predominant conditions, three children live together in 8.9% (n = 217) of the cases; in 30 homes (1.2%), there are four children, but there is also the case where 5, 6, and 7 children live together, which total 9 homes (0.3%). That is, their child, about whom they have responded in the booklet, is an only child or is the only child in the house 33.8% of the time (n = 820), lives with a sibling 55% of the time, and are among 3 or more children at home 11.2% of the time.

Regarding the children under 12 years of age for whom the participants responded to the items in the booklet, 50.9% are male (n = 1236), and 48.4% are female (n = 1174). Only 3.8% are 12 (n = 93), and 2-year-olds are 4.6% (n = 108). Thus, it can be considered that between 2–12 years, all ages are represented. The average age is 7.23 years [SD = 2.80; range 1–12 years]. Age is non-normally distributed [bias = −0.119 and kurtosis 1.039; K-S = 0.056, df = 3120, p = 0.000; $P_{25} = 5$, $P_{75} = 10$, $P_{50} = 7$).

The participants who were eliminated from the instrumental study (the 591 participants who submitted the booklet with little or no commitment to the research and the 124 we estimated who left items unanswered for MAR or NMAR reasons) did not differ in the sociodemographic characteristics from the 2427 parents who were part of the study.

2.3. Procedure

The researchers contacted 130 elementary schools (primary schools) in Spain, and 73 agreed to collaborate (characteristics of the schools, location, rural vs. urban, size, and participation are shown in Section S5 of the Supplementary Materials). A conference was organized in each of the 73 elementary schools aimed at all the students' families. All attendees were informed that research was being carried out to expand knowledge about parenting and coparenting, and they were shown the content of the answer booklet. All fathers and mothers with sons and daughters between 2 and 12 years old were invited to participate.

To ensure the maximum possible participation and response rate and avoid acquiescence in the response, extreme precautions were taken throughout the data collection process [54,55]. In this sense, the participants were warned that paying attention to the questions and answering honestly was necessary, only referring to the youngest of their children. Furthermore, due to the booklet length, they were informed that they would have one month to respond. They were also told that during that time, they could contact the project researchers to resolve any questions, and a telephone number and email address were provided. All attendees were informed that the school management team would send four reminders to avoid oblivion (one weekly reminder for four weeks in the school's usual way of communicating with students' families).

People who gave informed consent received the response booklet and an opaque envelope. To guarantee anonymity and discretion, an ad hoc mailbox was set up in each school where they had to insert the anonymous answer booklet inside the opaque envelope when they had completed it. The research respected all laws on protecting personal data and had permission from the Bioethics Committee of the University of Santiago de Compostela.

2.4. Measurements

The Coparenting Relationship Scale (CRS) [26]. The questionnaire consists of 35 items, divided into 7 dimensions of coparenting related to the four domains of Feinberg's model [9] as follows:

1. The domain of coparenting agreement with a subscale of the same name, Coparenting agreement (4 items);
2. The coparenting support/undermining domain was represented by 3 subscales, Coparenting Support (6 items), Endorsement of Partner's Parenting (7 items), and Coparenting Undermining (6 items);
3. The domain management of family relationships was assessed with the subscale Exposure to Conflict (5 items);
4. The domain division of childrearing work was made up of the subscale called Division of Labor (2 items).

Finally, Feinberg et al. [26] created a 5-item subscale measuring the degree to which coparenting enhanced intimacy and strengthened the couple's relationship, which they called Coparenting Closeness (5 items).

Feinberg et al. [26] concluded that "The overall Coparenting Relationship Scale demonstrated excellent internal consistency, with Cronbach's alphas ranging from 0.91 to 0.94 across gender and data collection time" [26] (p. 8).

All items have a 6-point response scale ranging from 0 "not true of us" to 6 "very true of us", except for the Exposure to Conflict subscale, where responses ranged from 0 "never" to 6 "very often". For correction, the mean score for the items of each of the subscales is calculated (14 items are inverse, see Sections S1 and S2, Table S1 of the Supplementary Materials). Example items are *I believe my partner is a good parent; My partner and I have the same goals for our child; My partner does not trust my abilities as a parent.*

Parenting and Family Adjustment Scales (PAFAS). Sanders et al. [56] developed and adapted to Spanish by Fariña et al. [57], resulting in a valid, reliable, brief, and comprehensive measure to evaluate Spanish parents' parenting styles and family adjustment. It consists of 20 items distributed in two subscales and five factors. The Parenting subscale is made up of the factors of Coercive parenting (5 items), Positive stimulation (3 items), and Maternal/Paternal filial relationships (4 items), and the Family Adjustment subscale is made up of the factors of Parental adjustment (4 items) and Adjustment family (4 items). The reliability coefficient was calculated using the coefficient H; in both subscales, it was 0.96. Participants respond to the extent that each statement is correct for their situation on a Likert-type scale, with 4 response alternatives (0 "never", 1 "rarely/sometimes", 2 "quite a few/many times", 3 "most of the time/always"). Example items in the Parenting subscale include *I shout or get angry with my child when they Misbehave; I give my child a treat, reward or fun activity for behaving well;* and *I give my child attention (e.g., a hug, wink, smile or kiss) when they behave well.* Example items in the Family Adjustment subscale include *I cope with the emotional demands of being a parent; I work as a team with my partner in parenting;* and *I feel happy.*

Parental Efficacy Scale (CAPES). It was built by Morawska et al. [58] and adapted with sound psychometric properties for the Spanish population by Seijo et al. [59]. The scale comprises 25 items grouped into two factors: Child's Competencies (10 items) and Behavioral and Emotional Problems (15 items). The reliability coefficient calculated using Cronbach's alpha was 0.94 and 0.84 in the respective scales. Participants respond to each item on a 4-point Likert-type scale, from 0, "not true at all", to 3, "true most of the time", depending on how true the statement was for their child in the past 4 weeks. Items are summed to yield a total intensity score (CAPES intensity scale) composed of a behavioral score and an emotional maladjustment score. Higher scores indicate higher levels of problems. Example items in the Child's Competencies factor include *Can keep busy without constant adult attention; Does what they are told to do by adults;* and *Talks about their views, ideas and needs appropriately.* Example items in the Behavioral and Emotional Problems include

Gets upset or angry when they don't get their own way; Loses their temper; and *Takes too long getting dressed*.

2.5. Data Analysis

We can summarize the axes that determine the data analysis in the process of adapting the CRS questionnaire [26] to the Spanish population of engaged parents (Eg) and separated or divorced parents (S&D) into two.

In the first axis, the response booklet indicated that items 31–35 (corresponding to the *Exposure to Conflict* scale) would only be answered if a couple was broken up, that is, separated or divorced. This was performed for four reasons. The first is because the same authors who constructed the questionnaire write, "However, we believe that coparenting relations may differ from one child to the next, and thus recommend that some subscales (e.g., exposure to conflict) be administered regarding each child separately" [26] (p. 12). Therefore, we understand that the authors contemplate a certain freedom in how these items are considered. The second is because the items that represent the *Exposure to Conflict* factor are ordered consecutively and not presented in random order among the set of scale items, as are the rest. Due to the influence that the order of presentation of the items has on the response of the participants, as highlighted in the previous section [60,61], we consider that it is possible that the response to the first item conditions the response to the others, even from the rest of the items (because there is no control over the order in which participants respond to the items), causing an unwanted response pattern in the questionnaire. Third, Feinberg et al. [26] found a mean value and a standard deviation less than 1 in this factor. This result indicates that the items that make up the factor are not discriminative in the population of parents to which the sample belongs [43]. Pinto et al. [30] decided to eliminate these items to find a good fit in the model, possibly for the same reason. The common denominator of these two investigations was the sample. In Feinberg et al. [26], the sample was heterosexual couples who were expecting their first child at the time of recruitment, and in Pinto et al. [30], the sample was the father's prenatal., Fourth, because Feinberg et al. [26] and all the research above that has adapted and validated the CRS questionnaire to other countries and/or other *sample particularities* have found a correlation ≥ 0.60 between the *Exposure to Conflict* and *Coparenting Undermining* scales, therefore, we estimate that the magnitude of the conflict that may exist between members who have children in common, whether they were together or separated or divorced, can also be captured with the items of the *Coparenting Undermining scale*, thus making the duration of the questionnaire shorter. Therefore, in this research, the 6-factor model is studied in a 30-item test, and we call this initial model CRS^{6F}.

As explained in the description of the procedure in Section 2.2, this research is part of a more extensive investigation on coparenting and parenting, and the added value of the *Exposure to Conflict* factor in the evaluation of coparenting exclusively in divorced and/or separated is the subject of future research.

In the second axis, Feinberg et al. end the article as follows: "We hope that this measure, or future refinements of it, will be useful for examining family relationships across various contexts. We look forward to further inquiries examining the reliability and validity of this measure in an array of families, with diverse sociodemographic backgrounds, levels of risk, and stages of family development" [26] (p. 12). This research has these words as its starting point, and what is pursued in achieving the two objectives stated above is to select those items from the CRS^{6F} that are useful and valid to evaluate coparenting both in parents who live together and in parents who do not live together and have separated or divorced, and in the same way for men and women. That is, we intend to select items that allow us to evaluate coparenting and that are invariant depending on the marital status and sex of the parent to study the coparenting relationship in depth. To this end, a core part of this research is the development of an exhaustive Exploratory Factor Analysis (before testing a theoretical model through Confirmatory Factor Analysis), where the relevance of the items is carefully examined in the different subsamples of parents and where emphasis is placed on the analysis of the replication of the results, as detailed below.

Data analysis was organized into three main blocks.

2.5.1. Block of Analysis 1: Analysis of the Factor Structure of the Questionnaire, Determination of Its Dimensionality, and Study of the Reliability of the Measure

The process of assessing the dimensionality structure of *The Coparenting Relationship Scale* (Feinberg et al. [26]) began by assessing whether the 6-factor model in a 30-item test (model CRS^{6F}) was valid in the Spanish population of engaged parents (Eg) and separated or divorced parents (S&D). This was conducted in two ways: by a Semiconfirmatory Factor Analysis (sCFA) using Procrustean rotations against a target matrix [62] and by the Confirmatory Factor Analysis (CFA). Both methods converge in that the original model does not fit the data. Thus, a study was conducted to determine which dimensional structures are appropriate and their compositions.

Following the required procedure for cross-validation [63], we used an *internal replicability analysis*, and the sample was randomly divided into two independent samples, taking extreme care so that the participants in both subsamples were balanced according to the variables sex and marital status.

With the calibration sample (n = 1239), a successive Exploratory Factor Analysis (EFA) was performed, and the most suitable items were selected. Previously, a descriptive study of the items in each subgroup defined by sex and marital status was carried out (see Section S2 of the Supplementary Materials), and it was determined to eliminate all inappropriate items. Experts consider items with the corrected homogeneity index (HIc) < 0.25 [43], skewness > 3 and kurtosis > 6 [64,65], standard deviation less than 1, and items that have a mean value close to the maximum or minimum value of the item response [39,43]. Next, in successive EFAs, the items without loading, the complex items, and the items loading less than 0.40 were eliminated one by one and in this order [66] until a simple, clear, and interpretable solution was obtained. The model best fitted by EFA was called model M1 and was composed of 21 items dimensioned in 2 correlated factors.

The sCFA was performed using the FACTOR program (V.11.04.02) [67], which examines the model fit based on the Root Mean Square Deviation (RMSD) [68]. If the RMSD < 0.05, the misfit is trivial; between 0.05 and 0.10, it is moderate, and if the RMSD > 0.10, the misfit is substantial [69,70]. The descriptive study of the items was carried out using IBM SPSS 27. The EFA was carried out with FACTOR and with JASP (V.0.14.1.0) (both provide complementary information), and CFA (described later) was carried out with JASP.

Because the items are ordinals and some items showed skewness and/or kurtosis values significantly far from normality, the polychoric correlation matrix was used in all the EFA and CFA models tested [62,71]. The ordinal nature of the items also determined the estimation method used. For all EFA models, the estimation procedure was Minimum Residuals in JASP and Robust Unweighted Least Squares (RULS) in FACTOR (both procedures are equivalent [72]). The number of factors to be retained was determined by taking into account the result of the optimal implementation of the Parallel Analysis (PA, [73]) and by considering eigenvalues above 1 (Kaiser's criterion) and the Scree Test. For the correlation between the factors to be expressed in their full magnitude, the direct solution was obliquely rotated using Promin robust rotation in FACTOR [74] and oblimin rotation in JASP. The models were evaluated with the Root Mean Square Error of Approximation (RMSEA), Tucker–Lewis index (TLI), and BIC. Satisfactory reference values are RMSEA $\leq$ 0.06, TLI $\geq$ 0.95 [66,75], and a lower BIC. The simplicity of the model was assessed using the S index [76].

Next, in the calibration sample, three aspects were evaluated. First, it was assessed whether the factor solution of M1 approaches unidimensionality. This was considered using the indices UniCo, ECV, and MIREAL. Data can be treated as essentially unidimensional when UniCo > 0.95, ECV > 0.85 or MIREAL < 0.30 [77]. Second, it was evaluated whether a second-order factor could exist. The Added-Value analysis [78] will allow us to decide by observing the mean squared error reduction (PRMSE) if a second-order factor better defines the dimensionality. Third, the strength of construct replication by the H index [77] was evaluated. High H values (>0.80) suggest a well-defined latent variable, which is more likely to be stable across studies. In contrast, low H values indicate a poorly defined latent variable, which is expected to change across studies.

Before performing the CFA in the validation sample (n = 1188), EFA also examined whether the items would be assigned to the same factors and whether the items' factor loadings would have an equivalent magnitude in both samples. The difference between the standardized factor loadings was calculated and squared for each item. The squared difference > 0.04 indicates that the factor loadings are volatile, and the construct will not be replicated in other samples [42]. It was verified that all items were positioned the same way as in the calibration sample and that no item was volatile. Thus, once the replication was confirmed in the validation sample, Model M1 was tested by CFA, showing a satisfactory fit. However, it was decided to eliminate one item because it had $R^2 < 0.20$ and a standardized factor loading < 0.50. This most parsimonious and best-fitting model is Model M2, which was tested to assess factorial invariance.

The CFA used the Diagonally Weighted Least Squares with Mean and Variance corrected (WLSMV) [79] estimation method. Based on the modification indices, the correlation between the errors was left free. The fit of the model was examined by 4 indices: RMSEA, Standardized Root Mean Square of Residuals (SRMR), the comparative fit measure concerning the null model of independence (Confirmatory Fit Index, CFI), and the χ^2/df ratio. Satisfactory reference values of the latter three indices were SRMR < 0.08, CFI $\geq$ 0.95 [75,80], and $\chi^2/gl < 3$ [81]. Next, the multi-group CFA according to sex groups and marital status was performed. The deviation of the metric, scalar and strict invariance models from the configurational invariance model was examined based on the magnitude of changes in fit indices in CFI, RMSR and RMSEA [82,83]. Chen [82] recommend using CFI for the invariance evaluation first, supplemented by RMSEA and SRMR. A change of −0.010 or more in the CFI combined with changes in RMSEA of 0.015 and SRMR of 0.03 (for metric invariance) or 0.015 (for scalar or residual invariance) was used as an indication of non-invariance. The internal structure analysis was concluded by examining composite reliability (CR) [66].

The reliability of the measure of the resulting scale, CRS-$S_{Eg\text{-}S\&D}$, was then estimated by analyzing internal consistency using Cronbach's standardized alpha and McDonald's ordinal omega. Values greater than 0.70 were considered acceptable [66].

2.5.2. Analysis Block 2: Study of the Evidence of Validity

Convergent and discriminant validity were analyzed using different estimators. On the one hand, it was examined on the basis of the correlation between the factors of the CRS-$S_{Eg\text{-}S\&D}$ and the factors of the PAFAS [57] and CAPES [59] questionnaires. This was performed independently for the total sample and for each marital status. Values of r $\geq$ 0.20, r $\geq$ 0.50 and r $\geq$ 0.80 express a weak, moderate and strong correlation, respectively [84]. On the other hand, convergent validity was examined by jointly analyzing the average variance extracted (AVE) and composite reliability (CR) derived from the CFA [85], and considering the standardized factor loadings [66,86].

Discriminant validity existed if the square root of AVE was greater than the square between the correlations of the latent factors [85], and convergent validity if AVE > 0.5.

2.5.3. Analysis Block 3: Evaluation of the Strength of the Total Coparenting Measure Calculated Using CRS-$S_{Eg\text{-}S\&D}$ to Classify the Sample Participants into Different Categories

A two-stage cluster analysis was carried out, randomizing the order of the participants on 20 occasions as a sensitivity analysis and as an evaluation of the replicability of the result. The quality of clusters was considered poor, sufficient, or good based on the work developed by Kaufman and Rousseeuw [87]. MANOVA was then performed to determine how different the resulting clusters were and how different they were in each of the two factors that make up the total measure of the CRS-S$_{Eg-S\&D}$. The analysis was completed by performing a stepwise discriminant analysis [88,89] to examine which dependent variable (Factor 1 or Factor 2) had the most strength to differentiate between the clusters, or if the discrimination strength resided in a combination of both, providing special attention to the standardized coefficients and the magnitude and sign of the centroids. Finally, in the clusters identified based on the total measure of the CRS-S$_{Eg-S\&D}$, the measure of the two dimensions in each group resulting from the combination Sex x Marital Status was represented graphically.

The correlation observed between the empirical scores of the 2 factors was r = 0.576 ($p < 0.001$). Therefore, it constituted an appropriate condition ($0.30 < r < 0.80$) to use MANOVA [90,91] and control the Type I error that could accumulate if independent ANOVAs were performed instead [66,92]. Because the covariance matrices were heterogeneous (Box's M = 181.66; $p = < 0.001$), the result was examined using Wilks' Lambda statistic [93], and resampling was used to estimate the parameters [94]. The level of significance was $\alpha = 0.05$, and the reference values $1 - \beta > 0.80$, and partial eta squared (η^2) of 0.01, 0.06, and 0.14 represented small, medium, and large, respectively [95,96].

3. Results

3.1. Evidence of Validity Based on the Internal Structure and Reliability of the Scale Score

The results are shown in Tables 1 and 2.

Table 1. Descriptive statistics of the items of *The Coparenting Relationship Scale* [26] that make up the questionnaire adapted to the Spanish population of engaged parents and separated or divorced parents, CRS-S$_{Eg-S\&D}$, and factor loadings of Model M1 in EFA, of Model M2 in CFA, and of the model invariant (Model M2, in CFA) to sex and to current marital status.

								Evaluation and Adjustment of CRS-S$_{Eg-S\&D}$ Dimensionality						Evaluation of Factorial Invariance of CRS-S$_{Eg-S\&D}$. [V] CFA M2, K = 20			
		Descriptive Statistics, IH$_C$, Alpha						[C] EFA M1; K = 21			[V] EFA M1; K = 21	[V] CFA M2; K = 20		[B] Factor Loading by [1] Sex and [2] Marital Status			
Factors in M1 and M2	Items [A]	M	SD	Skw	Kur	HI$_C$	[I] Alpha	F.Load.	Uniqu.	Com.	F.Load.	F.Load.	R^2	Male	Female	Eg	S&D
[D] F1 (k = 14)	2	4.45	1.74	−0.91	−0.42	0.59	0.932	0.667	0.565	0.647	0.697	0.621	0.386	0.596	0.629	0.562	0.595
	3	4.87	1.60	−1.34	0.60	0.69	0.931	0.657	0.470	0.834	0.732	0.769	0.591	0.756	0.770	0.708	0.785
	6	5.11	1.35	−1.60	1.76	0.69	0.931	0.628	0.471	0.789	0.680	0.739	0.546	0.629	0.758	0.664	0.763
	10	4.49	1.70	−0.85	−0.54	0.58	0.932	0.711	0.536	0.779	0.661	0.671	0.450	0.670	0.671	0.656	0.667
	14	4.91	1.56	−1.33	0.58	0.52	0.934	0.546	0.687	0.633	0.614	0.614	0.377	0.501	0.633	0.533	0.787
	17	5.03	1.55	−1.57	1.29	0.63	0.931	0.694	0.508	0.774	0.715	0.716	0.512	0.639	0.737	0.596	0.753
	18	4.39	1.60	−0.64	−0.79	0.61	0.932	0.656	0.553	0.750	0.664	0.714	0.510	0.634	0.729	0.659	0.811
	19	4.61	1.57	−1.00	−0.07	0.69	0.930	0.744	0.414	0.810	0.793	0.694	0.631	0.774	0.798	0.747	0.834
	23	4.72	1.69	−1.11	−0.09	0.66	0.931	0.713	0.481	0.834	0.723	0.728	0.530	0.642	0.743	0.641	0.822
	24	4.96	1.53	−1.47	1.18	0.75	0.929	0.843	0.297	0.911	0.877	0.847	0.717	0.855	0.845	0.790	0.852
	25	4.88	1.54	−1.32	0.65	0.75	0.929	0.894	0.248	0.897	0.862	0.850	0.722	0.884	0.844	0.803	0.895
	26	4.75	1.66	−1.16	0.10	0.78	0.929	0.869	0.251	0.955	0.870	0.891	0.794	0.901	0.889	0.856	0.899
	27	4.66	1.68	−1.10	−0.07	0.72	0.929	0.826	0.330	0.929	0.818	0.844	0.712	0.877	0.839	0.831	0.817
	30	4.44	1.78	−0.87	−0.56	0.55	0.933	0.652	0.603	0.690	0.687	0.632	0.389	0.602	0.632	0.573	0.536
[D] F2 (k = 6)	[i] 8	4.27	1.46	−1.59	1.69	0.54	0.934	0.584	0.605	0.659	0.617	0.730	0.532	0.861	0.703	0.636	0.765
	[i] 9	4.05	1.46	−1.41	1.34	0.64	0.933	0.774	0.356	0.799	0.610	0.764	0.583	0.695	0.755	0.723	0.905
	[i] 11	4.13	1.44	−1.46	1.48	0.51	0.935	0.735	0.506	0.748	0.726	0.649	0.421	0.608	0.659	0.602	0.717
	[i] 12 [D]	4.49	1.20	−2.06	4.48	0.52	0.939	0.664	0.566	0.693	0.688	0.575	0.331	0.533	0.579	0.585	0.609
	[i] 15	3.92	1.48	−1.21	0.70	0.52	0.934	0.637	0.575	0.592	0.654	0.627	0.393	0.564	0.634	0.588	0.625
	[i] 16	4.55	1.33	−2.25	4.62	0.44	0.936	0.617	0.665	0.715	0.581	-----	-----	-----	-----	-----	-----
	[i] 29	4.38	1.25	−1.81	3.49	0.53	0.934	0.531	0.651	0.657	0.588	0.637	0.406	0.600	0.650	0.632	0.561

Legend. [A] = The number of the items corresponds to the numbering of the original scale [26] presented in the Supplementary Materials; [i] = inverse item; M, SD, Skw., Kur., HIc and [I] Alpha = mean, standard deviation, skewness, kurtosis, and corrected homogeneity index, respectively, and Cronbach's alpha of the scale if the item is removed, respectively, found in the calibration sample; [C] = calibration sample (50% approx., n = 1239); [V] = validation sample (50% approx., N = 1188). [1,2] In the validation sample, male = 20.03% (n = 238), female = 79.96% (n = 950), and Eg = 90.067% (n = 1070), and S&D = 9.93% (n = 118); K = number of items in the tested model; k = number of items in the factor; F.Load. = factorial loadings; Uniqu. = uniqueness; Com. = comunalidad; ----- It was considered necessary to eliminate item 16 because $R^2 < 0.30$ ($R^2 = 0.234$) and standardized factorial loadings < 0.50 (F. Loading = 0.484); [B] = Standardized factorial loadings of M2 for male, female, Eg and S&D that were obtained in the configural invariance model are shown; [D] Crombach's alpha [in M1 EFA (F1 = 0.943, and F2 = 0.838 and total test = 0.935] [in M2 CFA (F1 = 0.943 and F2 = 0.829 and total test = 0.936].

Table 2. Dimensionality models tested using EFA and CFA of the *The Coparenting Relationship Scale* [22] in the adaptation process to the Spanish population of engaged parents and separated or divorced parents, $CRS\text{-}S_{Eg\text{-}S\&D}$.

	MODEL	χ^2 (*df*)	χ^2/df	BIC/ECVI	CFI [TLI]	RMSEA [90%CI]	SRMR	[1] S			
[T] CFA	CRS[6S] (K = 30)	2972.158 (390)	7.62	1312	0.968 [0.964]	0.052 [0.050–0.054]	0.071	0.195			
[C] EFA	CRS[6S] (K = 30)			−123.124	[0.881]	0.069 [0.066–0.071]		0.212			
[C] EFA	M1 (K = 21)			**−0.536**	**[0.912]**	0.071 [0.067–0.074]		**0.999**			
[V] CFA	M1 (K = 21)	203.218 (188) [H]	1.08	0.328	0.999 [0.999]	0.008 [0–0.016]	0.035				
[V] CFA	M2 (K = 20)	**176.660 (169)** [J]	**1.04**	**0.226**	**1 [1]**	**0.006 [0–0.015]**	**0.034**				
[V,3] **Invariance**	**M2 Sex**	χ^2 (*df*)	χ^2/df		CFI	RMSEA [90%CI]	SRMR	ΔCFI	ΔRMSEA	ΔSRMR	
Conf. Invar.		227.651 (338)	0.673		1	0 [0–0]	0.040				
Metr. Invar.		282.733 (356)	0.794		1	0 [0–0]	0.044	0	0	0.004	
Scal. Invar.		305.615 (374)	0.817		1	0 [0–0]	0.043	0	0	−0.001	
Strict Invar.		317.394 (394)	0.805		1	0 [0–0]	0.044	0	0	0.001	
Invariance	**M2 MS**										
Conf. Invar.		300.160 (338)	0.888		1	0 [0–0.005]	0.041				
Metr. Invar.		432.841 (356)	1.215		0.996	0.019 [0.012–0.025]	0.047	0.004	0.001	0.006	
Scal. Invar.		505.343 (374)	1.351		0.994	0.024 [0.019–0.030]	0.047	0.002	0.005	0	
Strict Invar.		594.265 (394)	1.508		0.991	0.029 [0.024–0.034]	0.050	0.003	0.005	0.003	

Legend. χ^2/df ratio [77]; BIC/ECVI = parsimony indices, BIC information criteria in EFA/expected cross-validation index in CFA; CFI [TLI] = comparative fit index [Tucker–Lewis index]; RMSEA = Root Mean Square Error of Approximation; SRMR = Standardized Root Mean Square of Residuals in CFA; S = Bentler's simplicity index; [1] S was obtained through FACTOR (JASP does not provide the value); CRS[6S] (K = 30), model found by Feinberg et al. [26], deleting the *Exposure to Conflict* scale. K = 30 items and 6 factors; [T] = total sample, N = 2427 participants; [C] = calibration sample (50% approx., n = 1239); [V] = validation sample (50% approx., N = 1188); M1 = best fitted model in the EFA (k = 21), where nine items were eliminated; M2 = the CFA of Model M1 fits well. However, it was considered necessary to eliminate item 16 (see the explanation in Table 1). [3] configural, metric, scalar, and strict invariance, respectively; Δ comparison of the increment of the observed value in CFI, SRMR and RMSEA; MS = marital status (Eg and S&D); [H] $p = 0.212$; [J] $p = 0.328$. The best-fitting models of the EFA and CFA are highlighted in bold. For the rest, see Table 1.

The model found by Feinberg et al. [26] of 30 items and six factors, Model CRS^{6F}, does not fit the data from the sample of Spanish engaged parents (Eg) and separated or divorced parents (S&D). Both methods, sCFA and CFA, allow us to conclude the same result. In the sCFA, the RMSD values for the six subscales were 0.207, 0.148, 0.128, 0.163, 0.188, and 0.086, indicating a moderate mismatch for the Coparenting Closeness subscale (0.086), and a substantial mismatch for the remaining five subscales, with the total mean mismatch being 0.158. The initial CFA showed a very unsatisfactory fit only in χ^2/df ($\chi^2/df = 7.62$; CFI [TLI] = 0.968 [0.964]; SRMR = 0.071 and RMSEA = 0.052) (see Table 2), and although all standardized factor loadings were statistically significant, the loadings of the items *The stress of being parents has distanced us as a couple* (item 28), *The other parent does not trust my abilities as a parent* (item 13), and *The other parent likes to play with the child but leaves the unpleasant work for me* (item 5), belonging to the subscales *Coparenting Closeness*, *Coparenting Undermining* and *The Division of Labor*, respectively, were lower than what experts [66,80] consider reasonable (0.410, 0.451, and 0.313, in the order cited). In addition, the R^2 values of the items *The stress of parenthood has caused my partner and me to grow* (item 28), *My partner doesn't like to be bothered by our child* (item 29), *My partner does not trust my abilities as a parent* (item 13), *My partner likes to play with our child and then leave dirty work to me* (item 5), and *El otro progenitor no asume la resposabilidad como padre/madre* (item 20), belonging to the subscales *Coparenting Closeness, Endorsement of Partner Parenting, Coparenting Undermining* and the *Division of Labor* were also notably low (0.168, 0.250, 0.204, 0.089, and 0.276, respectively). Even so, the internal consistency examined using the standardized Cronbach's alpha of the subscales *Coparenting Agreement, Coparenting Closeness, Coparenting Support, Endorsement of Partner Parenting, Coparenting Undermining* and *The Division of Labor*, and the total scale, was, respectively, 0.764, 0.780, 0.916, 0.866, 0.803, 0.282, 0.943. See the wording of the CRS items in both languages, English and Spanish, in Section S1 of the Supplementary Materials.

A modeling process was then initiated with the calibration sample (n = 1239) through successive EFAs. In the application of the CRS^{6F} Model found by Feinberg et al. [26], it was found that the dimensional structure was complex (S = 0.212) and the CFI was unsatisfactory (0.881) (see Table 2) because some items were represented in more than one factor, other items were not in none, and some factors were not represented (see Section S3 of the Supplementary Materials, Table S5). With resounding unity, PA, the Scree Test, and Kaiser's criterion indicated that two factors were appropriate to represent the dimensionality of the set of 30 items. Thus, first of all, based on the descriptive statistics of the items in the calibration sample (observed according to sex and marital status), items 1, 4, 7, 21, 22, and 5 were eliminated because they were inappropriate (the first five items, because they showed inadequate descriptive statistics to be part of an FA in the Eg subsample, male and female, and item 5 because the four subsamples showed a HIc value < 0.30; see Tables S1–S4 in Section S2 of the Supplementary Materials). Once the above analysis was performed, modeling using the EFA began, and items 20, 28, and 13 were eliminated (items 20 and 28 were then eliminated because they had a factor loading < 0.40; once the previous two were eliminated, item 13 showed no loading and was also eliminated). As a result, a total of nine items were eliminated. Thus, Model M1 by EFA sized with two factors consisting of a total of 21 items (F1 and F2 have 14 and 7 items, respectively) has a very satisfactory fit (BIC = −0.536; CFI = 0.912; RMSEA = 0.071; S = 0.999) (see Table 2). The uniqueness (<0.70), the communality (>0.50), and the standardized loadings factorials (>0.50) are appropriate for all items (see Table 1), and the model explains 63.89% of the variance (0.526% and 0.112%, F1 and F2, respectively). The data adequacy examined using the KMO sphericity and Bartlett's tests was satisfactory in all models examined.

On the other hand, the UniCo = 0.916 and ECV = 0.821 indexes show that the structure of the M1 model moves away from unidimensionality. The Added-Value analysis allows us to conclude that the model with two primary factors fits significantly better (PRMSE = 0.901 [0.888–0.910] and 0.967 [0.963–0.970] for F1 and F2, respectively) than a model with a second-order factor (PRMSE = 0.355 and 0.703 for F1 and F2, respectively). The H index indicated that the latent variables in F1 and F2 were well defined (latent H index = 0.901 and 0.967, for F1 and F2, respectively), and the squares of the difference between the standardized factor loadings of the EFA of M1 in the calibration and validation samples were less than 0.04, demonstrating that the dimensional structure was replicable in the same factors and the same items (see Table 1). Additionally, the internal consistency was very satisfactory (alpha = 0.943, 0.839, and 0.935 for F1, F2, and the entire scale, respectively).

Therefore, it was concluded that Model M1 sized by EFA is the simplest and the best-adjusted model. It has been replicated in the validation sample, the latent variables F1 and F2 are well defined, and the measures of F1 and F2 in the Spanish sample of Eg and S&D are reliable.

The CFA with the validation sample (n = 1188) corroborated a satisfactory fit of the M1 Model (χ^2/df = 1.08; CFI [TLI] = 0.999 [0.999]; SRMR = 0.035 and RMSEA = 0.008) (see Table 2). However, it was decided to eliminate item 16 because it showed an R^2 lower than 0.30 (R^2 = 0.234) and a standardized factor loading lower than 0.50 (F. loading = 0.484). The resulting Model, the M2 Model, has an even more satisfactory fit than M1 (χ^2/df = 1.04;

CFI [TLI] = 1 [1]; SRMR = 0.034 and RMSEA = 0.006) (see Table 2). The composite reliability is excellent, 0.946 and 0.826 for factors F1 and F2, respectively.

The factorial invariance of M2 as a function of sex and marital status was then tested. Based on the fit indexes χ^2/df, CFI, and RMSEA, and based on the fact that the magnitude of the changes in absolute values of CFI, RMSR, and RMSE [82,96] does not exceed the recommended limits [82,83,96], it could be concluded that there is strong configurational, metric, scalar and strict invariance for males and females and engaged parents and separated or divorced parents (see Table 2), and therefore, the items measure the same dimensions with the same structure, regardless of sex and marital status. This property is a prerequisite so that the empirical scores for each factor can be compared and interpreted validly [97].

In M2, the internal consistency evaluated by Cronbach's alpha test (0.913 and 0.829, for F1 and F2, respectively) and by McDonald's ordinal omega (0.943, 0.831 for F1 and F2, respectively) was adequate.

It is thus concluded that M2 sized with two factors consisting of a total of 20 items is the simplest, best adjusted model for the sample of Spanish parents, it is invariant according to sex and the marital status, and the measure derived from each of its factors is reliable. The new questionnaire for Spanish parents is called CRS-$S_{Eg\text{-}S\&D}$. The resulting factors were defined as *Positive Coparenting* (F1, 14 items) and *Negative Perception of Coparenting* (F2, 6 items), and both measure the construct that we call *Coparenting Vitality*.

3.2. Evidence for Convergent and Discriminate Validity

Some results are shown in Table 3. See Section S3 of the Supplementary Materials (Tables S7 and S8).

On the basis of the relationship between the factors of the CRS-$S_{Eg\text{-}S\&D}$. The correlation in the total sample between the direct scores of the factors F1 (*Positive Coparenting*) and F2 (*Negative Perception of Coparenting*) is r = 0.512 ($p < 0.001$), and this relationship is maintained in both samples of parents (Eg and S&D), although it is slightly lower with respect to that calculated in the total sample because the variability is less (see Table 3).

Based on the relationship between the empirical scores of the CRS-$S_{Eg\text{-}S\&D}$ *factors with the factors of the PAFAS and CAPES*. Table 3 shows that in the sample of Eg parents, there is a statistically significant correlation between F1 CRS-S with F22 PF and PF-T (r = 0.601 and r = 0.510, respectively) and also between CRS-S-T with F22 PF and PF-T (r = 0.599 and r = 0.516, respectively). On the other hand, in the subsample of S&D parents, there is only a statistically significant relationship between CRS-S-T and F22 PF (r = 0.522). The most notable thing is that in the S&D subsample, the link between F1 CRS-S and F22 PF disappears, which does appear in the Eg subsample. The magnitude of the correlation is an indicator of the existence of convergent validity, as expected. The divergence between what happens in the S&D and Eg subsamples is an indicator that F1 CRS-S is capable of identifying differences between S&D and Eg, and this was an objective of this research. These should be studied in future research because they are indicators of a solid practical implication.

It is also notable that, in the same way, in both subsamples, F2 CRS-S is not significantly related to any of the PAFAS or CAPES factors. This aspect is very relevant and also requires further investigation. A priori means that the PAFAS questionnaire does not evaluate a Negative Perception of Coparenting and that a Negative Perception of Coparenting is not related to the behavior of the children assessed through the CAPES.

On the basis of the relationship between the latent variables. The correlation between the latent factors is $r_l = 0.563$ ($p < 0.001$). AVE from F1 and F2 are 0.5627 and 0.444, respectively, indicating high convergent validity in F1 [85] and marginal convergent validity in F2. Anyway, given that CR is always greater than 0.6 for all latent constructs, convergent validity could also be concluded for F2 [85] (p. 46). Furthermore, in all cases, the square root of AVE is greater than the square between the correlations of the latent factors. Therefore, it can be concluded that discriminant validity exists too [85].

Table 3. Correlation between the factors of CRS-$S_{Eg\text{-}S\&D}$, PAFAS, and CAPES and between the total score of the questionnaires. The correlations are shown in the set of men and women (without distinguishing between sexes) in the subsamples of engaged parents and separated or divorced parents.

		F1 CRS-S	F2 CRS-S	F11 PF	F12 PF	F13 PF	F21 PF	F22 PF	F1 CP	F2 CP	CRS-S-T	PF-T	CP-T
Eg	F1 CRS-S	1	0.404 **	0.150 **	0.182 **	0.267 **	0.320 **	**0.601 ****	−0.108 **	−0.253 **	**0.860 ****	**0.510 ****	−0.212 **
	F2 CRS-S		1	0.266 **	0.014	0.221 **	0.110 **	0.394 **	−0.156 **	−0.280 **	**0.814 ****	0.349 **	−0.217 **
	F11 PF			1	−0.038	0.183 **	0.052 *	0.151 **	−0.142 **	−0.370 **	0.244 **	**0.508 ****	−0.301 **
	F12 PF				1	0.248 **	0.170 **	0.171 **	−0.107 **	0.075 **	0.123 **	**0.561 ****	−0.047 *
	F13 PF					1	0.308 **	0.374 **	−0.197 **	−0.243 **	0.293 **	**0.619 ****	−0.067 **
	F21 PF						1	0.413 **	−0.099 **	−0.147 **	0.265 **	**0.584 ****	−0.159 **
	F22 PF							1	−0.168 **	−0.247 **	**0.599 ****	**0.701 ****	−0.265 **
	F1 CP								1	0.133 **	−0.154 **	−0.228 **	**0.877 ****
	F2 CP									1	−0.316 **	−0.303 **	**0.593 ****
	CRS-S-T										1	**0.516 ****	−0.283 **
	PF-T											1	−0.338 **
S&D	F1 CRS-S	1	0.497 **	−0.052	0.131 *	0.007	0.139 *	0.481 **	−0.113	−0.076	**0.875 ****	0.302 **	−0.137 **
	F2 CRS-S		1	0.049	−0.021	0.033	0.125	0.435 **	−0.077	−0.051	**0.855 ****	0.274 **	0.093 **
	F11 PF			1	−0.008	0.280 **	0.098	0.112	−0.102	−0.443 **	−0.004	**0.517 ****	−0.282 **
	F12 PF				1	0.294 **	0.197 **	0.073	−0.145*	−0.077	0.067	**0.519 ****	−0.136 *
	F13 PF					1	0.376 **	0.137 *	−0.261 **	−0.366 **	0.023	**0.583 ****	−0.372 **
	F21 PF						1	0.333 **	−0.177 **	−0.295 **	0.152 *	**0.621 ****	−0.292 **
	F22 PF							1	−0.176 *	−0.209 **	**0.522 ****	**0.684 ****	−0.241 **
	F1 CP								1	0.274 **	−0.110	−0.310 **	**0.833 ****
	F2 CP									1	−0.074	−0.456 **	**0.694 ****
	CRS-S-T										1	0.328 **	−0.134 **
	PF-T											1	−0.452 **

Legend. Eg and S&D = engaged parents and separated or divorced parents, respectively; CRS-S, PF and CP, is the abbreviated way of referring to CRS-$S_{Eg\text{-}S\&D}$, PAFAS, and CAPES in this table (for reasons of space); F1 and F2 in CRS-S are *Coparentalidad Positiva* and *Percepción Negativa de la Coparentalidad*, respectively, F11, F12, F13, F21, and F22 in PAFAS are *Family adjustment, Positive encouragement, Parent-child relationship, Parental adjustment*, and *Family adjustment*, respectively; F1 and F2 in CAPES are *Child's competencies*, and *Behavioral and emotional problems*, respectively; CRS-S-T, PF-T and CP-T = total scores for the respective scales. All scores were transformed as indicated in the text (in PAFAS, each factor could achieve a maximum of 0.20, and in CRS-$S_{Eg\text{-}S\&D}$ and CAPES, each factor could achieve a maximum of 0.5, such that the total sum of each scale can reach a maximum value of 1); **,* = $p < 0.01$ and $p \leq 0.05$, respectively Correlations greater than 0.50 have been highlighted in bold.

3.3. *Evaluation of the Strength of the Total Coparenting Measure Calculated Using CRS-$S_{Eg\text{-}S\&D}$ to Classify the Sample Participants into Different Categories*

In all published works that use the CRS questionnaire [26], the calculation of the mean for each factor is proposed, and the calculation of the total mean of the set of items is proposed as an estimate of a total measure of coparenting. However, the factors found by Feinberg et al. [26] have a different number of items (there are factors with two, four, five, six, and seven items), and thus the factors that have more items have a greater weight in the total sum and therefore in the total average. Furthermore, a total average dissolves the particular contribution of each factor. In this research, we propose calculating the measure of each factor as a weighted adjusted measure in the following way. The sum of the items of each dimension is divided by the total sum possible in the factor. Because the CRS questionnaire adapted to the Spanish population comprises two factors, the previous result is multiplied by 0.5. Then, the value obtained from the two factors is added algebraically. The maximum possible measurement of each of the two factors will be 0.5, and the maximum value of the total measurement in CRS-$S_{Eg\text{-}S\&D}$ will be one. In this way, the measurement of both factors can be compared in different circumstances, and it will be possible to observe which factor contributes the most to the total measurement. However, when the measurements of each factor are compared, it can be performed with the average or with the result of this calculation. The results of the statistical analyses will be identical. However, when the total score for CRS-$S_{Eg\text{-}S\&D}$ is examined, it should be performed in this way that we propose to attribute equal weight to the two dimensions that make up the construct and not dissolve the variability contained in the dimensions it comprises.

The result of the two-stage cluster analysis is conclusive. The classification quality reaches a value of 0.7, which in the terminology of Kaufman & Rousseeuw [87] is good. Therefore, it can be concluded that the data reasonably or strongly evidence the structure of the clusters. The *Coparental Vitality* measure calculated using the total weighted measure of CRS-$S_{Eg\text{-}S\&D}$ allows the sample of participants to be divided into three differentiated clusters that we have called *Coparental Robustness* or *Robust Coparenting, Moderate Coparenting*, and *Coparenting Rickets* or *Inadequate Coparenting*. MANOVA revealed that the effect size of the variable that defines the clusters is very big [cluster: $\Lambda = 0.209$; F = 1438.64 (df_1; $df_2 = 4$; 4846); $p = 0.001$; $\eta^2 = 0.543$], and both dimensions were statistically significant with $\eta^2 = 0.656$ (F = 2306.41) and $\eta^2 = 0.534$ (F = 1391.14), respectively, for F1 CRS-Sp and F2 CRS-Sp (both df1 and df2 were 2 and 2424, and $p < 0.001$). Figures 1 and 2 show the graphic representation of the distribution of CRS-S Totalp in each cluster and the descriptive statistics of each dimension (F1 CRS-S and F2 CRS-S, and Total CRS-S), referring to its weighted value and average value.

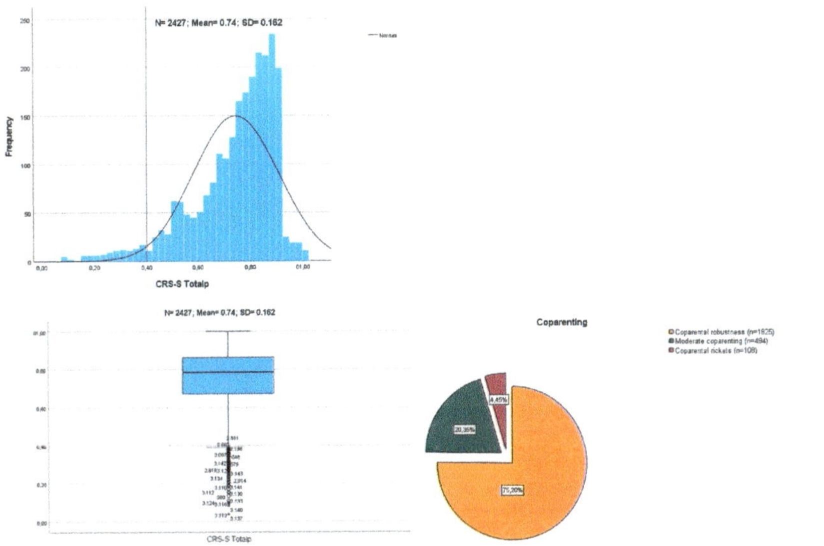

Figure 1. Distribution of the total weighted score for CRS-S in the group of participants: histogram, box plot, and percentage of participants in each of the three coparenting clusters derived from the result of the two-stage cluster analysis. *Note:* CRS-S = is the abbreviated way of naming CRS-$S_{Eg\text{-}S\&D}$. On the left chart, a dividing line is placed at 0.40. This value is the observed (approximate) value of the CRS-S Totalp distribution, below which are found the outliers and the extreme cases. The outliers (represented by circles) and extreme cases (represented by asterisks are visualized in the box plot graph in the center of Figure 1.

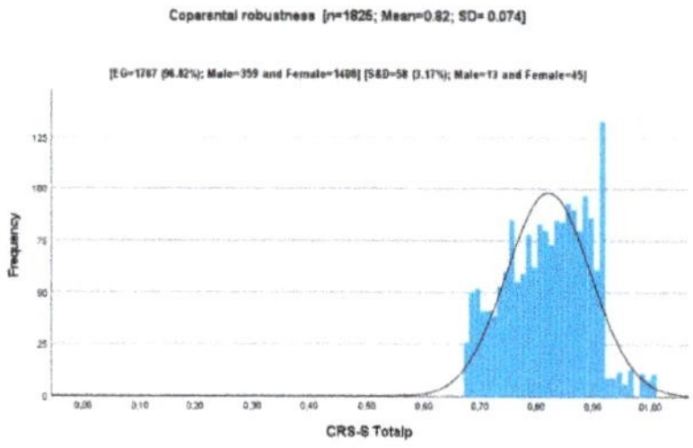

	EG			D&S		
	Mn	Mx	Mean (SD)	Mn	Mx	Mean (SD)
F1p	0.24	0.5	0.43 (0.05)	0.29	0.5	0.40 (0.06)
F2p	0.19	0.5	0.38 (0.04)	0.25	0.5	0.38 (0.05)
Tp	**0.67**	**1**	**0.82 (0.07)**	**0.68**	**0.96**	**0.78 (0.07)**
F1m	20.93	6	50.2 (0.59)	30.43	6	40.8 (0.71)
F2m	20.33	6	40.6 (0.56)	3	6	40.5 (0.64)
Tm	30.65	6	50.0 (0.47)	30.90	50.7	40.7 (0.52)

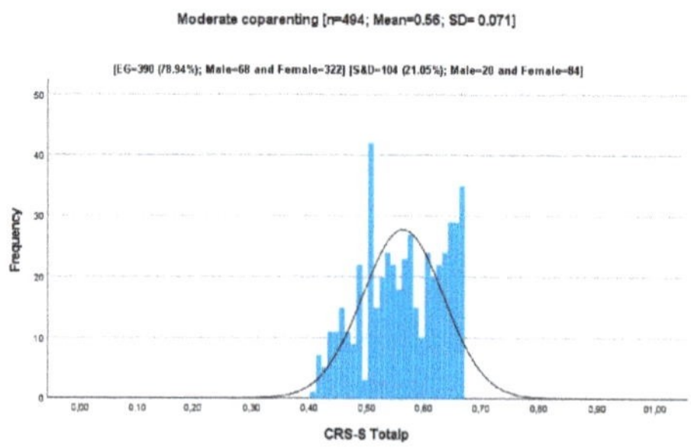

	EG			D&S		
	Mn	Mx	Mean (SD)	Mn	Mx	Mean (SD)
F1p	0	0.5	0.29 (0.08)	0	0.45	0.23 (0.08)
F2p	0	0.5	0.27 (0.08)	0	0.5	0.29 (0.07)
Tp	**0.41**	**0.67**	**0.57 (0.06)**	**0.41**	**0.66**	**0.53 (0.07)**
F1m	0	6	3.5 (0.96)	0	5.43	2.7 (1.04)
F2m	0	6	3.2 (0.98)	0	6	3.5 (0.92)
Tm	1.50	4.65	3.4 (0.53)	1.80	4.30	3.0 (0.60)

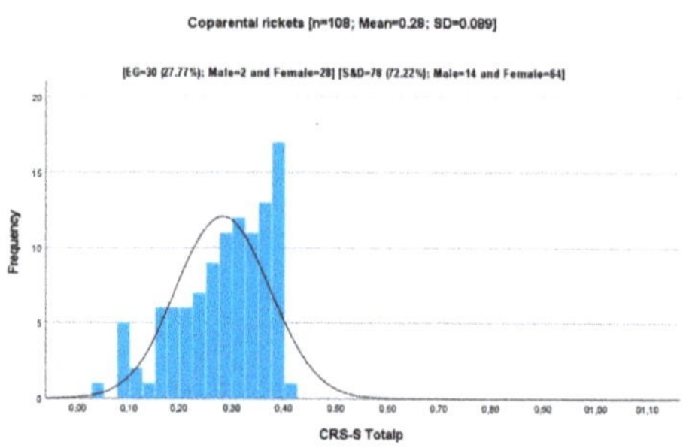

	EG			D&S		
	Mn	Mx	Mean (SD)	Mn	Mx	Mean (SD)
F1p	0.02	0.28	0.17 (0.06)	0.02	0.30	0.12 (0.05)
F2p	0.04	0.29	0.15 (0.06)	0.00	0.35	0.14 (0.07)
Tp	**0.10**	**0.40**	**0.33 (0.06)**	**0.04**	**0.40**	**0.26 (0.09)**
F1m	0.29	3.36	2.0 (0.81)	0.29	3.64	1.4 (0.62)
F2m	0.50	3.50	1.9 (0.77)	0.00	4.17	1.7 (0.89)
Tm	0.65	2.75	2.0 (0.51)	0.25	2.85	1.5 (0.50)

Figure 2. Left panel: For each of the three coparenting clusters, the distribution of the total weighted CRS-S score and description of demographic characteristics, sex, and marital status are shown. **Right panel**: For each of the three coparenting clusters, descriptive statistics of the two CRS-S dimensions and the total score (average and weighted scores) are shown. *Note*: In the tables, F1p, F2p, Tp, F1m, F2m and Tm = F1 CRS-Sp, F2 CRS-Sp, CRS-S Totalp, F1 CRS-Sm, F2 CRS-Sm, and CRS-S Totalm, respectively. The value of CRS-S Totalp is highlighted in bold because the distribution is represented in the graphs located in the middle part of this large table. For the rest, see Figure 1.

Figure 3 shows the representation of the F1 CSR-Sp, F2 CSRp, and CSR Totalp scores for the three *Coparental Vitality* profiles in each subsample defined by the crossing of levels of the variables sex and marital status (SxMS).

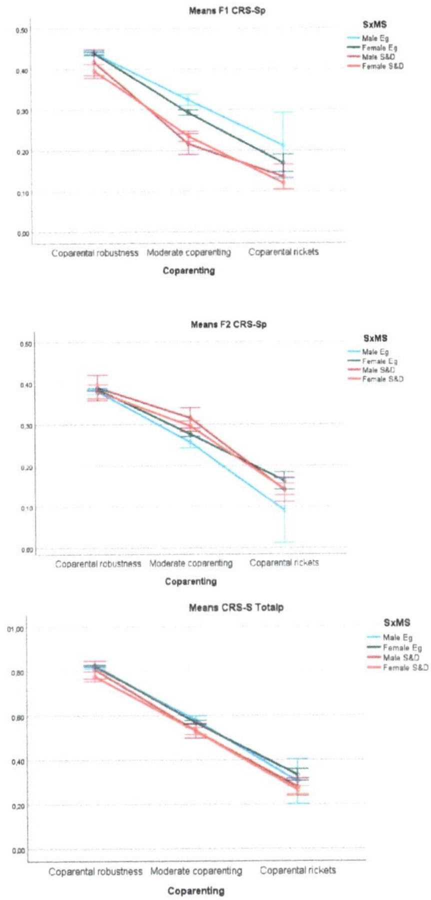

Figure 3. In order, representations of the scores F1 CSR-Sp, F2 CSRp, and CSR Totalp for the three profiles of coparental vitality in each subsample that is defined by the crossing of levels of the variables sex and marital status (SxMS). *Note:* See Figures 1 and 2.

To evaluate the importance or strength of each of the two dimensions in the discrimination of the three levels of *Coparental Vitality*, a discriminant analysis was carried out [the grouping variable was Coparenting, with three levels reached by the two-stage cluster, and the independent variables were F1 CRS-Sp and F2 CRS-Sp]. The discriminant analysis (see Figure 4) revealed that two discriminant functions contribute to the differentiation of the three degrees of *Coparental Vitality*, with the contribution of the first (%σ = 99.9%; Rc = 0.889) being much higher than the second. In the first function, both variables, F1 SRC-Sp and F2 SRC-Sp, to a greater extent F1 SRC-Sp, contribute significantly to establishing a strong differentiation between the three levels of coparental vitality (see centroids in Figure 4). The second function, whose contribution is statistically significant but residual in magnitude (%σ = 0.1%; Rc = 0.060), is very revealing for two reasons. One reason is because it only contributes to differentiating *Coparental Rickets* from the other two levels of coparenting (see the sizes of the centroids), and the other reason is because the variable F2 SRC-Sp exerts a similar influence to that exerted in Function 1, but F1 CSR-Sp shows a negative value, which it could be interpreted as the substantial weakening of the measurement of the F1 SRC-Sp dimension that contributes the most to reach the state of *Rickets Coparenting* or *Inadequate Coparenting*.

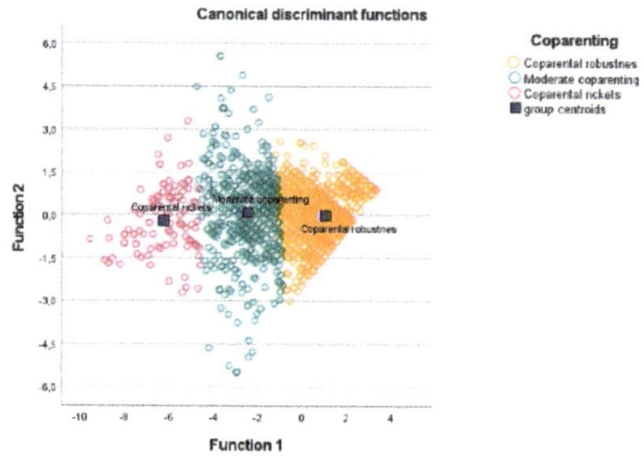

Discriminant function. Correct classification 97.3%	Centroids		
	Coparental robustness	Moderate coparenting	Coparental rickets
Function 1 [Av = 3.768; **%σ = 99.9%**; **Rc = 0.889**; Λ = 0.209; χ^2 = 3794.022; *gl* = 4; *p* = 0.000] [C. Std.: F1 CRS-Sp = **0.851**; F2 CRS-Sp = **0.718**]	1.035	−2.464	−6.221
Function 2 [Av = 0.004; **%σ = 0.1%**; **Rc = 0.060**; Λ = 0.996; χ^2 = 8.717; *gl* = 1; *p* = 0.003] [C. Std.: F1 CRS-Sp = **−0.562**; F2 CRS-Sp = **0.724**]	−0.013	0.091	−0.201

Figure 4. The upper part shows the graph of the distribution of the groups centroids of coparental vitality in the solution of the discriminant analysis carried out on the total sample. The bottom part shows a summary of the discriminant analysis (grouping variable = the three levels of coparental vitality derived from the two-stage cluster analysis; independent variables = F1 CRS-Sp and F2 CRS-Sp). *Note*: In the discriminant analysis, Av = eigenvalue; %σ = percentage of explained variance; Rc = canonical correlation; Λ = Wilks' Lambda test statistic; *df* = degrees of freedom; and C. Std. = standardized coefficients of the relevant variables in the discrimination of the 3 groups, *Coparental robustness*, *Moderate coparenting*, and *Coparental rickets*. For the rest, see Figures 1 and 2.

4. Discussion and Conclusions

"The advantages of this measure will also facilitate the assessment of the domains of coparenting in clinical practice, allowing intervention to capitalize on areas of strength and focus on improving areas of difficulty" [26] (p. 12). Due to the great usefulness of the coparenting measure, and because the adaptation of the Coparenting Relationship Scale for the Spanish population carried out by Plá [37] has severe limitations, as highlighted in the Introduction, an instrumental investigation was carried out to adapt and validate the CRS to the Spanish population of engaged parents (Eg) and separated or divorced parents (S&D), evaluating the strength of the total measure of coparenting to classify the sample participants into different categories.

The research design was carefully planned, and extreme precautions were taken throughout the research process to guarantee the results' replicability. An attempt has been made to avoid biases from the sample, the procedure, the data collection, and the bias caused by the analysis method. We think it is important to elaborate on the former in this Discussion section in three points.

First, it was verified through CFA and sCFA that the model found by Feinberg et al. [26] consisting of 30 items and six factors (Model CRS^{6S}) does not fit satisfactorily to the Spanish population of Eg and S&D parents. A detailed study was then initiated to determine its dimensional structure. In the process, special attention was paid to two aspects: one that selected from the set of items those that had the greatest strength to capture the variability in the coparenting measure between all parents and that was valid for both sexes and for all civil marital statuses in which coparenting can take place, and the other that prevented the bias induced by the method or the sample from being responsible for the result found. Technically, taking care of both aspects will ensure the replicability of the result, and to achieve this, the dimensionality study was carried out in five steps. Initially, the sample was divided into two to conduct the cross-validation analysis, ensuring that sex and marital status were correctly balanced. Second, based on the descriptive statistics, all inappropriate items to describe the sample were eliminated. Third, consecutive EFAs were performed until a good model fit was achieved. The best-fitting model was called M1. M1 was then compared with other possible models (unidimensional and second-order factor), and the strength of the latent construct and its replicability were examined. Fourth, having found that M1 was a satisfactory model, it was tested using AFC and adjusted again, resulting in Model M2. Fifth, the factorial invariance of the M2 model was examined, and it was found that the M2 model has strong configurational, metric, scalar, and strict invariance for males and females and engaged parents and separated or divorced parents.

Second, we consider it necessary to study the dimensionality of the CRS in this way in the process of adaptation and validation of the sample of Spanish parents for two fundamental reasons. One is because the dimensional study by Feinberg et al. [26] was carried out in a sample with very particular characteristics that do not represent the set of parents in the population, heterosexual couples who, at the time of recruitment, were expecting their first child, a limitation that the authors highlighted, and based on this, they urged researchers to examine this structure in other samples. We must add that the sample size of the number of items was tiny (ratio 6.40:1). The second reason is despite the adaptation of the CRS that has been performed on multiple occasions, as stated in the Introduction, only three of them, Costa et al. [26], Dumitriu et al. [36], and Favez et al. [35] (excluding the one carried out by Plá, for the reasons previously indicated), have been performed for the entire population, men and women, Eg and D&S. We consider this aspect fundamental, given that otherwise the adaptation could be extended *ad infinitum* to all imaginable sample singularities. Therefore, we believe that the three cited investigations are the reference to contrast the results of this investigation.

Third, experts in the method have shown that a good model fit does not prove that the model is theoretically sound [64,80], that larger samples produce more precise solutions [98,99], that replication (perform the analysis using cross-validation and by evaluating the difference between factor loadings) avoids overfitting of the models and adds value to the result of the factor analysis [38,96], and that the EFA should always be a prior step to the CFA [42,100].

In this research, the proportion of Eg parents is much higher than that of S&D parents, and in each marital status, women are represented in a greater proportion than men. This also happens in the three reference investigations. The percentage of women is 70%, 63.40% and 56.9%, respectively, in Costa et al. [34], Dumitriu et al. [36], and Favez et al. [35], and the percentage of Eg is 80% in Costa et al. [34] and 69% in Dumitriu et al. [36] (Favez et al. [35] do not indicate this detail). However, this research distances itself from the three reference investigations in critical methodological aspects, which we summarize in two points.

The first is that the ratio between the sample size and the number of items is very large (41.3:1), being far removed from the research carried out by Costa et al. [34], Favez et al. [35] and Dumitriu et al. [36], which was 19.20:1, 11.4:1 and 14.4:1, respectively (the same occurs in research with parents of samples with unique characteristics, as shown in Section S4 of the Supplementary Materials).

The second is that none of the three conducts the analysis through cross-validation, and the value given to the descriptive analysis of the items to examine their suitability is not part of the scale (it is only performed to decide on the estimation method). None of them previously carried out an EFT, and in all three, the model of Feinberg et al. [26] of seven factors was tested directly using CFA.

Favez et al. [35], despite observing that items 13, 16, 21, and 22 were strongly skewed and had very high kurtosis, despite watching that they had a mean value very close to the lowest response value for the item, specifically 0.57, 0.51, 0.63 and 0.75 in the total sample, respectively, and that their SD was less than 1, they decided not to dispense with any item and use robust tests.

Costa et al. [34] and Dumitriu et al. [36] considered reducing the number of items on the scale as appropriate. Costa et al. [34] eliminated four items (items 13, 28, 5, and 20), and Dumitriu et al. [36] eliminated seven items (items 6, 7, 8, 28, 29, 5, and 20). Both were performed based on the factor loading or R^2 observed in the CFA solution. Despite the eliminated items (only Costa et al. [34] decided to eliminate the Division of Labor factor), neither of the two investigations considered that the dimensionality was different due to removing items. In this research, ten items were eliminated, including the four eliminated by Costa et al. [34] and four (of seven) eliminated by Dumitriu et al. [36]. The Supplementary Materials (Section S4) describes the items destroyed in the investigations with singular samples.

Furthermore, Favez et al. [35] and Dumitriu et al. [36] conclude that the 7-factor Feinberg model fits their data, and Costa et al. [34] conclude that the model fits with six factors. However, in the three cases, the model is fitted tangentially (Costa et al. [34]: [$\chi^2/gl = 4.69$; CFI = 0 0.90; GFI = 0.85, RMSEA = 0.07], Dumitriu et al. [36] [$\chi^2/gl = 3.90$, RMSEA = 0 0.076] and Favez et al. [35] [$\chi^2/gl = 2.94$; CFI = 0.863; RMSEA = 0.07; SRMR = 0.078], and although experts emphasize that a well-fitted model does not indicate that the model is valid, none of these three investigations considered testing a different model. Feinberg et al. [26], Costa et al. [34], Favez et al. [35], and Dumitriu et al. [36], and the investigations carried out with singular samples too (see Section S4 in the Supplementary Materials) found a very high correlation between some factors, and that is a sufficient reason to think that another model perhaps fits better to the observed data.

Thus, it is concluded that the Model with 20 items sized in two factors is the simplest and best adjusted model for the sample of Spanish parents; it is invariant according to sex and marital status, and the measure derived from each of its factors is reliable and valid. The new questionnaire for Spanish parents is called CRS-$S_{Eg\text{-}S\&D}$. The resulting factors were defined as *Positive Coparenting* (F1, fourteen items) and *Negative Perception of Coparenting* (F2, six items), and their joint evaluation could indicate what we call *Coparental Vitality*.

The first factor has been called *Positive Coparenting* because it brings together items that refer to a parent's cognition, feelings, and behaviors about the type of parental relationship they maintain with the other parent and the behaviors of the other that are necessary or facilitating for the exercise of positive coparenting. The higher the score, the greater the perception of harmony of the person responding regarding the exercise of co-parenting they are carrying out, and the more positive the perception they have of the behaviors and attitudes of the other parent as a father. The 14 items that make up F1, numbered with the number of the original scale of Feinberg et al. [26], are as follows:

2—My relationship with my partner is stronger now than before we had a child.

3—My partner asks my opinion on issues related to parenting.

6—My partner and I have the same goals for our child.

10—My partner tells me I am doing a good job or otherwise lets me know I am being a good parent.

14—My partner is sensitive to our child's feelings and needs.

17—I feel close to my partner when I see him or her play with our child.

18—My partner has a lot of patience with our child.

19—We often discuss the best way to meet our child's needs.

23—My partner is willing to make personal sacrifices to help take care of our child.

24—We are growing and maturing together through experiences as parents.

25—My partner appreciates how hard I work at being a good parent.

26—When I'm at my wits end as a parent, my partner gives me extra support I need.

27—My partner makes me feel like I'm the best possible parent for our child.

30—Parenting has given us a focus for the future.

The second factor has been called *Negative Perception of Coparenting* because the items that compose it establish discrepancies in parenting and parental behaviors that are incompatible with adequate coparenting. The higher the score on this factor, the greater the negative perception about the coparenting exercise they are performing.

The six items that make up F2, listed with the number of the original scale of Feinberg et al. [26], are as follows:

8—It is easier and more fun to play with the child alone than it is when my partner is present too.

9—My partner and I have different ideas about how to raise our child.

11—My partner and I have different ideas regarding our child's eating, sleeping, and other routines.

12—My partner sometimes makes jokes or sarcastic comments about the way I am as a parent.

15—My partner and I have different standards for our child's behavior.

29—My partner doesn't like to be bothered by our child.

Factor 1 has items corresponding to four of the six factors contained in CRS^{6S} [*Coparenting Closeness*—items 2, 17, 24, and 30; *Endorse Partner Parenting*—items 14, 18, and 23; *Coparenting Support*—items 3, 10, 19, 25, 26, and 27, and *Coparenting Agreement*—item 6]. Factor 2 has items corresponding to three of the six factors contained in CRS^{6S} [*Coparenting Agreement*—items 9, 11, and 15; *Endorse Partner Parenting*—item 29, and *Coparenting Undermining*—items 8 and 12]. The only factor not represented is the *Division of Labor*, which also disappeared in the CRS adaptation process carried out by Costa et al. [34] (see Section 4 of the Supplementary Materials to see in which other investigations this factor disappeared too). Therefore, given that the two factors contain the items of five scales in Feinberg et al. [26], we consider that the theoretical model of Feinberg et al. [26] is correct. Still, the dimensional structure differs from the one they found.

On the other hand, Feinberg et al. [26] found that the *Exposure to Conflict* factor was positively related to the *Coparenting Undermining* factor (0.40 and 0.60 in the subsamples of fathers and mothers, respectively). They also found it was negatively associated with the *Coparenting Closeness* factor (−0.46 and −0.26 in the subsamples of fathers and mothers, respectively). The fact that the items that make up the *Coparenting Undermining* factor in Feinberg et al. [26] are part of Factor 2 and that the items that make up the *Coparenting Closeness* factor in Feinberg et al. [26] are part of Factor 1 supports, a priori, the argument presented in Section 2.5 *Data analysis* to avoid introducing the *Exposure to Conflict* factor was correct. However, this aspect must be studied in depth, as indicated below. Finally, research on the *Division of Labor* scale should be conducted to determine whether it truly adds value to the construct.

The *Coparental Vitality* measure calculated using the total weighted measure of CRS-$S_{Eg\text{-}S\&D}$ allows the sample of participants to be divided into three differentiated clusters that we have called *Coparental Robustness* (or *Robust Coparenting*), *Moderate Coparenting*, and *Coparenting Rickets* (or *Inadequate Coparenting*). Since this measure gives equal weight to both factors, it will allow the coparenting status of the parents to be evaluated more effectively.

Thus, considering that coparenting is a mediating factor between the couple's relationship and the parents' ability to adapt to their new roles and responsibilities [9], the result of the study presented here should be considered a starting point that requires future research on at least the following questions: (1) Study the differences between Eg and S&D parents in *Positive Coparenting* and *Negative Perception of Coparenting*, and examine if sex is a moderating variable of the differences (the proven factorial invariance allows this analysis to be carried out with guarantee). It is necessary to know if the total score resulting from the sum of the score achieved in the two factors (using the weighted measure) is capable of faithfully capturing the state of *Coparental Vitality* that a person describes and experiences, or on the contrary, the position reached should be taken into account in each of the two factors (the result of the discriminant analysis supports this last aspect more than the first). The analysis of the added value of the *Exposure to Conflict* scale must accompany the analysis described in this first point. As was made clear at the beginning of Section 2.5 *Data analysis*, only S&D people responded to the five items of this scale. It is necessary to examine whether the *Coparental Vitality* of S&D people can be expressed with the same depth with these items and without them. This is expected to be the case, among other things, due to the distribution of the factors found by Feinberg et al. [26] in the two factors found in this research, as described before. (2) Examine to what extent different variables (e.g., sexual orientation, culture, years divorced, number of children, religion or training received for parenting, being in child–parent reunification processes, and being adoptive parents) exert an added moderating effect on the previous differences [10,11,18]. (3) Evaluate the practical validity of the measure and its predictive validity to determine its usefulness as a diagnostic or assessment measure in different conditions (separation, divorce, adoption, child–parent reunification, the effectiveness of intervention programs for the exercise of positive coparenting with independence of the particularity of the family, such as parenting coordination, etc.) [1,2,26,30,101–106]. (4) Delve into the possibility of identifying a cut-off point based on which to determine when a coparenting relationship enters a state of risk [2,29]. (5) Determine how the coparenting relationship changes as the age of the children changes and with the passage of time [107,108]. (6) Determine how coparenting is different depending on the children's problems (gifted children, autistic children, etc., in relation to children who do not have serious physical, cognitive, mental, or behavioral issues) [5,102,105].

Despite the control carried out throughout the research process, avoiding limitations has not been possible. The most notable is the asymmetry of participation based on sex. Although all parents, fathers, and mothers had the opportunity to participate in the study, self-selection could have occurred, affecting the results since this is a voluntary behavior.

However, based on the strength of the results found, despite the limitations, it can be concluded that the CRS-$S_{Eg\text{-}S\&D}$ questionnaire is reliable and valid for the study of coparenting in Spanish parents with children aged between 2 and 12 years.

Supplementary Materials: The following supporting information can be downloaded at https://www.mdpi.com/article/10.3390/children11050535/s1. Section S1: The Coparenting Relationship Scale (CSR) developed by Feinberg et al., (2012) [26], and translated to the Spanish adult population by Plá (2015) [37] (adapting the wording to our research to facilitate reading and responding). Section S2: The descriptive statistics of the items of six scales of the CRS questionnaire (Feinberg et al., 2012 [26]) in the responses of Spanish parents with children between the ages of 2 and 12 years (the Conflict Exposure scale is excluded). Due to the involvement of engaged parents (Eg) and separated or divorced parents (S&D) of both sexes, the results are presented independently for men and women of each marital status in the total sample (N = 2427) (Table S1), in the calibration subsample (n = 1239; 51.05%, approximately 50% of N) (Table S2), and in the validation subsample (n = 1188; 48.94%; approximately, 50% of the remaining sample of N, once the calibration sample has been extracted) (Table S3). The descriptive statistics are also presented for the total sample and the calibration and validation subsamples without differentiating between sexes or marital status (Table S4). Section S3: Table S5. Descriptive statistics of the items of six scales (the Exposure to Conflict scale is excluded) of the CRS questionnaire (Feinberg et al., 2012 [26]) in the calibration subsample (n = 1239), and pattern of factor loadings of the rotated matrix obtained through the EFA, requesting the same dimensionality of the six factors found by (Feinberg et al., 2012 [26]) (Table S5). The examination of the convergent and discriminant validity of the resulting dimensions in the adapted and validated questionnaire, CRS-SEg-S&D, examined through an empirical evaluation of the linear correlation with the factors that dimension the PAFAS questionnaires is also shown (Fariña et al., 2021 [57] and CAPES (Seijo et al., 2021 [59])) (Tables S6–S8). Section S4: This section shows the information that completes some paragraphs of the Discussion and Conclusions section of the article text. This added information is highlighted in red in for a better location. Section S5: Identification data of the participation of educational centers. Table S9. Exhaustive distribution of participation in schools is shown in the graph (left panel), and the distribution is ordered in participation intervals in a tabular way (right panel).

Author Contributions: Conceptualization, F.F., D.S. and R.A.; research design, M.P.F.; research planning, F.F., D.S. and R.A.; data analysis, M.P.F.; writing of the Data analysis and Results sections, M.P.F.; writing—original draft preparation, F.F., D.S. and R.A.; supervision of the entire research process, F.F. and D.S.; final writing of the article, F.F., D.S. and R.A.; review and editing, D.S. All authors have read and agreed to the published version of the manuscript.

Funding: This research has been funded by the Consellería de Cultura, Educación, Formación Profesional y Universidades (ED431B 2023/09).

Institutional Review Board Statement: This study was approved on 23 June 2016, by the Bioethics Committee of the University of Santiago de Compostela (Spain). The study was conducted according to the Declaration of Helsinki.

Informed Consent Statement: Informed consent was obtained from all subjects involved in the study.

Data Availability Statement: The data presented in this study are available upon request from the corresponding authors. The data are not publicly available due to privacy reasons.

Acknowledgments: We would like to express our gratitude to the anonymous reviewers, the Assistant Editor, and the Production Editor for their constructive and valuable comments that substantially improved the paper.

Conflicts of Interest: The authors declare no conflicts of interest.

References

1. Fariña, F.; Seijo, D.; Novo, M.; Castro, B. Assessing a parental break up family program from a Therapeutic Jurisprudence approach. *Rev. Investig. Educ.* **2023**, *21*, 96–113.
2. Saini, M.; Belcher-Timme, R.; Nau, D. A multidisciplinary perspective on the role, functions, and effectiveness of parenting coordination. *Fam. Court. Rev.* **2020**, *58*, 658–672. [CrossRef]
3. Seijo, D.; Fariña, F.; Fernández, M.P.; Sánchez, V. Vivencia de la parentalidad: Diagnóstico de la parentalidad experimentada e intensidad de sentimientos. [Parenting experience: Diagnosis of experienced parenting and intensity of feelings]. *Rev. Investig. Educ.* **2023**, *21*, 6–30.
4. Sun, Y. The role of family on internet addiction: A model analysis of co-parenting effect. *Cogent Soc. Sci.* **2023**, *9*, 2163530. [CrossRef]
5. Posada, D.; López-Larrosa, S. Parentalidad positiva: Afecto, control y justicia del trato parental hacia díadas fraternas y su relación con los problemas socio-emocionales de los hijos adolescentes [Positive parenting: Parental affect, control and justice towards siblings' dyads and their relationships with adolescent children's socio-emotional problems]. *Rev. Investig. Educ.* **2023**, *21*, 48–61.
6. Rivas, S.; Beltramo, C. Presentación. In *Parentalidad Positiva: Una Mirada a una Nueva Época*; Rivas, S., Beltramo, C., Eds.; Pirámide: Madrid, Spain, 2022; pp. 21–26.
7. Ronaghan, D.; Gaulke, T.; Theule, J. The association between marital satisfaction and coparenting quality: A meta-analysis. *J. Fam. Psychol.* **2023**, *38*, 236–245. [CrossRef] [PubMed]
8. Caldera, Y.M.; Lindsey, E.W. Coparenting, mother-infant interaction, and infant-parent attachment relationships in two-parent families. *J. Fam. Psychol.* **2006**, *20*, 275–283. [CrossRef] [PubMed]
9. Feinberg, M. The Internal Structure and Ecological Context of Coparenting: A Framework for Research and Intervention. *Parent. Sci. Pract.* **2003**, *3*, 95–131. [CrossRef] [PubMed]
10. McHale, J.P.; Lauretti, A.; Talbot, J.; Pouquette, C. Retrospect and prospect in the psychological study of coparenting and family group process. In *Retrospect and Prospect in the Psychological Study of Families*; McHale, P., Grolnick, W.S., Eds.; Lawrence Erlbaum Associates Publishers: New York, NY, USA, 2002; pp. 127–165.
11. Pilkington, P.; Rominov, H.; Brown, H.K.; Dennis, C.L. Systematic review of the impact of coparenting interventions on paternal coparenting behaviour. *J. Adv. Nurs.* **2019**, *75*, 17–29. [CrossRef]
12. Xiao, X.; Loke, A.Y. The effects of co-parenting/intergenerational co-parenting interventions during the postpartum period: A systematic review. *Int. J. Nurs. Stud.* **2021**, *119*, 103951. [CrossRef]
13. Eira Nunes, C.; De Roten, Y.; El Ghaziri, N.; Favez, N.; Darwiche, J. Co-parenting programs: A systematic review and meta-analysis. *Fam. Relat.* **2021**, *70*, 759–776. [CrossRef]
14. Favez, N.; Widmer, E.D.; Frascarolo, F.; Doan, M.-T. Mother-stepfather co-parenting in stepfamilies as predictor of child-adjustment. *Fam. Process.* **2019**, *58*, 446–462. [CrossRef] [PubMed]

15. McHale, J.P.; Lindahl, K.M. *Coparenting: A Conceptual and Clinical Examination of Family Systems*; American Psychological Association: Washington, DC, USA, 2011.
16. Fariña, F.; Arce, R.; Tomé, D.; Seijo, D. Validación del Cuestionario Actitud ante el Conflicto Parental: Autoinformada y Referenciada (ACPar) [Validation of the Attitude to Parental Conflict Questionnaire: Self-reported and Referenced (ACPar)]. *Rev. Iberoam. Psicol. Salud* **2020**, *11*, 1–14.
17. Feinberg, M.E.; Kan, M.L.; Hetherington, E.M. The longitudinal influence of coparenting conflict on parental negativity and adolescent maladjustment. *J. Marriage Fam.* **2007**, *69*, 687–702. [CrossRef] [PubMed]
18. Schoppe-Sullivan, S.J.; Mangelsdorf, S.C. Parent characteristics and early coparenting behavior at the transition to parenthood. *Soc. Dev.* **2013**, *2*, 363–383. [CrossRef]
19. Jiménez-Granado, A.; Hoyo-Bilbao, J.D.; Fernández-González, L. Interaction of Parental Discipline Strategies and Adolescents' Personality Traits in the Prediction of Child-to-Parent Violence. *Eur. J. Psychol. Appl. Leg. Context* **2023**, *15*, 43–52. [CrossRef]
20. Martínez-Gómez, J.A.; Rey-Anacona, C.A.; Bolívar-Suárez, Y.; Rodríguez-Díaz, F.J.; Álvarez-Arregui, E. Effects of negative communication on family dynamic and dating violence. *Rev. Iberoam. Psicol. Salud* **2023**, *14*, 83–91. [CrossRef]
21. Pineda, D.; Muris, P.; Martínez-Martínez, A.; Piqueras, J.A. Prevalence of Child Sexual Abuse in Spain: A Survey Study. *Eur. J. Psychol. Appl. Leg. Context* **2023**, *15*, 8–88. [CrossRef]
22. Molla Cusi, L.; Günther-Bel, C.; Vilaregut Puigdesens, A.; Camprecios Orriols, M.; Matali Costa, J.L. Instruments for the Assessment of Coparenting: A Systematic Review. *J. Child. Fam. Stud.* **2020**, *29*, 2487–2506. [CrossRef]
23. Abidin, R.R.; Brunner, J.F. Development of a parenting alliance inventory. *J. Clin. Child. Psychol.* **1995**, *24*, 31–40. [CrossRef]
24. McHale, J.P. Overt and covert coparenting processes in the family. *Fam. Process.* **1997**, *36*, 183–201. [CrossRef] [PubMed]
25. Teubert, D.; Pinquart, M. The Coparenting Inventory for Parents and Adolescents (CI-PA): Reliability and validity. *Eur. J. Psychol. Assess.* **2011**, *27*, 206–215. [CrossRef]
26. Feinberg, M.; Brown, L.D.; Kan, M.L. A multi-domain self-report measure of coparenting. *Parent-Sci. Pract.* **2012**, *12*, 1–21. [CrossRef] [PubMed]
27. McHale, J.P. *Charting the Bumpy Road of Coparenthood Understanding the Challenges of Family Life. Zero to Three*; American Psychological Association: Washington, DC, USA, 2007.
28. Van Egeren, L.A.; Hawkins, D.P. Coming to terms with coparenting: Implications of definition and measurement. *J. Adult Dev.* **2004**, *11*, 165–178. [CrossRef]
29. Lamela, D.; Figueiredo, B.; Bastos, A.; Feinberg, M. Typologies of post-divorce coparenting and parental well-being, parenting quality and children's psychological adjustment. *Child. Psychiatry Hum. Dev.* **2016**, *47*, 716–728. [CrossRef]
30. Pinto, T.M.; Figueiredo, B.; Feinberg, M.E. The coparenting relationship scale—Father's prenatal version. *J. Adult Dev.* **2019**, *26*, 201–208. [CrossRef]
31. Lee, J.; Feinberg, M.; Wells, M. The Swedish Brief Coparenting Relationship Scale: Psychometrics and Concurrent Validity Among Primiparous and Multiparous Fathers. *Fam. Relat.* **2020**, *70*, 823–839. [CrossRef]
32. Lamela, D.; Morais, A.; Jongenelen, I. Psychometric Validation of the Coparenting Relationship Scale in Portuguese Mothers. *Av. Psicol. Latinoam.* **2018**, *36*, 585–601. [CrossRef]
33. Leal, D.; Gato, J.; Coimbra, S.; Tasker, F.; Tornello, S. The Prospective Co-Parenting Relationship Scale (PCRS) for Sexual Minority and Heterosexual People: Preliminary Validation. *Int. J. Environ. Res. Public Health* **2022**, *19*, 6345. [CrossRef]
34. Costa, P.A.; Garcia, I.Q.; Tasker, F.; Leal, I. Adaptação das versões completa e breve da Escala de Relação Coparental (ERC) em uma amostra comunitária de pais e mães Portugueses (Adaptation of the complete and brief version of the Coparenting Relationship Scale in a community sample of Portuguese fathers and mothers). *Rev. Psicol.* **2020**, *34*, 236–248.
35. Favez, N.; Tissot, H.; Golay, P.; Max, A.; Feinberg, M.E.; Bader, M. French adaptation of the Coparenting Relationship Scale: A scale for the assessment of the interparental relationship. *Eur. J. Psychol. Assess.* **2021**, *37*, 433–439. [CrossRef]
36. Dumitriu, G.; Dudu, A.; Butac, L.M. Validation of the Romanian version of coparenting relationship scale. *Int. J. Environ. Res. Public Health* **2022**, *9*, 24–34. [CrossRef]
37. Plá, M. La Coparentalidad: El rol que Desempeña en la Aparición de Problemas de Conducta en la Adolescencia. Ph.D. Thesis, Universidad Pontificia Comillas, Madrid, Spain, 2015.
38. Bornstein, M.H. Cultural approaches to parenting. *Parent-Sci. Pract.* **2012**, *12*, 212–221. [CrossRef] [PubMed]
39. Ferrando, P.J.; Anguiano-Carrasco, C. El análisis factorial como técnica de investigación en psicología. *Pap. Psicol.* **2010**, *31*, 18–33.
40. Gorsuch, R.L. Exploratory factor analysis: Its role in item analysis. *J. Pers. Assess.* **1997**, *68*, 532–560. [CrossRef]
41. Gorsuch, R.L. New procedure for extension analysis in exploratory factor analysis. *Educ. Psychol. Meas.* **1997**, *57*, 725–740. [CrossRef]
42. Osborne, J.W. *Best Practices in Exploratory Factor Analysis*; Create Space Independent Publishing: Scotts Valley, CA, USA, 2014.
43. Nunnally, J.C.; Bernstein, I.J. *Teoría Psicométrica*; McGraw-Hill: Madrid, Spain, 1995.
44. Whiteside, S.P.; Lynam, D.R. The Five Factor Model and impulsivity: Using a structural model of personality to understand impulsivity. *Pers. Indiv Differ.* **2001**, *30*, 669–689. [CrossRef]
45. Goretzko, D.; Pham, T.T.H.; Bühner, M. Exploratory factor analysis: Current use, methodological developments and recommendations for good practice. *Curr. Psychol.* **2021**, *40*, 3510–3521. [CrossRef]
46. Hancock, G.R.; Stapleton, L.M.; Mueller, R.O. *The Reviewer's Guide to Quantitative Methods in the Social Sciences*, 2nd ed.; Routledge: New York, NY, USA, 2018.

47. American Educational Research Association; American Psychological Association; National Council on Measurement in Education. *Standards for Educational and Psychological Testing*; American Psychological Association: Washington, DC, USA, 2014.
48. Muñiz, J.; Fonseca-Pedrero, E. Ten steps for test development. *Psicothema* **2019**, *31*, 7–16.
49. Cronbach, L.J. Further evidence on response sets and test design. *Educ. Psychol. Meas.* **1950**, *10*, 3–31. [CrossRef]
50. Berry, D.T.R.; Wetter, M.W.; Baer, R.A.; Larsen, L.; Clark, C.; Monroe, K. MMPI-2 random responding indices: Validation using self-report methodology. *Psychol. Assess.* **1992**, *4*, 340–345. [CrossRef]
51. Meier, S.T. *The Chronic Crisis in Psychological Measurement and Assessment: A Historical Survey*; Academic: Cambridge, MA, USA, 1994.
52. Osborne, J.W.; Blanchard, M.R. Random responding from participants is a threat to the validity of social science research results. *Front. Psychol.* **2011**, *2*, 12. [CrossRef] [PubMed]
53. Wise, S.L. An Investigation of the Differential Effort Received by Items on a Low-Stakes Computer-Based Test. *Appl. Meas. Educ.* **2006**, *9*, 95–114. [CrossRef]
54. Fernández, P.; Vallejo, G.; Livácic, P.; Tuero, E. The (ir)responsibility of (under)estimating missing data. *Front. Psychol.* **2018**, *9*, 556. [CrossRef]
55. Fernández, P.; Vallejo, G.; Livacic, P.; Tuero, E. Validez Estructurada para una investigación cuasi-experimental de calidad. Se cumplen 50 años de la presentación en sociedad de los diseños cuasi-experimentales. *An. Psicol.* **2014**, *30*, 756–771.
56. Sanders, M.R.; Morawska, A.; Haslam, D.M.; Filus, A.; Fletcher, R. Escalas de ajuste familiar y de crianza (PAFAS): Validación de una medida breve de informe de los padres para su uso en la evaluación de las habilidades de crianza y las relaciones familiares. *Child. Psychiatry Hum. Dev.* **2014**, *45*, 255–272. [CrossRef] [PubMed]
57. Fariña, F.; Seijo, D.; Tomé, D.; Castro, B. Adaptación española y propiedades psicométricas de la Escala de Parentalidad y Ajuste Familiar (PAFAS). *Rev. Psicol. Clín. Niños Adolesc.* **2021**, *8*, 40–46. [CrossRef]
58. Morawska, A.; Sanders, M.R.; Haslam, D.; Filus, A.; Fletcher, R. Child Adjustment and Parent Efficacy Scale: Development and Initial Validation of a Parent Report Measure. *Aust. Psychol.* **2014**, *49*, 241–252. [CrossRef]
59. Seijo, D.; Tomé, D.; Sanmarco, J.; Morawska, A.; Fariña, F. Spanish adaptation and validation of the child adjustment and parent efficacy scale. *Sustainability* **2021**, *13*, 4647. [CrossRef]
60. Şahin, M.D. Effect of Item Order on Certain Psychometric Properties: A Demonstration on a Cyberloafing Scale. *Front. Psychol.* **2021**, *12*, 590545. [CrossRef]
61. Weinberg, M.K.; Seton, C.; Cameron, N. The measurement of subjective wellbeing: Item-order effects in the personal wellbeing index—Adult. *J. Happiness Stud.* **2018**, *19*, 315–332. [CrossRef]
62. Ferrando, P.J.; Lorenzo-Seva, U. Exploratory item factor analysis: Additional considerations. *An. Psicol.* **2014**, *30*, 1170–1175.
63. Thompson, B. *Exploratory and Confirmatory Factor Analysis: Understanding Concepts and Applications*; American Psychological Association: Washington, DC, USA, 2004.
64. Byrne, B.M. *Structural Equation Modeling with AMOS: Basic Concepts, Applications, and Programming*; Routledge: London, UK, 2010.
65. Bentler, P.M. *EQS 6, Structural Equations Program Manual*; Multivariate Software Inc.: Encino, CA, USA, 2006.
66. Hair, J.F., Jr.; Black, W.C.; Babin, B.J.; Anderson, R.E.; Tatham, R.L. *Multivariate Data Analysis*, 6th ed.; Pearson Education International: London, UK, 2006.
67. Lorenzo-Seva, U.; Ferrando, P.J. FACTOR: A computer program to fit the exploratory factor analysis model. *Behav. Res. Methods* **2006**, *38*, 88–91. [CrossRef] [PubMed]
68. Levine, M.S. *Canonical Analysis and Factor Comparison*; Sage: New York, NY, USA, 1977.
69. Curran, P.J.; West, S.G.; Finch, J.F. The robustness of test statistics to nonnormality and specification error in confirmatory factor analysis. *Psychol. Methods* **1996**, *1*, 16–29. [CrossRef]
70. Kaplan, D. Evaluating and modifying covariance structure models: A review and recommendation. *Multivar. Behav. Res.* **1990**, *25*, 137–155. [CrossRef] [PubMed]
71. Muthen, B.; Kaplan, D. A comparison of some methodologies for the factor analysis of non-normal Likert variables: A note on the size of the model. *Br. J. Math. Stat. Psychol.* **1992**, *45*, 19–30. [CrossRef]
72. Jöreskog, K.G. *Factor Analysis by MINRES*; Technical Report. 2003. Available online: https://ssicentral.com/wp-content/uploads/2021/04/lis_minres.pdf (accessed on 22 April 2024).
73. Timmerman, M.E.; Lorenzo-Seva, U. Dimensionality assessment of ordered polytomous items with parallel analysis. *Psychol. Methods* **2011**, *16*, 209. [CrossRef]
74. Lorenzo-Seva, U.; Ferrando, P.J. Robust Promin: A method for diagonally weighted factor rotation. *Liberabit* **2019**, *25*, 99–106. [CrossRef]
75. Hu, L.; Bentler, P.M. Cutoff criteria for fit indexes in covariance structure analysis: Conventional criteria versus new alternatives. *Struct. Equ. Model.* **1999**, *6*, 1–55. [CrossRef]
76. Bentler, P.M. Factor simplicity index and transformations. *Psychometrika* **1977**, *42*, 277–295. [CrossRef]
77. Ferrando, P.J.; Lorenzo-Seva, U. Assessing the quality and appropriateness of factor solutions and factor score estimates in exploratory item factor analysis. *Educ. Psychol. Meas.* **2018**, *78*, 762–780. [CrossRef]
78. Ferrando, P.J.; Lorenzo-Seva, U. On the added value of multiple factor score estimates in essentially unidimensional models. *Educ. Psychol. Meas.* **2019**, *79*, 249–271. [CrossRef] [PubMed]

79. DiStefano, C.; Morgan, G.B. A comparison of diagonal weighted least squares robust estimation techniques for ordinal data. *S Struct. Equ. Model.* **2014**, *21*, 425–438. [CrossRef]
80. Kline, R.B. *Principles and Practice of Structural Equation Modelling*, 4th ed.; Guilford Publications: New York, NY, USA, 2016.
81. Schermelleh-Engel, K.; Moosbrugger, H.; Muller, H. Evaluating the fit of structural equation models: Tests of significance and goodness-of-fit models. *Psychol. Methods* **2003**, *8*, 23–74.
82. Chen, F.F. Sensitivity of goodness of fit indexes to lack of measurement invariance. *Struct. Equ. Model.* **2007**, *14*, 464–504. [CrossRef]
83. Luong, R.; Flake, J.K. Measurement invariance testing using confirmatory factor analysis and alignment optimization: A tutorial for transparent analysis planning and reporting. *Psychol. Methods* **2023**, *28*, 905–924. [CrossRef] [PubMed]
84. Ferguson, C.J. An effect size primer: A guide for clinicians and researchers. In *Methodological Issues and Strategies in Clinical Research*; Kazdin, A.E., Ed.; American Psychological Association: Washington, DC, USA, 2016; pp. 301–310.
85. Fornell, C.; Larcker, D.F. Evaluating Structural Equation Models with Unobservable Variables and Measurement Error. *J. Mark. Res.* **1981**, *18*, 39–50. [CrossRef]
86. Cheung, G.W.; Wang, C. Current approaches for assessing convergent and discriminant validity with SEM: Issues and solutions. *Acad. Manag.* **2017**, *1*, 12706. [CrossRef]
87. Kaufman, L.; Rousseeuw, P.J. *Finding Groups in Data: An Introduction to Cluster Analysis*; John Wiley & Sons: Hoboken, NJ, USA, 2009.
88. Enders, C.K. Performing Multivariate Group Comparisons Following a Statistically Significant MANOVA. *Meas. Eval. Couns. Dev.* **2003**, *36*, 40–56. [CrossRef]
89. Smith, K.N.; Lamb, K.N.; Henson, R.K. Making meaning out of MANOVA: The need for multivariate post hoc testing in gifted education research. *Gift. Child. Q.* **2020**, *64*, 41–55. [CrossRef]
90. Bray, J.H.; Maxwell, S.E. *Multivariate Analysis of Variance*; Sage: Thousand Oaks, CA, USA, 1985; Volume 54.
91. Tabachnick, B.G.; Fidell, L.S. *Using Multivariate Statistics*; Harper & Row, Publishers: New York, NY, USA, 1989.
92. Maxwell, S.E.; Delaney, H.D. *Designing Experiments and Analyzing Data: A Model Comparison Perspective*, 2nd ed.; Lawrence Erlbaum Associates: Mahwah, NJ, USA, 2004.
93. Ateş, C.; Kaymaz, Ö.; Kale, H.E.; Tekindal, M.A. Comparison of Test Statistics of Nonnormal and Unbalanced Samples for Multivariate Analysis of Variance in terms of Type-I Error Rates. *Comput. Math. Methods Med.* **2019**, *2019*, 2173638. [CrossRef]
94. Vallejo, G.; Ato, M.; Fernández, P. A robust approach for analyzing unbalanced factorial designs with fixed levels. *Behav. Res. Methods* **2010**, *42*, 607–617. [CrossRef] [PubMed]
95. Cohen, J. A power primer. *Psychol. Methods* **1992**, *112*, 155–159. [CrossRef] [PubMed]
96. Jiang, N. Investigating Performance of Model Fit Indices In Multiple-Group Confirmatory Factor Analysis: Complications with Ordinal Data. Ph.D. Thesis, University of South Carolina, Columbia, SC, USA, 2022.
97. Millsap, R.E.; Meredith, W. Factorial invariance: Historical perspectives and new problems. In *Factor Analysis at 100: Historical Developments and Future Directions*; Cudeck, R., McCallum, R., Eds.; Lawrence Erlbaum Associates Publishers: New York, NY, USA, 2007; pp. 131–152.
98. Costello, A.B.; Osborne, J.W. Best Practices in Exploratory Factor Analysis: Four recommendations for getting the most from your analysis. *Pract. Assess.* **2005**, *10*, 1–9.
99. Guadagnoli, E.; Velicer, W.F. Relation of sample size to the stability of component patterns. *Psychol. Bull.* **1988**, *103*, 265–275. [CrossRef] [PubMed]
100. Kyriazos, T.A. Applied Psychometrics: The 3-Faced Construct Validation Method, a Routine for Evaluating a Factor Structure. *Psychology* **2018**, *9*, 2044–2072. [CrossRef]
101. Fagan, J.; Henson, A.; Pearson, J. Low-income mothers' participation in the Understanding DadsTM intervention and changes in self-reported coparenting. *J. Fam. Soc. Work* **2021**, *24*, 199–218. [CrossRef]
102. González-Pasarín, L.; Bernedo, I.M. Programa de apoyo a la parentalidad positiva dirigido a familias biológicas y acogedoras durante el acogimiento familiar. [Positive parenting support programme for birth and foster families in foster care]. *Rev. Investig. Educ.* **2023**, *21*, 80–95.
103. Hammock, A.C.; McKillop, A.J.; Hayward, R.A.; Kohli, E.; Bessaha, M.L. Coparenting communication and hybrid masculinity in a fatherhood program. *Fam. Relat.* **2022**, *71*, 1122–1141. [CrossRef]
104. Novo, M.; Fariña, F.; Seijo, D.; Vázquez, M.J.; Arce, R. Assessing the effects of an education program on mental health problems in separated parents. *Psicothema* **2019**, *31*, 284–291.
105. Petrucci, P.C. First They Have to Show Up: How Dads Back! Academy Successfully Engaged Formerly Incarcerated Fathers in a Responsible Fatherhood Program. *Rev. Investig. Educ.* **2023**, *21*, 114–133.
106. Fariña, F.; Fernández, P.; Seijo, D. Programas de parentalidad desde la óptica y el análisis de los progenitores españoles. *Acción Psicol.* **2023**, *20*, 89–112.

107. Fernández, P.; Livacic, P.; Vallejo, G. Cómo elegir la mejor prueba estadística para analizar un diseño de medidas repetidas. *Int. J. Clin. Health Psychol.* **2007**, *7*, 153–175.
108. Livacic, P.; Vallejo, G.; Fernández, P. Procedimientos estadísticos alternativos para evaluar la robustez utilizando diseños de medidas repetidas. *Rev. Latinoam. Psicol.* **2006**, *38*, 579–598.

children

MDPI

Article

Managing Major Life Changes: An Exploratory Study Using the Bridges Transitions Framework to Help Foster Youth Prepare for Discharge

Ande A. Nesmith

School of Social Work, University of St. Thomas, St. Paul, MN 55105, USA; nesm3326@stthomas.edu

Abstract: Background: Adolescents in foster care endure frequent disruptive transitions, often culminating in discharge to independent living rather than reunification or adoption. Former foster youth fare poorly once on their own, with high rates of homelessness and social disconnection. This study explored the use of the Bridges Transitions Framework near the end of placement to help youth cope with the transition to adulthood. Methods: In this exploratory study, the framework was integrated into a foster agency's programming; then, we assessed outcomes using administrative data and youth interviews. Thirty-five youth participated. Status of employment, education, and social support was collected 18 months after exposure to the framework. Results: The participants reported moderate to high levels of social support, which is often limited or absent among foster care leavers. Relative to rates reported in state-level foster care data, participants had substantially higher rates of school enrollment after discharge. With very few empirically assessed models available for this population that specifically address internal coping with such substantial life changes, the Transitions Framework offers a tool that may help foster youth navigate aging out of care. Securing lasting and meaningful social support and employment and completing education remain elusive for former foster youth. Conclusions: To confirm the utility of the Transitions Framework, it is recommended to assess it with a large sample and matched comparison group over time.

Keywords: foster youth; transitions to adulthood; Bridges Transitions Framework; youth transitions

1. Introduction

Older youth in child welfare placements experience high rates of living situation changes throughout their foster care stays, culminating in discharge from care [1,2]. The first transition from their family home into foster care can be traumatic in the life of adolescents, who are still developing their sense of identity [3].

One of the first in-depth and well-designed prospective longitudinal studies of older foster youth and their transitions to adulthood was conducted in the U.S. Midwest: the "Midwest Evaluation of the Adult Functioning of Former Foster Youth", known as "The Midwest Study" [4,5]. Although their work began nearly twenty years ago, the findings continued to be used and referenced widely and have since been replicated in other regions [6]. Courtney and colleagues' research found that placement moves during foster care can have a cumulative effect on youth once they transition out of foster care into independent living, impacting education, employment, housing stability, and social support in early adulthood [4,5]. Similar findings have been found in other studies [7,8]. This

https://doi.org/10.3390/children12010022

represents no small subset of foster children. In the U.S., 23% of children enter care as adolescents (13+ years), and 28% of all children currently in care are placed during their adolescent years [9]. Rather than being reunified with their families or adopted, as many as 9% of youth who leave the system each year do so by aging out of the system [9]. The impact of placement into care is long-lasting and may be compounded by additional changes that occur during placement spells (especially moves to different homes) [10,11]. Social service providers may be faced with helping youth cope with their admission into care and transitions during placement, while simultaneously preparing them for the transition out of care.

U.S. federal policies require that the child welfare system attends to the impact of these major disruptions at both admission and discharge. For example, the Fostering Connections to Success Act (2008) [12] prioritizes stable kin relationships and connections to original communities and schools when children are first placed. It requires that, when possible, children remain in their current schools to enhance educational stability. Looking toward discharge, the Foster Care Independence Act (1999) [13] appropriates substantial funds to independent living programs to provide education, training, employment services, and financial support for foster youth aged 16 to 18. However, as will be discussed here, adhering to these policies has proven challenging in practice, and outcomes for former foster youth continue to be poor.

There is very little research evidence that points to improved outcomes for youth aging out of foster care [14,15]. The California Evidence-based Clearinghouse for Child Welfare [14] examines and rates programs for scientific evidence of positive outcomes. In their category regarding youth transitioning to adulthood to live independently, only one program was identified as being supported by scientific evidence. Three programs were described as having promising evidence, and the remainder could not be assessed. The program with scientific evidence, Better Futures, sought to increase post-secondary education among those who were not opposed to continuing their education by providing a 3-day training, community-based coaching, and relationship support. Greeson and colleagues (2020) [15] examined 79 programs and interventions for youth aging out and found only three that were supported with robust research evidence that they affected outcomes within six months to a year post-intervention. These focused on mental health, post-secondary education, and/or building supportive relationships.

Absent from most of these interventions is attention to the impact of major life changes on the youth, their internal response to them, and external reactions that, without some guidance, may lead to behaviors that can make such transitions difficult. The present study explores the application of a framework designed specifically to help individuals cope with difficult life transitions. This study explores the utility of the Bridges Transitions Framework [16] to help older foster youth navigate transitions and determine if there were signs of improved education, social support, or employment at least in the short-term—18 months later.

1.1. Transitions While in Foster Care Placement

Those who enter foster care as adolescents typically undergo several placement transitions until they exit the system, most often by reaching the age of majority rather than by adoption or family reunification [2]. The earliest moves tend to be among foster homes; however, with continued disruptions, youth placements increasingly transition away from family-like settings and into congregate care, group homes, residential treatment centers, or juvenile justice settings. In fact, among those entering care at age 13 or older, about half will move from family-like settings into congregate care [17]. This can be a self-perpetuating situation because placement instability can also exacerbate existing behavioral issues [18,19].

Youth in foster care often have limited control over important decisions such as placement moves, which can affect their ability to cope with substantial transitions [10,20]. These decisions represent major life changes such as admission to foster care or moves to new placements, neighborhoods, and schools, yet youth often have little say in them. In turn, high rates of moves can negatively impact education, employment, housing, and social support.

1.2. Education

The more moves a youth experiences, the more likely their education is also disrupted, which can have a lasting impact that extends into adulthood [2,21]. Despite federal law, the necessary resources and coordination between schools and child welfare organizations are frequently lacking. Transcripts and Individual Educational Plans (IEPs) often do not transfer with placement moves, slowing academic progress and contributing to the low high school graduation rates observed among foster youth [21]. Moreover, the level of educational attainment decreases with each additional move during a foster care spell. By age 23, about a quarter of former foster youth still do not have a high school diploma or GED [5].

1.3. Employment and Housing

Former foster youth struggle to secure employment and housing. Independent living services that coach foster youth in concrete skills such as money management or resume and job interviewing training are essential but not enough to bring stability to these youth post-discharge [22]. Courtney and colleagues' (2005) [4] Midwest Study found that fewer than half of discharged foster youth were employed by age 19. This is also true on a broader level: the National Youth in Transition Database reveals that, among former foster youth across the U.S., only 35% are employed at least part-time [9].

Stable housing remains elusive for many former foster youth. In the years following discharge, periods of homelessness are common. By 19 years old, 19% of former foster youth experienced at least one episode of homelessness nationally, and 32% experienced at least one episode of homelessness in the same state as the present study [9,20].

1.4. Social Support

Independent living services also do not adequately address the socio-emotional needs of youth [16,23]. A growing body of research points to the critical role of social and emotional support—particularly from a supportive adult—that any young person needs during transition to adulthood, yet this is minimal or absent for foster youth [11].Transitions during placement can impact the support youth are able to secure as they exit care [24]. Recurring placement moves can result in a sense of rejection, especially when they occur repeatedly. Youth may respond by "emotionally shutting down", withdrawing, or behaving in ways that increase the chances of another transition. This, in turn, can further impede their ability to connect with future caregivers or supportive adults [10]. These are among the behaviors that the Transitions Framework aims to ameliorate.

This study examined employment, social support, and education among young people who were placed in foster care as adolescents 18 months after they were trained in applying the Transitions Framework to their own lives.

1.5. Conceptual Framework: Bridges' Transitions

The Transitions Framework [16] draws a distinction between external changes one experiences and internal transitions that are responses to those changes. Change is situational, typically events that occur outside an individual's control, such as the death of a loved one, losing a job, or in this context, aging out of foster care. Transitions are internal psychological reactions to external changes. Substantial changes tend to yield more difficult transitions. Though the framework was originally developed for use in organizational management, it has been applied to other settings [25,26]. While it has not generally been applied to child welfare, one study examined its use with 34 Romanian foster youth leaving foster care to understand their social and psychological transitions and how they were both distinct and interconnected [27]. This study used the framework to help service providers, rather than the youth themselves, recognize the transition process for youth. To date, there has been little to no empirical research in which youth were taught about the framework to give them insight into their own experience of changes and potentially develop coping strategies as they enter and exit foster care.

The theory of change using this framework has several components to help youth cope with change. First, it provides youth with tools to recognize and understand their own internal transition responses and how the related behaviors may be received by others. This helps them to make sense of their own behaviors and anticipate their reactions, opening opportunities for changing their behavior. Second, it helps youth to normalize their emotional reactions to external change and increase their own patience as they adjust. For example, the framework includes a concept called "The Marathon Effect", which explains that people will move at different paces toward a similar end or goal, that coping with change takes time, and there will be moments in which it feels like they are making faster progress than at other times. Understanding that setting goals works best after they have allowed themselves to grieve the past sets them up for success regarding those goals. Finally, the framework involves reinforcing the concepts and processes of the adults in their lives. This includes training their social workers/caseworks and foster parents and allows them to reinforce new learning and behaviors amongst the youth. Managing their own emotions and behaviors, in turn, can lead to more stable relationships at home and in the workplace.

1.6. The Present Study

This exploratory study examined how youth who were trained in the Transitions Framework fared 18 months later in three key wellbeing outcomes that historically are challenging for this group: social support, educational involvement, and employment. The findings presented here draw from the third and final wave of data collection from a multi-year evaluation of the Transitions Framework implemented in a non-profit U.S. Midwestern foster care provider (hereon referred to as "the agency"). The agency integrated the Bridges Transitions Framework into their programming to prepare adolescents in foster care adjust to their transitions into foster care, as well as to prepare older youth to age out of the system as young adults. Unlike other prior work, in addition to service providers, foster youth and their foster parents were trained.

1.7. Training Components and Application of Transitions Framework

Transitions Framework trainings aimed to help participants normalize emotional responses to change, become familiar their own internal transition process, and develop effective coping strategies. This knowledge is also important for the adults caring for youth, to understand what drives observable behaviors following a change in youth's lives. The framework organizes reactions to change into phases called Endings, the Neutral Zone, and New Beginnings [16]. Though this generally represents a particular order, an individual may encounter aspects of more than one phase simultaneously. Critical to the framework is the focus on process rather than goals and moving at one's own natural pace through the phases. Participants learned to understand and recognize the three transitions phases in their own lives, as described below.

Endings are triggered by loss, which for foster youth often includes separation from family and friends, connection to community and school, a shift to a new living situation with different people and rules, or discharge from foster care. The internal response may be experienced as a range of emotions such as anger, mourning, regret, sadness, regret, or nostalgia and wistfulness. The framework encourages reflection on the past and cautions against asking youth to set goals or develop new plans during this time. Problems with adjustment can occur if the past is not honored, or if youth are urged to focus on future plans while they still grieve. In this phase, social workers and caregivers are encouraged to help youth sustain meaningful memories by engaging in discussions about family or past events and listening when youth broach the subject, without attempting to move the conversation to the present or future.

During the Neutral Zone, endings are honored, and while youth accept the reality of their new situation, they may still feel unsettled in their living arrangement, ambivalent about new commitments, and untrusting of new relationships. In this phase, youth may exhibit disruptive or resistant behaviors or strong emotional reactions to people and situations. Caregivers and social workers are encouraged to exercise patience and recognize the underlying feelings that drive those actions rather than responding to the behaviors.

Finally, in New Beginnings, youth can imagine the future, establish goals, and embark on new relationships. This phase is marked by confidence and renewal. This is the phase where most people want to be, but, according to Bridges (2009) [16], they cannot attain it without first experiencing the first two phases. Here, foster parents and social workers help youth identify new paths toward goals and celebrate successes.

1.8. Implementation

The agency worked with a Transitions Framework expert consultant who conducted several two-day interactive trainings with all 10 agency social workers and supervisors, using a "train-the-trainer" approach. The social workers then conducted trainings with foster parents and adolescent foster youth served through the agency. The trainings were comprised of small groups (5–8 youths and their foster parents) and were conducted in four-session sequences, repeatedly offered over the course of the study. A rolling enrollment allowed youth aged as young as 13 (though the youngest participant was 15 years old) to participate shortly after they were admitted to foster care over the course of three years. Some of the trained youth participated in future trainings as "Transitions Coaches", co-leading new trainings and sharing their own transitions experiences to demonstrate how the framework worked in real situations.

The structure was highly interactive. Participants mapped their transition processes on paper, shared stories, and practiced assessing their own and others' transitional phases. Both youth and foster parents were provided with concrete behaviors and strategies to experiment with at home and then discuss in subsequent sessions for feedback and direction. For their part, foster parents were encouraged to value and honor the losses youth endured and to identify triggers and recognize underlying factors that drive challenging youth behaviors. They then practiced effective response strategies taught in the trainings.

To support continued use of the framework, the social workers integrated the transitions concepts in meetings with foster parent meetings and during youth programming. When behavioral problems were discussed, social workers asked youth and foster parents to first identify recent and past changes that might contribute to the behaviors and to identify the youth's stage of transitions.

2. Methods

The findings here report on findings 18 months after foster youth were initially trained in the Transitions Framework. In this exploratory study, participants were interviewed in person, answering questions about their current living situation, future plans, social support, education, and employment.

2.1. Human Subjects Review

The research activities for this study were reviewed and approved by two research ethics boards: the primary investigator's university IRB as well as the county human services IRB that oversaw the children in the foster care agency. All participants underwent an informed consent process; for minors, legal guardian consent and age-appropriate child assents were obtained prior to enrolling in the study.

2.2. Sampling

The participants were drawn from a pool of 54 youths who were trained in the Transitions Framework and took a post-test 6–9 months later. The original training included 63 youths who provided pre-test baseline data. Eighteen months post-training, all 54 youths were invited to participate in a final interview, and 35 (64.8%) enrolled. Most of the 19 youths who did not participate in the final interview (84%, $n = 16$) did not respond to invitations. For the remaining three, their legal guardians declined continued involvement for the youth.

While there are no data available across all categories for those who did not participate in the final interview, there were some demographic and placement data available that did not reveal substantial differences. An examination of demographics and placement information revealed that those who did not continue to third wave of data collection (Wave 3) were quite similar to those who participated, with very slight variations (6% or less) in race distributions, gender breakdown, age, proportion who were discharged, age at discharge, and reason for placement. For the 19 who did not continue, due to very small numbers in each subcategory and for confidentiality reasons, the specific subcategory breakdowns are not provided here.

2.3. Measurement and Data Collection

The data were collected to assess indicators of stability 18 months later. This study used the Medical Outcomes Study Social Support Survey (MOS) and agency administrative data from the youth's placement records for demographic and placement information.

2.3.1. Medical Outcomes Study Social Support Survey (MOS)

The MOS is a 19-item standardized tool found to be reliable and valid and has been used with foster youth in prior research [28]. It contains four social support subscales, including emotional-informational, tangible, affectionate, and positive social interaction. These were assessed with a five-point Likert scale, in which a score of 5 represents the most support ("all of the time") and 1 represents the least support ("none of the time").

2.3.2. Administrative Data

Placement data were extracted from the youth's placement records collected when the youth first enrolled in the study. These were data that were input into the data system contemporaneously by social service providers. To protect privacy, a data request for the following variables was submitted, and the foster agency staff pulled the information for the research: placement information included prior placement history, placement reasons, and permanency plans. For those who left foster care, discharge data that were routinely tracked and stored in the foster care database system were entered at the time of discharge, and information was pulled by agency staff. For those remaining in care 18 months later, placement records were used to collect updated information. These data included discharge date (if relevant), employment and educational status, living arrangement plans, and current living situation.

2.3.3. Open-Ended Question

As part of the interview, participants were asked to share whether or not the transitions training continued to make a difference to them (and if so, in what ways) and to provide an example.

2.4. Analysis

Descriptive statistics were used to analyze the primary data from the 34 participants on employment status, living situation, educational status, the MOS social support responses, and demographics. The open-ended question was not intended to collect extensive or in-depth qualitative data but rather shed some light on whether or not the participants were still thinking about or using transitions concepts and if they perceived it as useful. The responses were fairly brief and organized according to the type of example they provided (if any) using a content analysis approach that assessed specific words and phrases in line with the type of impact.

3. Findings

3.1. Participants

All 35 youths were admitted to their most current placement as adolescents—at 16 years old on average. By 18 months post-training, 57% (n = 20) were discharged. The youth averaged 17 years old at the start of the study and 18.5 years old at Wave 3. Gender identity was nearly split between male and female, with one youth who identified as transgender. About three-fourths (74.3%) of the youth had a prior placement, and most (92.5%) were in non-relative foster care at the start of the study (Table 1). Consistent with national figures, the most common reason for placement was neglect (68.6%), followed by physical abuse (54.3%) and parental substance abuse (48.6%). Seventy percent of the youth had a permanency plan to remain in care until they aged out at 18 or 21, though a notable minority had plans for family reunification (15.8%). A large share of the youth had some visits with parents, with 55% occurring often. However, nearly a third did not have any parental visits

Table 1. Placement variables.

Variable	Percent
Non-relative placement (at time of programming)	92.5
Reason for placement *	
Neglect	68.6
Physical abuse	54.3
Parental substance abuse	48.6
Other reason	20.0
Permanency plan	
Reunification	15.8
Remain in care until age out	71.4
Adoption	5.7
Other	7.1

Table 1. *Cont.*

Variable	Percent
Parental visits	
Frequent	54.2
Occasionally/irregular	14.4
None	31.4
Prior placement	74.3
Age at prior placement (years)	10.8

* Does not sum to 100% because they can fall into more than one category.

On average, the participants were 18.5 years old, and those discharged were 18.6 years old (Table 2). In terms of the racial and ethnic breakdown, it is not surprising that the foster care group is more ethnically diverse than national rates. This reflects the racial disproportionalities that exist in foster care nationally and even more heavily in the midwestern state where this study was conducted, where Black children are twice as likely as White children to enter a child welfare placement [29].

Table 2. Ethnicity and age *.

Demographic	%
African Amer./Black/African	55.4
Asian or Pacific Islander	8.6
Caucasian	20.0
Native American	0.0
Hispanic	10.8
Multiracial *	10.8
Mean age (years)	18.5
Age range (years)	16.4–19.8

* Columns do not add to 100% due to overlapping categories.

3.2. Still in Care, Plans for Discharge

Fifteen of the youth were still in care. Seven were scheduled to exit care within the year. Another six expected to leave within the next two years, and two planned to remain in care until they were 21. About three-quarters (n = 11) of the youth planned to enroll in college or technical school upon discharge, while two hoped to enroll in the military and two wanted to finish high school. In terms of employment plans, which could coincide with educational plans, eight youths planned to continue working at their current job and six expected to look for a job; the remaining youth was unsure.

3.3. Post-Discharge

Post-discharge, we examined the status of the participants' education, employment, and relationship status (Table 3). They had a high rate of educational enrollment (80%) compared to 43% of 19-year-olds in the same state [30]. At this time, 5% were married and 10% were cohabitating.

Table 3. Education and employment.

	All n = 35	Discharged n = 20
Education: Enrolled in school	88.6%	80%
Enrolled in high school or GED program	74.3%	30%
Enrolled in post-secondary ed./vocation	14.3%	50%
Employment (part-time, post-discharge)	-	35%

Looking at high school or GED, 74.3% were enrolled, reflecting some of the younger participants who were still living in care. Post-discharge, only 35% of the participants reported employment, likely a factor of school enrollment.

Lastly, we turn to the measures of perceived social support. The MOS survey provided four scales to assess tangible, emotional, social, and affectionate support (Table 4). One the whole, the youth reported ratings in the mid to higher end of the five-point range. The mean scale scores ranged from 3.7 (tangible support) to 4.1 (positive social interaction and affection).

Table 4. Perceived social support (n = 35).

Subscales and Items How Often Do You Have Someone to...	Mean Score *
Emotional/Informational Support, Scale Score	3.8
listen to you	3.9
confide in	4.0
share your worries with	3.5
understand your problems	3.7
give you information	3.7
give you advice you really want	4.1
turn to for suggestions	4.0
Tangible Support, Scale Score	3.7
help you if you were confined to bed	3.4
take you to the doctor	3.8
prepare your meals if you were unable to do it yourself	3.9
help with daily chores if you were sick	3.7
Positive Social Interaction Support, Scale Score	4.1
have a good time with	4.2
get together with for relaxation	3.8
do something enjoyable with	4.2
Affectionate Support, Scale Score	4.1
shows you love and affection	4.1
love you and make you feel wanted	4.1
who hugs you	4.2

* 1 = none of the time; 5 = all the time.

While the data cannot tell us whether transitions explicitly played a part in these high social support scores, the open-ended question responses aligned with the MOS results. All the participants named at least one aspect of the Transitions Framework training that they believed they benefitted from and retained 18 months later. The most common category and one in which most of the participates referenced regarded managing their emotions and the resulting impact on relationships. One participant explained the importance of understanding the root causes of their feelings.

"With Transitions, it has helped me understand like how I'm feeling and what I can do because I'm feeling that certain way and I don't always have to blow up because I'm mad. I might be mad, but there's something deeper that's making me mad".

Others used their new self-knowledge to temper how they kept lines of communication open with others when they were unhappy.

"It really helped me a lot knowing when I was angry, frustrated, and grieving. I know how to communicate that towards to people, instead of usually what I do is shut down and be off on my own".

Several participants specifically named learning about the "Marathon Effect" as useful to them. Understanding the marathon effect made some youth feel better equipped to understand where others were and how to speak with them about their transitions,

"The marathon effect... I loved the idea that you don't have to be rushed into anything, like you don't have to feel like you should be at a certain point".

Another explained, "The marathon effect is like if someone's in Endings, you don't necessarily be like, Oh, everything's going to be okay, everything's going to be good. Because they're not ready to look at that kind of stuff yet".

One component of the Transitions training is helping youth recognize the difference between reacting versus responding to stressful situations. Reacting, they learned, is behaving in a heated way without thought of consequence, whereas responding is a more thoughtful and careful way of responding. One participant shared,

"And then (the Transitions program) taught me like how to actually control my emotions, too. Well, Transitions mostly helped me on my anger, because before I was in the Transitions (program), I had a lot of anger issues. Like, if I get mad at someone, I pretty much get into a fight. I just learned that, you know, by fighting him, like by fighting a person like this is bad, it's only going to make the problem bigger".

4. Limitations

This study has several limitations. As an exploratory study, it does not include a control group, which would allow for the investigation of the counterfactual: what outcomes might look like in the absence of exposure to the intervention. To truly claim scientific evidence of change, there must be some sort of control group that offers a reasonable opportunity to compare based on key variables and is a way to rule out extraneous competing variables. Without a control group, it cannot be claimed that the framework was responsible for the findings. The sample size is small and represents youth from a single agency, limiting both the degree of analysis that can be conducted and generalizability. It is possible that the more motivated youth or foster parents attended the trainings, leading to more positive findings, though all foster parents are required to maintain continuing education credits, which were an incentive beyond simple motivation.

5. Discussion

The Transitions Framework offers a new approach to addressing a key source of stress and anxiety for youth in non-relative foster care: critical and monumental life changes that are not in their control but can alter everything that is familiar to them. There is some evidence that the framework may have positive short-term impacts on youth perceptions of change [26]. This study examined whether there were differences in longer-term well-being outcomes for education, employment, housing, and social support. This study found that 80% of the young people who were discharged were enrolled in school. Such a small sample, of course, does not permit much extrapolation. However, this is a positive sign, especially when state-level data show that only 43% of similar-aged youth exiting care were enrolled in school [29,31].

All foster youth experience transitions that can be difficult if not traumatizing—for example, the beginning of the day they are first placed in out-of-home care, which yields long-lasting negative impacts on their early adulthood [8,18]. Implemented in a foster care context, the Transitions Framework aims to help youth and their caregivers understand the link between external change, the internal experience of it (transitions) and how this influences behavior, emotions, and relationships [16]. The framework offers clear concepts in lay language that are accessible to young people, as well as concrete strategies to apply them.

Employment post-discharge was 35%, while it was 46% in the rest of the state among care leavers. This may be an artifact of their high level of school enrollment (80% overall; 50% post-secondary), though it cannot be determined with these data.

The youth, including those discharged, reported fairly positive support across all four MOS scales. The responses to the open-ended question indicate that participants were applying learnings from the framework in their everyday lives, contributing to better social relationships. We know that social support and connectedness have been a longstanding concern amongst foster care leavers who aged out [8,22,32]. While this study was not able to determine causal effect, as the first foster care agency to apply this framework throughout their programming, the findings are at least promising and point to the value of further research in a larger, controlled study.

6. Conclusions

It is evident from the extant research in the U.S. that the child welfare system needs to improve the stability and quality of care for youth residing in out-of-home placements and better prepare them for their transition to adulthood (e.g., [9]). This is a longstanding intractable problem in child welfare, yet there exist scant evidenced-based interventions that have addressed the issue. In particular, it is critical to attend to foster youth's educational, employment, and socio-emotional needs as they move toward discharge and independent living. At the same time, youth need strategies to manage the emotional trauma of admission into care and repeated placement moves during placement. In turn, this may help them build healthier and sustained relationships. Educating youth and those who care for them about the process of adjusting to transitions can normalize youth reactions to change, raise personal awareness about past traumas and emotional responses, foster psychological wellbeing, and enhance healthy relationships [11,16]. Introducing these strategies prior to discharge, in conjunction with programming traditional independent living skills, allows youth to practice new ways of coping while they are still in a safe setting.

Funding: This research received no external funding.

Institutional Review Board Statement: The study was conducted in accordance with the Declaration of Helsinki and approved by Ethics Committee of Hennepin County Human Services and Public Health Department for studies involving humans (protocol code 296859-1, 5 March 2018).

Informed Consent Statement: Informed consent was obtained from all adult subjects involved in this study. For adolescents under the age of 18, legal guardian consent was obtained, and youth assent was obtained for those participants. Written informed consent to publish this paper was obtained from the subjects.

Data Availability Statement: The dataset presented in this article are not readily available because of privacy and ethic restrictions in regard to the study participants. Requests to access the datasets should be directed to nesm3326@stthomas.edu.

Conflicts of Interest: The author declares no conflicts of interest.

References

1. Konijn, C.; Admiraal, S.; Baart, J.; van Rooij, F.; Stams, G.; Colonnes, C.; Lindauer, R.; Assink, M. Foster care placement instability: A meta-analytic review. *Child. Youth Serv. Rev.* **2019**, *96*, 483–499. [CrossRef]
2. White, C.R.; O'Brien, K.; Pecora, P.; Buher, A. Mental health and educational outcomes for youth transitioning from foster care in Michigan. *Fam. Soc. J. Contemp. Soc. Serv.* **2015**, *96*, 17–24. [CrossRef]

3. Mitchell, M. "No One Acknowledged My Loss and Hurt": Non-death Loss, Grief, and Trauma in Foster Care. *Child Adolesc. Soc. Work. J.* **2018**, *35*, 1–9. [CrossRef]
4. Courtney, M.E.; Dworsky, A.; Ruth, G.; Keller, T.; Havlicek, J.; Bost, N. *Midwest Evaluation of the Adult Functioning of Former Foster Youth: Outcomes at Age 19*; Chapin Hall Center for Children at the University of Chicago: Chicago, IL, USA, 2005.
5. Courtney, M.; Dworsky, A.; Lee, J.; Raap, M. *Midwest Evaluation of the Adult Functioning of Former Foster Youth: Outcomes at Age 23 and 24*; Chapin Hall at the University of Chicago: Chicago, IL, USA, 2009.
6. Havlicek, J.; Courtney, M.E. Maltreatment histories of aging out foster youth: A comparison of official investigated reports and self-reports of maltreatment prior to and during out-of-home care. *Child Abus. Negl.* **2016**, *52*, 110–122. [CrossRef] [PubMed]
7. Havlicek, J. Lives in motion: A review of former foster youth in the context of their experiences in the child welfare system. *Child. Youth Serv. Rev.* **2011**, *33*, 1090–1100. [CrossRef] [PubMed]
8. Curry, S.R.; Abrams, L.S. Housing and social support for youth aging out of foster care: State of the research literature and directions for future inquiry. *Child Adolesc. Soc. Work. J.* **2015**, *32*, 143–153. [CrossRef]
9. Children's Bureau. *National Youth in Transitions Database Outcomes Data Snapshot: National*; Administration for Children and Families: Washington, DC, USA, 2022.
10. Hébert, S.T.; Lanctôt, N.; Turcotte, M. "I didn't want to be moved there": Young women remembering their perceived sense of agency in the context of placement instability. *Child. Youth Serv. Rev.* **2016**, *70*, 229–237. [CrossRef]
11. Nesmith, A.; Christophersen, K. Smoothing the Transition to Adulthood: Creating Ongoing Supportive Relationships among Foster Youth. *Child. Youth Serv. Rev.* **2014**, *37*, 1–8. [CrossRef]
12. Fostering Connections to Success and Increasing Adoptions Act. H.R.6893—110th Congress. 2008. Available online: https://www.congress.gov/bill/110th-congress/house-bill/6893 (accessed on 25 October 2024).
13. Foster Care Independence Act. H.R.3443—106th Congress. 1999. Available online: https://www.congress.gov/bill/106th-congress/house-bill/3443 (accessed on 25 October 2024).
14. CEBC. Youth Transitioning to Adulthood Programs: California Evidence-Based Clearinghouse for Child Welfare. 2024. Available online: https://www.cebc4cw.org/program/better-futures/ (accessed on 25 October 2024).
15. Greeson, J.K.P.; Garcia, A.R.; Tan, F.; Chacon, A.; Oritz, A.J. Interventions for youth aging out of foster care: A state of the science review. *Child. Youth Serv. Rev.* **2020**, *113*, 105005. [CrossRef]
16. Bridges, W. *Transitions: Making Sense of Life's Changes*; Da Copo Press: Cambridge, MA, USA, 2009.
17. DHHS. *A National Look at the Use of Congregate Care in Child Welfare*; U.S. Department of Health and Human Services: Washington, DC, USA, 2015.
18. Casey Family Programs. What Affects Placement Stability? Strong Families Issue Brief. 2023. Available online: https://www.casey.org/placement-stability-impacts/ (accessed on 25 October 2024).
19. Maguire, D.; May, K.; McCormack, D.; Fosker, T. A Systematic Review of the Impact of Placement Instability on Emotional and Behavioural Outcomes Among Children in Foster Care. *J. Child Adolesc. Trauma* **2024**, *17*, 641–655. [CrossRef] [PubMed]
20. Children's Bureau. *National Youth in Transitions Database Outcomes Data Snapshot: State*; Administration for Children and Families: Washington, DC, USA, 2022.
21. Scannapieco, M.; Smith, M.; Blakeney-Strong, A. Transition from foster care to independent living: Ecological predictors associated with outcomes. *Child Adolesc. Soc. Work. J.* **2016**, *33*, 293–302. [CrossRef]
22. Greeson, J.K.P.; Garcia, A.R.; Kima, M.; Thompson, A.E.; Courtney, M.E. Development & maintenance of social support among aged out foster youth who received independent living services: Results from the Multi-Site Evaluation of Foster Youth Programs. *Child. Youth Serv. Rev.* **2015**, *53*, 1–9.
23. Fowler, P.J.; Marcal, K.E.; Zhang, J.; Day, O.; Landsverk, J. Homelessness and aging out of foster care: A national comparison of child welfare-involved adolescents. *Child. Youth Serv. Rev.* **2017**, *77*, 27–33. [CrossRef] [PubMed]
24. Seita, J.; Day, A.; Carrella, A.; Pugh, G.L. Assessing the Help-Seeking Behaviors of Foster Care Alumni within their Own Social Networks. *J. Sociol. Soc. Work.* **2016**, *4*, 1–10. [CrossRef]
25. Anghel, R. Transition within Transition: How young people learn to leave behind institutional care whilst their carers are stuck in neutral. *Child. Youth Serv. Rev.* **2011**, *33*, 2526–2531. [CrossRef]
26. Van Ryzin, M.J.; Mills, D.; Kelban, S.; Vars, M.R.; Chamberlain, P. Using the Bridges transition framework for youth in foster care: Measurement development and preliminary outcomes. *Child. Youth Serv. Rev.* **2011**, *33*, 2267–2272. [CrossRef]
27. Dima, G.; Skehill, C. Making sense of leaving care: The contribution of Bridges model of transition to understanding the psycho-social process. *Child. Youth Serv. Rev.* **2011**, *33*, 2532–2539. [CrossRef]
28. Sherbourne, C.D.; Stewart, A.L. The MOS Social Support Survey. *Soc. Sci. Med.* **1991**, *32*, 705–714. [CrossRef] [PubMed]
29. Minnesota Dept. of Human Services. Foster Care 2021 Statistics 2021. Available online: https://chlss.org/blog/infographic-foster-care-in-minnesota-2021-statistics/ (accessed on 25 October 2024).

30. ACF. Percent Enrolled and Attending School by State. U.S. Administration for Children and Families. 2019. Available online: https://www.acf.hhs.gov/sites/default/files/documents/cb/percent_enrolled_attending_school.pdf (accessed on 25 October 2024).
31. Minnesota Dept. of Human Services. Foster Care: Temporary Out-of-Home Care for Children. 2024. Available online: https://www.co.brown.mn.us/DocumentCenter/View/330/Minnesota-Department-of-Human-Services-Foster-Care-Flyer-PDF (accessed on 25 October 2024).
32. Marion, E.; Paulsen, V.; Goyette, M. Relationships matter: Understanding the role and impact of social networks at the edge of transition to adulthood from care. *Child Adolesc. Soc. Work. J.* **2017**, *34*, 573–582. [CrossRef]

children

MDPI

Article

The Impact of Parental Monitoring on Exposure to Multiple Substances and Bullying in Croatian Students

Maja Valentic [1,*], Luka Simetin [2], Dijana Mayer [1,3], Filip Simetin [2] and Ivana Pavic [1]

1 Croatian Institute of Public Health, 10000 Zagreb, Croatia; dijana.mayer@hzjz.hr (D.M.); ivana.pavic@hzjz.hr (I.P.)
2 School of Medicine, University of Zagreb, 10000 Zagreb, Croatia; lsimetin@mef.hr (L.S.); fsimetin@mef.hr (F.S.)
3 School of Medicine, Catholic University of Zagreb, 10000 Zagreb, Croatia
* Correspondence: maja.valentic@hzjz.hr

Abstract: Background/Objectives: Adolescence is a critical period for experimenting with a wide range of risky behaviors, which are often influenced by family dynamics, including parental monitoring. This study aims to analyze the patterns of exposure to multiple substances and bullying among Croatian students by age and gender in 2022 and examine the association of exposure to multiple substances and bullying with maternal and paternal monitoring. **Methods**: The data were obtained from the 2022 Health Behaviour in School-aged Children (HBSC) study conducted in Croatia among students aged 11, 13, and 15. Two multinomial logistic regressions were performed separately by age and gender. **Results**: Exposure to multiple instances of bullying is more common among boys than girls in all three age groups, while exposure to multiple substances varies depending on age. The analysis revealed the strong protective effect of maternal monitoring against both substance use and bullying. Paternal monitoring showed less consistent effects but still indicated that lower paternal monitoring was associated with higher exposure to multiple substances and bullying, particularly at age 13. **Conclusions**: The patterns of multiple substance use and bullying vary by gender and age, emphasizing the need for tailored intervention strategies. Programs that strengthen parental monitoring, particularly maternal monitoring, should be prioritized.

Keywords: parental monitoring; substance use; bullying; students

1. Introduction

Adolescence is a dynamic and critical development period characterized by many social, physical, physiological, and psychological changes [1]. Its defining characteristics include independence from parents and family, valuing friendships and peer groups, exploring one's identity, and experimenting with a wide range of behaviors, some of which are risky and inappropriate [1].

Adolescent multiple substance use is a significant and growing problem today, as it is linked to poor mental health as well as negative educational and social outcomes [2–4]. The early initiation of substance use and the use of multiple substances are strong indicators of future substance use problems and disorders [4]. Patterns of using multiple substances may identify different groups of adolescents with unique risk factors and future outlooks [2].

School bullying is a major social problem affecting children and adolescents worldwide [5]. It involves repeated negative actions over a period of time and can be direct, such as physical and verbal violence, or indirect, such as social exclusion [6]. Bullying is characterized by harmful intent and an imbalance of power that makes it hard for the victim to defend themselves [6]. A relatively new form of bullying is called cyberbullying, i.e., bullying via mobile phone or the Internet [7]. Many children who are involved in bullying, either as perpetrators or as victims, run the risk of facing psychological difficulties later in life [6–13].

Family dynamics is one of the key factors for shaping behaviors such as adolescent substance use and bullying [14–16]. Throughout adolescence, parents play a critical role in promoting healthy development, partly through parental monitoring [17–20]. Parental monitoring is a set of parenting behaviors that involves attention to and tracking youth's whereabouts, activities, and friendships [21].

The existing research on adolescent substance use emphasizes the importance of parental monitoring as a protective factor in its prevention [20,22–26]. Some studies suggest that parental monitoring has a protective effect against bullying and its negative outcomes, while other studies indicate it may be unrelated or even positively related to bullying perpetration and victimization [18,27–31]. Moreover, some studies suggest that maternal monitoring or maternal knowledge reduces adolescent substance use and bullying behaviors, while other studies highlight the additional protective effects of paternal knowledge and father–youth connectedness [32–36].

However, research that focuses on multiple substance use as well as exposure to multiple instances of bullying and its association with parental monitoring is still missing. Besides, there is a lack of research on these dynamics in Croatia, where cultural nuances may affect these associations despite their recognized importance.

This study aims to analyze the patterns of exposure to multiple substances and multiple instances of bullying among Croatian students by age and gender in 2022. Additionally, we aim to investigate the association of exposure to multiple substances as well as multiple instances of bullying with parental monitoring, both maternal and paternal. Exposure to multiple substances and bullying reveals particularly vulnerable students, which is why it is especially important to understand the characteristics of their parents to form appropriate preventive activities.

2. Materials and Methods

2.1. Sample

The data used for analysis were obtained from the 2022 Health Behaviour in School-aged Children (HBSC) study conducted in Croatia. The HBSC study is a WHO cross-sectional study that takes place every four years in various countries across Europe and North America. It comprises data from students aged 11, 13, and 15, and follows an internationally standardized protocol.

The Croatian sample was selected based on the official list of schools provided by the Ministry of Science and Education. The sampling unit used was the school class. School classes were chosen randomly at the national level and, for 15-year-olds, they were categorized by the type of high school. The sample consisted of 5338 students, with 51.69% girls (2759) and 48.31% boys (2579), and had a response rate of 64.60%. The sample included 1763 students aged 11 (average age 11.07), 1940 aged 13 (average age 12.96), and 1635 aged 15 (average age 14.99).

2.2. Measures

An internationally standardized questionnaire, translated into Croatian by back-translation, was used as the research instrument. Data collection occurred in the spring of 2022, between March and May. The survey was carried out anonymously and voluntarily, with passive parental consent. The online questionnaire was self-administered by students in the classroom under the supervision of a teacher, using the LimeSurvey online platform (https://community.limesurvey.org/; Version 3.28.26+220829).

2.2.1. Exposure to Multiple Substances

We created a new exposure to multiple substances variable, which we used as the dependent variable. We composed exposure to multiple substances from the following four variables at the age of 11 and 13: got drunk, smoked cigarettes, tried e-cigarettes, and drank energy drinks at least once in a lifetime. The question about lifetime cannabis use was posed only to pupils at age 15. This newly created exposure to multiple substance variable was split into three categories where those who used no substance (no exposure) were compared with those who used 1 or 2 substances (low exposure) and those who used 3 or 4 substances at the age of 11 and 13 and 3–5 substances at the age of 15 (high exposure).

Lifetime drunkenness was assessed with the question "Have you ever drunk so much alcohol that you were really drunk in life?" Response options were on a five-point scale ranging from "never" to "more than 10 times (or more)".

Lifetime cigarette smoking was measured with the question "How many days did you smoke cigarettes in life?". Response options were on a seven-point scale ranging from "never" to "30 (or more) days".

Lifetime e-cigarette use was evaluated using the question "How many days have you used electronic cigarettes (e.g., e-cigarettes, Wiip, e-hookah)? Please do not include products that 'heat, not burn' (e.g., IQOS, Glo, TEEPS)". Response options were on a seven-point scale ranging from "never" to "30 (or more) days".

Lifetime energy drinks use was evaluated using the question "Currently, how often do you drink energy drinks (e.g., Red Bull, Burn, Monster)? Also count taking small amounts". Response options were on a five-point scale ranging from "never" to "every day".

Lifetime cannabis use was evaluated using the question "Have you ever used cannabis?". Response options were on a seven-point scale ranging from "never" to "30 (or more) days".

2.2.2. Exposure to Multiple Instances of Bullying

We formed a new exposure to multiple instances of bullying variable, which we used as the dependent variable. We determined exposure to multiple instances of bullying from the following four variables: bullying perpetration, bullying victimization, cyberbullying perpetration, and cyberbullying victimization. This newly created exposure to multiple instances of bullying variable was split into three categories, where the category "no exposure" includes those who did not participate in bullying, including cyberbullying, neither as victims nor as perpetrators. The category of "low exposure" includes the response "once or twice" regarding 1 to 4 bullying variables combined with none, and 1 response of "2 or 3 times a month", combined with 3 negative answers. All other responses to at least one of four bullying variables ("2 or 3 times a month" in more than one bullying variable, "about once a week", and "several times a week") are classified in the "high exposure" category.

Bullying perpetration was assessed with the question "How often have you taken part in bullying another student(s) at school in the past couple of months?".

Bullying victimization was measured with the question "How often have you been bullied at school in the past couple of months?".

Cyberbullying perpetration was evaluated using the question "In the past couple of months how often have you taken part in cyberbullying (e.g., sent mean instant messages, email or text messages, wall postings, created a website making fun of someone, posted unflattering or inappropriate pictures without permission and posted them online or sent them to others)?".

Cyberbullying victimization was assessed with the question "In the past couple of months how often have you been cyberbullied (i.e., someone sent mean instant messages, email or text messages, wall postings, created a website making fun of me or someone took unflattering or inappropriate pictures of me without permission and posted them online)?".

Response options for all four bullying variables were not once, once or twice, two or three times a month, about once a week, and several times a week.

2.2.3. Parental Monitoring

We assessed parental monitoring with two created variables: maternal and paternal monitoring. The parental monitoring variables were independent in the analysis. We derived these two new variables from the answer to an identical question about mother and father with the following sub-questions: "How much does your mother/father know about...? who your friends are, how you spend your money, where you are after school, where do you go at night, and what you do on the internet". Response options were as follows: mother/father "knows a lot", "knows a little", "doesn't know anything", and "doesn't have or doesn't see mother/father". These newly created parental monitoring variables were split into three categories. The category "high monitoring" included the responses "knows a lot" to all five sub-questions and combinations of one response "knows a little" with four responses "knows a lot". Other responses fell into categories "low mother/father monitoring" or "no monitoring" ("don't have or don't see mother/father").

2.3. Statistical Analysis

Descriptive statistics was used to present the sample characteristics. Gender differences in dependent and independent variables were examined and tested using Pearson's chi-squared test. Two multinomial logistic regressions were performed separately for boys and girls in three age categories: 11, 13, and 15 years. First, a multinomial logistic regression was performed with exposure to multiple substances as a dependent variable and two mutually independent variables/factors: monitored by the mother and monitored by the father. Second, a multinomial logistic regression was performed with exposure to multiple instances of bullying as the dependent variable and two mutually independent variables/factors: monitored by the mother and monitored by the father.

The results of the logistic regression were presented as odds ratios with 95% confidence intervals.

The statistical significance level was set at $p < 0.05$.

IBM SPSS version 28 (IBM, Armonk, NY, USA) was used for conducting the statistical analyses.

3. Results

The results section is organized as follows: first, we present the findings related to exposure to multiple substances by age and gender, followed by the analysis of exposure to multiple instances of bullying. Lastly, we examine the associations between parental monitoring and exposure to both substances and bullying.

As presented in Table 1, high exposure to multiple substances was more prevalent among boys at age 11 (6.6%) compared to girls (4.6%), with a significant gender difference ($p < 0.001$). By age 15, girls started to show higher exposure than boys (40.5% vs. 34.2%, $p = 0.025$). Substance use increased with age for both genders, with girls surpassing boys in cigarette (42.7% vs. 34.8%) and e-cigarette (42.7% vs. 34.8%) use at age 15 ($p < 0.001$ for both). Drunkenness was more common among boys at age 11 (11.9% vs. 7.1%, $p = 0.001$), but by age 15, the rates were almost identical for both genders (45.3% vs. 45.9%). Similarly, boys at age 11 were more likely to consume energy drinks (33.4% vs. 25.6%, $p < 0.001$), but by age 15, the gender gap narrowed (64.4% of boys and 61.1% of girls). For cannabis use, no significant gender differences were found at age 15 (15.9% for boys and 16.5% for girls).

Table 1. Exposure to multiple substances by age and gender.

Exposure to Multiple Substances	Age 11				Age 13				Age 15			
	Boys	Girls	χ^2	p	Boys	Girls	χ^2	p	Boys	Girls	χ^2	p
Exposure to multiple substances												
High exposure	58	41	16	<0.001	160	180	1.1	0.580	256	359	7.5	0.025
	6.6%	4.6%			16.7%	18.3%			34.2%	40.5%		
Low exposure	279	223			392	385			317	326		
	32.0%	25.1%			40.9%	39.2%			42.4%	36.8%		
No exposure	536	626			406	416			175	202		
	61.4%	70.3%			42.4%	42.4%			23.4%	22.8%		

Table 1. *Cont.*

Exposure to Multiple Substances	Age 11				Age 13				Age 15			
	Boys	**Girls**	χ^2	p	**Boys**	**Girls**	χ^2	p	**Boys**	**Girls**	χ^2	p
Lifetime drunkenness												
At least once	104	63	12	0.001	202	185	1.5	0.220	339	407	0.1	0.820
	11.9%	7.1%			21.1%	18.9%			45.3%	45.9%		
Never	769	827			8	796			409	480		
	88.1%	92.9%			78.9%	81.1%			54.7%	54.1%		
Lifetime cigarette smoking												
At least once	72	55	2.8	0.093	171	197	1.6	0.21	260	379	10.8	0.001
	8.2%	6.2%			17.8%	20.1%			34.8%	42.7%		
Never	801	835			787	784			488	508		
	91.8%	93.8%			82.2%	79.9%			65.2%	57.3%		
Lifetime e-cigarette use												
At least once	75	63	1.4	0.237	204	239	2.6	0.108	265	410	19.5	<0.001
	8.6%	7.1%			21.3%	24.4%			35.4%	46.2%		
Never	798	827			754	742			483	477		
	91.4%	92.9%			78.7%	75.6%			64.6%	53.8%		
Lifetime energy drink use												
At least once	292	228	12.9	<0.001	490	497	0.1	0.831	482	542	1.9	0.165
	33.4%	25.6%			51.1%	50.7%			64.4%	61.1%		
Never	581	662			468	484			266	345		
	66.6%	74.4%			48.9%	49.3%			35.6%	38.9%		
Lifetime cannabis use												
At least once									119	146	0.1	0.763
									15.9%	16.5%		
Never									629	741		
									84.1%	83.5%		

As presented in Table 2, exposure to bullying was more frequent among boys at age 11 (9.4% vs. 6.4%, $p < 0.001$), and boys remained more involved in bullying perpetration and victimization across all age groups. At age 15, boys were more likely to be victims of bullying 2–3 times per month (10.8% vs. 5.3%, $p < 0.002$), and cyberbullying perpetration was higher among boys compared to girls at age 15 as well (7.3% vs. 1.8%, $p < 0.001$).

As shown in Table 3, at age 11, 34.0% of boys reported high maternal monitoring compared to 27.1% of girls ($p = 0.004$). By age 15, the figures increased to 53.5% for boys and 44.9% for girls ($p < 0.001$). More girls than boys at age 15 reported that their mothers knew about their friends (76.5% vs. 66.9%, $p < 0.001$). Moreover, 85.3% of boys and 90.8% of girls at age 11 stated their mothers knew where they went at night ($p < 0.001$), decreasing to 71.6% for boys and 81% for girls at age 15 ($p < 0.001$). When it comes to spending money, 62.8% of boys and 71.2% of girls aged 15 stated that their mother knows a lot about how they spend their money ($p = 0.005$). More girls compared to boys reported that the mother knows about where they are after school at the age of 11 (89.5% vs. 84.7%, $p = 0.002$) and at the age of 15 (79.7% vs. 73.6%, $p = 0.022$). In terms of internet use, statistical significance was found at the age of 11 (53.8% of boys and 58.6% of girls) and the age of 13 (33.6% of boys and 37.9% of girls, $p = 0.019$). For paternal monitoring, high monitoring was indicated by 50.5% of boys and 50.1% of girls at age 11, with a statistically significant difference found at age 13, where 54.0% of boys reported high monitoring compared to 60.4% of girls ($p = 0.024$).

Table 2. Exposure to multiple instances of bullying by age and gender.

Exposure to Multiple Instances of Bullying	Age 11				Age 13				Age 15			
	Boys	Girls	χ^2	p	Boys	Girls	χ^2	p	Boys	Girls	χ^2	p
Exposure to multiple instances of bullying												
High exposure	69	49			95	72			73	31		
	9.4%	6.4%			11.7%	8.2%			11.3%	3.8%		
Low exposure	307	249	23.5	<0.001	377	338	23	<0.001	216	230	40	<0.001
	41.9%	32.5%			46.5%	38.7%			33.4%	28.4%		
No exposure	357	467			338	464			357	549		
	48.7%	61.0%			41.7%	53.1%			55.3%	67.8%		
Bullying perpetration												
Never	649	713			675	778			558	761		
	81.5%	87.3%			77.5%	85.4%			81.7%	91.8%		
Once or twice per month	107	68	13.7	0.008	121	84	19	0.001	58	43	42	<0.001
	13.4%	8.3%			13.9%	9.2%			8.5%	5.2%		
2–3 times per month or more	40	36			75	49			67	25		
	5.0%	4.4%			8.6%	5.4%			9.8%	3.0%		
Bullying victimization												
Never	613	634			656	656			555	707		
	77.1%	77.8%			75.7%	72.2%			81.3%	84.9%		
Once or twice per month	99	101	1.6	0.816	107	143	5.7	0.219	54	82	17	0.002
	12.5%	12.4%			12.3%	15.7%			7.9%	9.8%		
2–3 times per month or more	83	80			104	109			74	44		
	10.4%	9.8%			12.0%	12.0%			10.8%	5.3%		
Cyberbullying perpetration												
Never	659	731			650	781			537	754		
	87.3%	91.9%			79.5%	87.6%			81.7%	92.0%		
Once or twice per month	67	42	12	0.018	117	93	27	<0.001	72	51	42	<0.001
	8.9%	5.3%			14.3%	10.4%			11.0%	6.2%		
2–3 times per month or more	29	22			51	18			48	15		
	3.8%	2.8%			6.2%	2.0%			7.3%	1.8%		
Cyberbullying victimization												
Never	682	709			703	727			562	706		
	86.5%	86.4%			81.5%	79.9%			81.8%	85.0%		
Once or twice per month	59	62	0.3	0.99	82	118	13	0.014	51	80	16	0.003
	7.5%	7.6%			9.5%	13.0%			7.4%	9.6%		
2–3 times per month or more	47	50			78	65			74	45		
	6.0%	6.1%			9.0%	7.1%			10.8%	5.4%		

Table 3. Parental monitoring by age and gender.

Parental Monitoring	Age 11				Age 13				Age 15			
	Boys	**Girls**	χ^2	p	**Boys**	**Girls**	χ^2	p	**Boys**	**Girls**	χ^2	p
Maternal monitoring												
High monitoring	249	214	11.3	0.004	378	342	16	<0.001	356	369	24	<0.001
	34.0%	27.1%			45.4%	38.4%			53.5%	44.9%		
Low monitoring	465	565			429	536			279	436		
	63.5%	71.4%			51.6%	60.2%			41.9%	53.1%		
No monitoring	18	12			25	13			31	16		
	2.5%	1.5%			3.0%	1.5%			4.7%	1.9%		
Mother knows a lot about...												
Who student's friends are	632	708	6.1	0.109	646	744	11	0.011	448	629	22	<0.001
	84.3%	88.5%			76.3%	82.6%			66.9%	76.5%		
How student spends his/her money	541	613	6.9	0.074	581	647	5.4	0.148	422	586	13	0.005
	72.6%	76.7%			69.0%	72.1%			62.8%	71.2%		
Where student is after school	629	714	14.9	0.002	676	746	4.9	0.178	493	656	9.6	0.022
	84.7%	89.5%			80.3%	83.2%			73.6%	79.7%		
Where student goes at night	631	724	18.7	<0.001	675	753	6.4	0.094	480	666	19	<0.001
	85.3%	90.8%			80.1%	83.9%			71.6%	81.0%		
What student does on the internet	401	468	9.4	0.024	283	341	9.9	0.019	186	249	6.9	0.077
	53.8%	58.6%			33.6%	37.9%			27.6%	30.3%		
Paternal monitoring												
High monitoring	369	393	3.9	0.146	450	537	7.4	0.024	381	503	3.1	0.213
	50.5%	50.1%			54.0%	60.4%			57.6%	61.3%		
Low monitoring	327	369			340	308			235	256		
	44.7%	47.0%			40.8%	34.6%			35.5%	31.2%		
No monitoring	35	23			43	44			46	62		
	4.8%	2.9%			5.2%	4.9%			6.9%	7.6%		
Father knows a lot about...												
Who student's friends are	505	483	17.4	0.001	496	430	22	<0.001	364	373	19	<0.001
	67.3%	60.1%			58.2%	47.7%			54.5%	45.3%		
How student spends his/her money	459	481	0,8	0.838	481	471	11	0.010	364	393	13	0.005
	61.5%	60.4%			56.9%	52.4%			54.4%	47.6%		
Where student is after school	510	552	4.2	0.238	529	518	8.5	0.036	380	424	7.6	0.054
	68.5%	69.1%			62.5%	57.9%			56.9%	51.5%		
Where student goes at night	534	587	5.2	0.158	560	567	7.9	0.048	390	480	3.9	0.270
	72.1%	74.1%			66.5%	63.3%			58.3%	58.2%		
What student does on the internet	355	382	2.4	0.493	275	256	9	0.030	176	182	9.2	0.026
	47.7%	48.0%			32.5%	28.6%			26.2%	22.1%		

More boys than girls at age 11 reported that their fathers knew about their friends (67.3% vs. 60.1%, $p = 0.001$), with 54.5% of boys and 45.3% of girls at age 15 indicating the same ($p < 0.001$). At age 15, 54.4% of boys and 47.6% of girls responded that their fathers know how they spend their money ($p = 0.005$). Also, more 13-year-old boys compared to girls stated that their father knows about where they are after school (62.5% vs. 57.9%, $p = 0.036$). Regarding paternal monitoring and internet use, statistical significance was found at the age of 13 (32.5% of boys and 28.6% of girls, $p = 0.030$) and age 15 (26.2% of boys and 22.1% of girls, $p = 0.026$).

Table 4 shows that boys aged 11 with no maternal monitoring had 23.21 times higher odds (CI 4.71–114.32) of high substance exposure compared to those with high maternal monitoring. Low maternal monitoring was also associated with increased odds for both high (4.23, CI 1.63–10.95) and low substance exposure (2.19, CI 1.46–3.27).

Table 4. Multinomial logistic regressions by age and gender on the association between parental monitoring and exposure to multiple substances.

Age	Substance Exposure	Parental Monitoring	Boys				Girls			
			Sig.	OR	95% Confidence Interval		Sig.	OR	95% Confidence Interval	
					Lower Bound	Upper Bound			Lower Bound	Upper Bound
11	High vs. no substance exposure	No vs. high maternal monitoring	0	23.21	4.71	114.32	0.07	1.23	0.98	1.53
		Low vs. high maternal monitoring	0	4.23	1.63	10.95	0.02	4.65	1.3	16.58
		No vs. high paternal monitoring	0.99	1.01	0.2	5.05	0.12	1.08	0.98	1.2
		Low vs. high paternal monitoring	0.49	0.72	0.28	1.84	0.25	2.4	0.54	10.65
	Low vs. no substance exposure	No vs. high maternal monitoring	0.36	1.82	0.5	6.61	0.76	0.78	0.15	4.01
		Low vs. high maternal monitoring	0	2.19	1.46	3.27	0	1.94	1.3	2.91
		No vs. high paternal monitoring	0.36	1.48	0.64	3.43	0.04	2.64	1.07	6.56
		Low vs. high paternal monitoring	0.88	1.03	0.69	1.54	0.01	1.65	1.11	2.44
13	High vs. no substance exposure	No vs. high maternal monitoring	0.08	3.52	0.85	14.55	0	14.04	2.61	75.55
		Low vs. high maternal monitoring	0	3.23	1.81	5.78	0	3.87	2.4	6.25
		No vs. high paternal monitoring	0.2	1.98	0.7	5.61	0.03	2.81	1.1	7.25
		Low vs. high paternal monitoring	0.31	1.38	0.74	2.56	0.01	2.27	1.27	4.06
	Low vs. no substance exposure	No vs. high maternal monitoring	0.03	3.11	1.09	8.83	0.11	3.9	0.73	20.82
		Low vs. high maternal monitoring	0	1.82	1.25	2.64	0	2.08	1.46	2.96
		No vs. high paternal monitoring	0.78	0.89	0.41	1.95	0.96	0.98	0.45	2.13
		Low vs. high paternal monitoring	0.96	0.99	0.68	1.45	0.05	1.43	1.01	2.02

Table 4. *Cont.*

Age	Substance Exposure	Parental Monitoring	Boys				Girls			
			Sig.	OR	95% Confidence Interval		Sig.	OR	95% Confidence Interval	
					Lower Bound	Upper Bound			Lower Bound	Upper Bound
15	High vs. no substance exposure	No vs. high maternal monitoring	0.02	4.63	1.34	16.01	0.27	2.25	0.54	9.44
		Low vs. high maternal monitoring	0	2.74	1.48	5.06	0	3.9	2.48	6.13
		No vs. high paternal monitoring	0.12	2.41	0.79	7.39	0	5.08	1.94	13.32
		Low vs. high paternal monitoring	0.31	0.72	0.39	1.35	0.01	1.87	1.16	2.99
	Low vs. no substance exposure	No vs. high maternal monitoring	0.73	0.79	0.21	3.01	0.43	1.74	0.44	6.91
		Low vs. high maternal monitoring	0.7	1.11	0.65	1.91	0	2.16	1.37	3.4
		No vs. high paternal monitoring	0.13	2.36	0.78	7.19	0.06	2.48	0.96	6.39
		Low vs. high paternal monitoring	0.22	1.41	0.81	2.45	0.73	0.93	0.61	1.42

Among 13-year-old boys, low maternal monitoring was associated with 3.23 times higher odds of high substance exposure (CI 1.81–5.78), while no monitoring was linked to 3.11 times higher odds of low substance exposure (CI 1.09–8.83). Low maternal monitoring also increased the odds of low substance exposure (OR 1.82, CI 1.25–2.64).

For 15-year-old boys, no maternal monitoring resulted in 4.63 times higher odds of high substance exposure (CI 1.34–16.01), and low monitoring led to 2.74 times higher odds (CI 1.48–5.06).

In 11-year-old girls, low maternal monitoring increased the odds of high substance exposure by 4.65 times (CI 1.30–16.58) and, for low exposure, by 1.94 times (CI 1.30–2.91). No paternal monitoring was linked to 2.64 times higher odds for low substance exposure (CI 1.07–6.56), and low paternal monitoring was associated with a 1.65 times increase (CI 1.11–2.44).

For 13-year-old girls, high odds of substance exposure were linked to no maternal monitoring (OR 14.04, CI 2.61–75.55), low maternal (OR 3.87, CI 2.40–6.25), no paternal (OR 2.81, CI 1.10–7.25), and low paternal monitoring (OR 2.27, CI 1.27–4.06). Higher odds of low exposure were associated with low maternal (OR 2.08, CI 1.46–2.96) and low paternal monitoring (OR 1.43, CI 1.01–2.02).

For girls aged 15, higher odds of high substance exposure were linked to low maternal monitoring (OR 3.90, CI 2.48–6.13), no paternal monitoring (OR 5.08, CI 1.94–13.32), and low paternal monitoring (OR 1.87, CI 1.16–2.99). Low maternal monitoring was also associated with higher odds of low substance exposure (OR 2.16, CI 1.37–3.40).

As shown in Table 5, in 11-year-old boys, low maternal monitoring was associated with a 4.28 times increase (CI 2.11–8.67) in exposure to bullying, while no paternal monitoring increased odds by 6.85 times (CI 2.15–21.81). Low maternal monitoring was linked to a 2.35 times higher risk (CI 1.54–3.58) for low exposure to bullying.

Table 5. Multinomial logistic regressions by age and gender on the association between parental monitoring and exposure to multiple instances of bullying.

Age	Exposure to Bullying	Parental Monitoring	Boys				Girls			
			Sig.	OR	95% Confidence Interval		Sig.	OR	95% Confidence Interval	
					Lower Bound	Upper Bound			Lower Bound	Upper Bound
11	High vs. no exposure to bullying	No vs. high maternal monitoring	0.1	3.23	0.76	13.71	0.5	2.27	0.21	23.99
		Low vs. high maternal monitoring	0	4.28	2.11	8.67	0.05	2.09	1.01	4.36
		No vs. high paternal monitoring	0	6.85	2.15	21.81	0.04	4.54	1.05	19.68
		Low vs. high paternal monitoring	0.9	1.02	0.5	2.1	0.02	2.54	1.15	5.61
	Low vs. no exposure to bullying	No vs. high maternal monitoring	0.3	0.39	0.07	2.08	0.61	1.51	0.32	7.14
		Low vs. high maternal monitoring	0	2.35	1.54	3.58	0	1.83	1.21	2.78
		No vs. high paternal monitoring	0.3	1.82	0.64	5.16	0.15	2	0.78	5.13
		Low vs. high paternal monitoring	0.3	1.24	0.83	1.84	0.01	1.66	1.14	2.44
13	High vs. no exposure to bullying	No vs. high maternal monitoring	0	10.32	2.66	40.13	0	16.13	3.29	79.01
		Low vs. high maternal monitoring	0	2.34	1.21	4.5	0	3.13	1.65	5.92
		No vs. high paternal monitoring	0	3.29	1.06	10.25	0.01	5.8	1.54	21.88
		Low vs. high paternal monitoring	0.1	1.68	0.84	3.36	0.01	3.14	1.32	7.45
	Low vs. no exposure to bullying	No vs. high maternal monitoring	0.8	1.16	0.31	4.38	0.88	0.87	0.14	5.55
		Low vs. high maternal monitoring	1	1	0.68	1.47	0	1.91	1.35	2.71
		No vs. high paternal monitoring	0.1	1.91	0.82	4.44	0	4	1.85	8.64
		Low vs. high paternal monitoring	0	1.48	1.01	2.18	0	1.89	1.31	2.73

Table 5. *Cont.*

Age	Exposure to Bullying	Parental Monitoring	Boys				Girls			
			Sig.	OR	95% Confidence Interval		Sig.	OR	95% Confidence Interval	
					Lower Bound	Upper Bound			Lower Bound	Upper Bound
15	High vs. no exposure to bullying	No vs. high maternal monitoring	0	9.06	2.78	29.47	0.91	1.01	0.84	1.21
		Low vs. high maternal monitoring	0	3.09	1.33	7.18	0.16	1.86	0.78	4.47
		No vs. high paternal monitoring	0.2	2.01	0.64	6.31	0.29	2.27	0.5	10.25
		Low vs. high paternal monitoring	0.4	0.7	0.3	1.63	0.43	1.54	0.53	4.5
	Low vs. no exposure to bullying	No vs. high maternal monitoring	0.5	0.67	0.19	2.37	0	5.19	1.7	15.84
		Low vs. high maternal monitoring	0.1	1.61	0.98	2.63	0	1.92	1.33	2.77
		No vs. high paternal monitoring	0.2	1.86	0.78	4.43	0	2.94	1.52	5.68
		Low vs. high paternal monitoring	0.9	0.98	0.59	1.64	0	2.11	1.34	3.33

Among boys aged 13, no maternal monitoring was associated with 10.32 higher odds (CI 2.66–40.13), and low maternal monitoring with 2.34 higher odds (CI 1.21–4.50) for high exposure to bullying. Similarly, no paternal monitoring was linked to 3.29 higher odds (CI 1.06–10.25), and low paternal monitoring to 1.48 higher odds (CI 1.01–2.18) for low exposure to bullying.

For boys aged 15, no maternal monitoring was associated with 9.06 higher odds (CI 2.78–29.47), and low maternal monitoring with 3.09 higher odds (CI 1.33–7.18) for high exposure to bullying.

Among girls aged 11, low maternal monitoring was associated with 2.09 higher odds (CI 1.01–4.36), no paternal monitoring with 4.54 higher odds (CI 1.05–19.68), and low paternal monitoring with 2.54 higher odds (CI 1.15–5.61) for high exposure to bullying. Additionally, low maternal monitoring was associated with 1.83 higher odds (CI 1.21–2.78), and low paternal monitoring with 1.66 higher odds (CI 1.14–2.44) for low exposure to bullying.

For girls aged 13, no maternal monitoring was associated with 16.13 higher odds (CI 3.29–79.01), and low maternal monitoring with 3.13 higher odds (CI 1.65-5.29) for high exposure to bullying. No paternal monitoring increased the odds by 5.80 (CI 1.54–21.88), while low paternal monitoring increased the odds by 3.14 (CI 1.32–7.45). For low exposure to bullying, low maternal monitoring was associated with 1.91 higher odds (CI 1.35–2.71), no paternal monitoring with 4.00 higher odds (CI 1.85–8.64), and low paternal monitoring with 1.89 higher odds (CI 1.31–2.73).

Among girls aged 15, low exposure to bullying was associated with 5.19 higher odds (CI 1.70–15.84) for no maternal monitoring, 1.92 higher odds (CI 1.33–1.77) for low maternal monitoring, 2.94 higher odds (CI 1.52–5.68) for no paternal monitoring, and 2.11 higher odds (CI 1.34–3.33) for low paternal monitoring.

4. Discussion

This study examined distinct age patterns in exposure to multiple substances and bullying among boys and girls in Croatia. The proportions of multiple substance use increased with age for both boys and girls, while exposure to multiple instances of bullying is most common at the age of 13. Exposure to multiple instances of bullying is more common among boys than girls in all three age groups, while there is no clear gender pattern with exposure to multiple substances, which varies depending on age.

Even at the age of 11, a significant proportion of girls, and especially boys, are already exposed to multiple psychoactive substances and bullying. This indicates that prevention programs are already necessary in the lower grades of elementary school and that these programs should be comprehensive, rather than focused on a single substance or one form of violence.

The results of this study reveal significant associations between parental monitoring (both maternal and paternal) and multiple substance use as well as exposure to bullying among adolescents in Croatia. Patterns of substance use and bullying vary by gender and age, emphasizing the need for gender- and age-specific intervention strategies.

This study showed the strong protective effect of parental monitoring against both substance use and bullying, which aligns with previous research [18,20,22–26,28,29,31]. High levels of maternal monitoring were consistently associated with lower odds of both exposure to multiple substances and bullying involvement, confirming the critical role mothers play in adolescent behavioral development [37,38]. The findings are consistent with previous research showing that when mothers are more involved and emotionally connected with their children, they have a greater influence on reducing risky behaviors [32–34,36].

On the other hand, the level of paternal monitoring appeared to be more inconsistent. Although high paternal monitoring was generally associated with reduced exposure to substances and bullying, the protective effect was less consistent compared to maternal monitoring. This might be due to the traditional roles and expectations of mothers and fathers in Croatian society, where mothers may take on a more active role in adolescent everyday activities [39,40]. However, the strong association between the absence of paternal monitoring and higher substance use and bullying at the age of 13 indicates that fathers' involvement becomes particularly crucial during early adolescence when adolescents are more susceptible to peer influence and external pressures [41].

5. Conclusions

This study shows the need for designing preventive strategies to reduce substance use and bullying among adolescents. Programs that strengthen parental monitoring, particularly maternal monitoring, should be prioritized. However, the results also indicate a need for greater paternal involvement, especially as children enter adolescence. Parenting interventions should encourage fathers to actively monitor their children's social interactions and online activities to reduce risky behaviors.

It is demonstrated that boys and girls have different needs when it comes to preventing substance use and bullying, so interventions need to be designed specifically for each gender. For example, girls might need programs that address cigarette and e-cigarette use during their late adolescence, while boys might benefit more from earlier interventions aimed at reducing alcohol and energy drink consumption.

While this study provides valuable insights by focusing on the combined effects of multiple risk behaviors (substance use and bullying) and their associations with parental monitoring, it is not without limitations. This study relies on self-reported data, which may be subject to reporting bias and memory inaccuracies. The cross-sectional design of the research disables establishing causal relationships between variables. Future research could use longitudinal designs to track changes in parental monitoring and adolescent behavior over time.

Author Contributions: Conceptualization, M.V. and I.P.; Data Curation, M.V.; Formal Analysis, M.V. and L.S.; Investigation, M.V. and L.S.; Methodology, M.V., L.S. and F.S.; Project Administration, M.V. and L.S.; Resources, L.S. and F.S.; Software, M.V. and L.S.; Supervision, D.M. and I.P.; Validation, M.V., L.S., D.M. and F.S.; Visualization, M.V. and F.S.; Writing—Original Draft, M.V.; Writing—Review and Editing, M.V., L.S., D.M. and F.S. All authors have read and agreed to the published version of the manuscript.

Funding: This research received no external funding.

Institutional Review Board Statement: This study was conducted in accordance with the Declaration of Helsinki, and approved by the Ethics Committee of the Croatian Institute of Public Health on 10 March 2022. The ethical approval code is 381-15-22-2.

Informed Consent Statement: Participation was voluntary (with passive parental consent), and the answers were strictly confidential.

Data Availability Statement: The raw data supporting the conclusions of this article will be made available by the authors upon request.

Conflicts of Interest: The authors declare no conflicts of interest.

References

1. Smetana, J.G.; Campione-Barr, N.; Metzger, A. Adolescent Development in Interpersonal and Societal Contexts. *Annu. Rev. Psychol.* **2006**, *57*, 255–284. [CrossRef] [PubMed]
2. Halladay, J.; Woock, R.; El-Khechen, H.; Munn, C.; MacKillop, J.; Amlung, M.; Ogrodnik, M.; Favotto, L.; Aryal, K.; Noori, A.; et al. Patterns of Substance Use Among Adolescents: A Systematic Review. *Drug Alcohol Depend.* **2020**, *216*, 108222. [CrossRef] [PubMed]
3. Chau, K.; Mayet, A.; Legleye, S.; Beck, F.; Hassler, C.; Khlat, M.; Choquet, M.; Falissard, B.; Chau, N. Association Between Cumulating Substances Use and Several School, Violence, and Mental Health Difficulties in Early Adolescents. *Psychiatry Res.* **2019**, *280*, 112480. [CrossRef] [PubMed]
4. Steinhoff, A.; Bechtiger, L.; Ribeaud, D.; Eisner, M.P.; Quednow, B.B.; Shanahan, L. Polysubstance Use in Early Adulthood: Patterns and Developmental Precursors in an Urban Cohort. *Front. Behav. Neurosci.* **2022**, *15*, 797473. [CrossRef]
5. Cosma, A.; Molcho, M.; Pickett, W. *A Focus on Adolescent Peer Violence and Bullying in Europe, Central Asia and Canada;* Health Behaviour in School-Aged Children International Report From the 2021/2022 Survey; WHO Regional Office for Europe: Copenhagen, Denmark, 2024.
6. Tatnall, A. School Bullying. In *Encyclopedia of Education and Information Technologies*; Springer: Berlin/Heidelberg, Germany, 2020; p. 1454.
7. Rajan, A.; Singh, A.; Pragathi, R.; Rashmitha Soumya Sindu, R.; Shilpa Reddy, K. Cyberbullying Detection. *Int. J. Innov. Res. Adv. Eng.* **2022**, *9*, 236–239. [CrossRef]
8. Bhatia, R. The Impact of Bullying in Childhood and Adolescence. *Curr. Opin. Psychiatry* **2023**, *36*, 461–465. [CrossRef]
9. Yoon, D.; Shipe, S.L.; Park, J.; Yoon, M. Bullying Patterns and Their Associations with Child Maltreatment and Adolescent Psychosocial Problems. *Child. Youth Serv. Rev.* **2021**, *129*, 106178. [CrossRef]
10. Lee, J. Pathways from Childhood Bullying Victimization to Young Adult Depressive and Anxiety Symptoms. *Child Psychiatry Hum. Dev.* **2021**, *52*, 129–140. [CrossRef]
11. Zych, I.; Farrington, D.P.; Llorent, V.J.; Ribeaud, D.; Eisner, M.P. Childhood Risk and Protective Factors as Predictors of Adolescent Bullying Roles. *Int. J. Bullying Prev.* **2021**, *3*, 138–146. [CrossRef]
12. Vrijen, C.; Wiertsema, M.; Ackermans, M.A.; van der Ploeg, R.; Kretschmer, T. Childhood and Adolescent Bullying Perpetration and Later Substance Use: A Meta-analysis. *Pediatrics* **2021**, *147*, e2020034751. [CrossRef]
13. Plexousakis, S.S.; Kourkoutas, E.; Giovazolias, T.; Chatira, K.; Nikolopoulos, D. School Bullying and Post-Traumatic Stress Disorder Symptoms: The Role of Parental Bonding. *Front. Public Health* **2019**, *7*, 75. [CrossRef] [PubMed]
14. Huang, Y.; Procházková, M.; Lu, J.; Riad, A.; Macek, P. Family Related Variables' Influences on Adolescents' Health Based on Health Behaviour in School-Aged Children Database, an AI-Assisted Scoping Review, and Narrative Synthesis. *Front. Psychol.* **2022**, *13*, 871795. [CrossRef] [PubMed]
15. Ingram, K.M.; Espelage, D.L.; Davis, J.P.; Merrin, G.J. Family Violence, Sibling, and Peer Aggression During Adolescence: Associations With Behavioral Health Outcomes. *Front. Psychiatry* **2020**, *11*, 472213. [CrossRef] [PubMed]
16. Arcadepani, F.B.; Eskenazi, D.Y.G.; Fidalgo, T.M.; Hong, J.S. An Exploration of the Link Between Bullying Perpetration and Substance Use: A Review of the Literature. *Health Educ. Behav.* **2019**, *22*, 207–214. [CrossRef]
17. Lionetti, F.; Palladino, B.E.; Passini, C.M.; Casonato, M.; Hamzallari, O.; Ranta, M.; Dellagiulia, A.; Keijsers, L. The Development of Parental Monitoring During Adolescence: A Meta-analysis. *Eur. J. Dev. Psychol.* **2019**, *16*, 552–580. [CrossRef]
18. Doty, J.L.; Lynne, S.D.; Metz, A.S.; Yourell, J.L.; Espelage, D.L. Bullying Perpetration and Perceived Parental Monitoring: A Random Intercepts Cross-Lagged Panel Model. *Youth Soc.* **2021**, *53*, 1287–1310. [CrossRef]

19. Rodríguez-Meirinhos, A.; Vansteenkiste, M.; Soenens, B.; Oliva, A.; Brenning, K.; Antolín-Suárez, L. When Is Parental Monitoring Effective? A Person-centered Analysis of the Role of Autonomy-Supportive and Psychologically Controlling Parenting in Referred and Non-Referred Adolescents. *J. Youth Adolesc.* **2020**, *49*, 352–368. [CrossRef]
20. Dittus, P.J.; Li, J.; Verlenden, J.V.; Wilkins, N.J.; Carman-McClanahan, M.N.; Cavalier, Y.; Mercado, M.C.; Welder, L.E.; Roehler, D.R.; Ethier, K.A. Parental Monitoring and Risk Behaviors and Experiences Among High School Students—Youth Risk Behavior Survey, United States, 2021. *MMWR Suppl.* **2023**, *72*, 37–44. [CrossRef]
21. Dishion, T.J.; McMahon, R.J. Parental Monitoring and the Prevention of Child and Adolescent Problem Behavior: A Conceptual and Empirical Formulation. *Clin. Child Fam. Psychol. Rev.* **1998**, *1*, 61–75. [CrossRef]
22. Gajewski, J.; Małkowska-Szkutnik, A. Family and Peer Factors Related to Alcohol Abuse and Smoking by 15-Year-Old Youth. *Med. Wieku Rozw.* **2012**, *16*, 322–328.
23. Zaborskis, A.; Sirvyte, D. Familial Determinants of Current Smoking Among Adolescents of Lithuania: A Cross-Sectional Survey 2014. *BMC Public Health* **2015**, *15*, 889. [CrossRef] [PubMed]
24. Šumskas, L.; Zaborskis, A. Family Social Environment and Parenting Predictors of Alcohol Use Among Adolescents in Lithuania. *Int. J. Environ. Res. Public Health* **2017**, *14*, 1037. [CrossRef] [PubMed]
25. Pedroni, C.; Dujeu, M.; Lebacq, T.; Desnouck, V.; Holmberg, E.; Castetbon, K. Alcohol Consumption in Early Adolescence: Associations with Sociodemographic and Psychosocial Factors According to Gender. *PLoS ONE* **2021**, *16*, e0245597. [CrossRef] [PubMed]
26. Puupponen, M.; Tynjälä, J.; Tolvanen, A.; Välimaa, R.; Paakkari, L. Energy Drink Consumption Among Finnish Adolescents: Prevalence, Associated Background Factors, Individual Resources, and Family Factors. *Int. J. Public Health* **2021**, *66*, 620268. [CrossRef] [PubMed]
27. Georgiou, S.N.; Stavrinides, P. Parenting at Home and Bullying at School. *Soc. Psychol. Educ.* **2013**, *16*, 165–179. [CrossRef]
28. Elsaesser, C.; Russell, B.; Ohannessian, C.M.; Patton, D. Parenting in a Digital Age: A Review of Parents' Role in Preventing Adolescent Cyberbullying. *Aggress. Violent Behav.* **2017**, *35*, 62–72. [CrossRef]
29. Jantzer, V.; Haffner, J.; Parzer, P.; Resch, F.; Kaess, M. Does Parental Monitoring Moderate the Relationship Between Bullying and Adolescent Nonsuicidal Self-Injury and Suicidal Behavior? A Community-Based Self-Report Study of Adolescents in Germany. *BMC Public Health* **2015**, *15*, 1–8. [CrossRef]
30. Meter, D.J.; Bauman, S. Moral Disengagement About Cyberbullying and Parental Monitoring: Effects on Traditional Bullying and Victimization via Cyberbullying Involvement. *J. Early Adolesc.* **2018**, *38*, 303–326. [CrossRef]
31. Çevik, Ö.; Ata, R.; Çevik, M. Bullying and Victimization Among Turkish Adolescents: The Predictive Role of Problematic Internet Use, School Burnout, and Parental Monitoring. *Educ. Inf. Technol.* **2021**, *26*, 3203–3230. [CrossRef]
32. Farrell, A.H.; Provenzano, D.A.; Dane, A.V.; Marini, Z.A.; Volk, A.A. Maternal Knowledge, Adolescent Personality, and Bullying. *Personal. Individ. Differ.* **2017**, *104*, 413–416. [CrossRef]
33. Lippold, M.A.; Greenberg, M.T.; Graham, J.W.; Feinberg, M.E. Unpacking the Effect of Parental Monitoring on Early Adolescent Problem Behavior: Mediation by Parental Knowledge and Moderation by Parent-Youth Warmth. *J. Fam. Issues* **2014**, *35*, 1800–1823. [CrossRef] [PubMed]
34. Villarreal, D.L.; Nelson, J.A. Parental Monitoring and Adolescent Risk Behaviors: The Moderating Role of Adolescent Internalizing Symptoms and Gender. *J. Child Fam. Stud.* **2018**, *27*, 3627–3637. [CrossRef]
35. Luk, J.W.; Wang, J.; Simons-Morton, B.G. The Co-Occurrence of Substance Use and Bullying Behaviors Among U.S. Adolescents: Understanding Demographic Characteristics and Social Influences. *J. Adolesc.* **2012**, *35*, 1351–1360. [CrossRef] [PubMed]
36. Hong, J.S.; Ryou, B.; Piquero, A.R. Do Family-Level Factors Associated With Bullying Perpetration and Peer Victimization Differ by Race? Comparing European American and African American Youth. *J. Interpers. Violence* **2020**, *35*, 4327–4349. [CrossRef] [PubMed]
37. Konowitz, L.; Lund, T.; Chia, S.W.C.; Reed, M.; Wood, W.; Liang, B.; Blustein, D.; Barnett, M. The Powerful Role of Mothers in Adolescent Purpose Development. *J. Psychol. Res.* **2023**, *5*, 1–16. [CrossRef]
38. Van Lissa, C.J.; Keizer, R.; Van Lier, P.A.C.; Meeus, W.H.J.; Branje, S. The Role of Fathers' Versus Mothers' Parenting in Emotion-Regulation Development From Mid-Late Adolescence: Disentangling Between-Family Differences From Within-Family Effects. *Dev. Psychol.* **2019**, *55*, 377–389. [CrossRef]
39. Ljubicic, M. Normative and Functional Dimension of Intergenerational Solidarity in the Narratives of Young Mothers. *Sociologija* **2016**, *58* (Suppl. S1), 306–323. [CrossRef]
40. Maskalan, A. In the Name of the Father: A Discussion on (New) Fatherhood, Its Assumptions and Obstacles. *Revija za socijalnu politiku* **2016**, *23*, 397–398. [CrossRef]
41. Sumter, S.R.; Bokhorst, C.L.; Steinberg, L.; Westenberg, P.M. The Developmental Pattern of Resistance to Peer Influence in Adolescence: Will the Teenager Ever Be Able to Resist? *J. Adolesc.* **2009**, *32*, 1009–1021. [CrossRef]

children

MDPI

Article

Family Dynamics, Socioeconomic Hardships, and Health Risk Behaviours of Bulgarian Adolescents during the COVID-19 Pandemic

Elitsa Dimitrova * and Anna Alexandrova-Karamanova

Institute for Population and Human Studies—Bulgarian Academy of Sciences, 1000 Sofia, Bulgaria; annaalexandrova@yahoo.com
* Correspondence: e.dimitrova@iphs.eu

Abstract: Background/Objectives: This study aims to explore family dynamics and the economic hardships experienced by families during the COVID-19 pandemic and their associations with adolescents' health risk behaviours (HRBs). Methods: Based on a representative study of adolescents aged 11–16 conducted in Bulgaria during the COVID-19 pandemic and HBSC data from the pre-pandemic period, logistic regression models were applied, assessing cigarette smoking, vaping, alcohol use, drunkenness, and cannabis use. The independent variables included demographics, Family Affluence Scale (FAS III), family structure, ease of communication with parents, and the authors' developed questions on parents' income and economic status change, family conflicts, and missing contact with extended family due to the pandemic. Results: Material status of the family showed increasing differentials in adolescents' HRBs during the pandemic. Parental unemployment, income reduction, and temporary lay-offs were associated with a higher risk of substance use. Family conflicts, missing contact with extended family, and difficulties in communication with the mother were related to a higher risk of substance use. Communication with the father was significantly associated with alcohol use and drunkenness. Boys had lower odds of vaping and higher odds of alcohol use, drunkenness, and cannabis use. Higher age and minority status were associated with an increase in adolescents' HRBs. Conclusions: This study highlights the need for special family-focused interventions in times of health and economic crises.

Keywords: cigarette smoking; e-cigarette use (vaping); alcohol use; drunkenness; cannabis use; COVID-19 pandemic; adolescents; socioeconomic hardships; family dynamics; Bulgaria; HBSC

1. Introduction

Bulgarian adolescents had some of the highest rates of cigarette smoking, alcohol consumption, drunkenness, and cannabis use in the pre-pandemic period among 45 countries, participating in the 2017/2018 wave of the Health Behaviour in School-aged Children (HBSC) study [1]. Significant differences were uncovered by sociodemographic characteristics such as age, gender, family structure, and material status of the family, with young people from affluent families being more prone to health risk behaviours (HRBs) [2]. A systematic review of the factors associated with adolescents' HRBs before the pandemic shows that peer influence, parental substance use, living in a single-parent family, easy access to harmful substances, parental styles (overprotection or loose parental control), and poor parental attachment were related to increased risk of alcohol use and drunkenness [3]. The factors significantly associated with cannabis use were peer influence, prior engagement in substance use (cigarette smoking and alcohol consumption), low parental monitoring, delinquent behaviours, and higher time spent in bars [3]. Depression, stress, poor academic achievements, parental and peer smoking, problems in family, conflicts with parents, and single parenting were identified as factors influencing cigarette smoking and vaping among young people. The use of nicotine products (regular cigarettes and heated tobacco products) was influenced also by restrictive policies and prohibitions of smoking in public places and easy access to nicotine products [3].

The COVID-19 pandemic reshaped everyday life, health, and wellbeing of adolescents and their families. In the case of Bulgaria, the pandemic was followed by an economic downturn related to lockdowns and restriction measures imposed during three major epidemic waves recorded in the country at the end of 2020 and 2021 and in early 2022 [4,5]. At that period, many families experienced economic hardships related to unemployment and the reduction in income and paid work of adult members [6,7]. The government implemented measures such as wage compensation schemes for companies and self-employed persons, aiming to support the economy in the period of imposed restrictions and interruption or reduction in work and business activities. Measures directly focused on families with (unemployed) adult members with dependent children were quite limited and included, for example, means-tested benefits for parents with children above 12 years who were at least 20 days in unpaid leave due to the pandemic and the provision of electronic devices for online schooling for children from ethnic minorities. Research shows that in families with increased financial strains during the pandemic, young people reported higher anxiety and depressive symptoms, decreased physical activity, unhealthy eating and higher engagement in substance use, prolonged screening time, and decreased academic performance [8–12]. In families with good relationships, the economic difficulties were less impactful, but in poor-functioning families experiencing financial difficulties, the lockdowns and stay-at-home measures restricted access to informal and formal support and exacerbated family conflicts, negatively affecting parents' and children's (mental) health [13–18].

Studies uncover different substance use patterns among adolescents during the COVID-19 pandemic. In certain contexts, the pandemic increased young people's vulnerability and stress, making them more susceptible to substance -use, while in other contexts the imposed restrictions and stay-at-home measures were associated with a reduction in HRBs, explained manly with the limited access to substances, and decreased frequency of outdoor activities [19,20]. Substance use among adolescents depends also on the pre-pandemic history of use, changes in the contacts with peers and friends, and increased tensions and conflicts in the family during the pandemic [21–25].

The theoretical framework of the present study is based on Bowen's Family Systems Theory [26,27]. According to this theory, the family system is an emotional entity featured by interconnectedness and mutual influence between family members. Changes in the emotional state of one family member influence the other family members. For example, parental anxiety and stress due to different life circumstances (e.g., unemployment, pressure at work, loss of income) might affect children's emotional state and levels of anxiety. The theory takes into account not only the internal dynamics of family systems but also external system dynamics. Family is connected to a hierarchy of living systems, including individual, family, neighbourhood, community, society, and supranational system. The concept of the Societal Emotional Process developed by Bowen [26] posits that different societal processes affect the family. Periods of societal regression and progression affect family as an emotional unit and the relationships between family members. In periods of regression (e.g., in conditions of societal health crises caused by the COVID-19 pandemic and the following economic downturn), family dynamics might be negatively affected, causing emotional and behavioural problems in young people and problematic relationships with parents. Following this framework, the present study aims to explore the association between individual characteristics, family dynamics, and the socioeconomic hardships experienced by the families in Bulgaria during the COVID-19 pandemic and their associations with adolescents' HRBs. We hypothesise that worsened family dynamics (family conflicts and limited contacts with close relatives due to the pandemic as well as difficulties in communication with parents) are associated with heightened risk of substance use (cigarette smoking, e-cigarette use [vaping], alcohol use, drunkenness, and cannabis use) among young people (H1). We expect also that the socioeconomic hardships (measured by the material status of the families, parental unemployment, temporary lay-offs, and decreases in income due to the pandemic) are associated with higher engagement of young people in substance use (H2). Our third hypothesis focuses on the interdependence between family dynamics (family conflicts) and the economic hardships experienced by the families during the pandemic. We expect that, in low-material-status families, frequent family conflicts will have a stronger negative effect on young people's HRBs (H3).

2. Materials and Methods

2.1. Survey Design and Sampling Strategy

We use data from the Health Behaviour in School-aged Children (HBSC) study conducted in 2018 in Bulgaria. HBSC is a cross-national school-based study of adolescent health and wellbeing conducted in 51 countries at present. It aims to explore young people's health and wellbeing, their determinants, and to inform youth policies [28]. The sample of HBSC-2018 is representative for the schoolchildren at ages 11, 13, and 15. After random selection of schools in all districts of the country, the survey was administered in class by an online questionnaire after obtaining parental consent. The national sample includes 4548 pupils (51.6% girls; mean age 13.5 (SD ± 1.65).

The study on adolescents' lives, (mental) health, and wellbeing is a school-based survey that aims to explore the implications of the pandemic on adolescents' (mental) health and wellbeing through young people's self-reports. The implementation of the survey began at the end of school year 2021/2022 (June 2022) and continued in school year 2022/2023 after relaxation of the public health measures and reopening of the schools in Bulgaria from March 2022. The national representative sample includes 3345 students aged 11–16 years selected from a random school sample in the 28 districts of the country. The mode of data collection includes an online questionnaire completed by students in the schools after obtaining parental consent. The mean age of the students is 13.5 years (SD ± 1.74, girls—49.2%).

Both surveys have similar design and sampling strategy, with a slight difference in the covered age groups. This allows for group-level comparisons. More information about the design of the surveys, the sampling procedures, and the main variables can be found elsewhere [29].

2.2. Modelling Procedure and Variables Used in the Analysis

We apply logistic regression models in order to study the relationship between adolescents' HRBs, family dynamics, and the socioeconomic hardships experienced by the families in Bulgaria during the COVID-19 pandemic. For comparison with the pre-pandemic period, we use logistic regression models applied to data from HBSC-2018 in order to outline the associations between selected sociodemographic and family-related variables and adolescents' HRBs at that period. In addition, we explore the interaction between family affluence and family conflicts during the pandemic with an additional set of logistic regression models. The dependent variables in the models are cigarette smoking, e-cigarette use (vaping), alcohol use, excessive alcohol consumption (drunkenness), and cannabis use. We created a separate category for the missing values and controlled for them in the models.

Measures developed and validated within the HBSC study [28] were used to measure the prevalence of adolescents' HRBs (dependent variables in the logistic regression models). Cigarette smoking is assessed by the question on how often a student smokes tobacco at present. The constructed variable includes the response option "I do not smoke" vs. combined response options, ranging from "Every day" to "Less than once a week". The measure is identical in both surveys.

E-cigarette use (vaping) is assessed by the question of how many days (if any) an adolescent vaped (used e-cigarettes) in the past 30 days. The constructed variable includes the response option "Never" and "1–2 days" vs. the options, ranging from "3–5 days" to "30 days (or more)". The measure of vaping is available only in the survey on adolescents' lives, (mental) health, and wellbeing during the pandemic.

The composite variable, measuring alcohol consumption among young people, is assessed by the question on how often at present the student drinks anything alcoholic (beer, wine, spirits, alcopops, or any other alcoholic drink). The constructed variable includes the responses "Never", "Rarely", and "Every month" vs. the responses "Every day" and "Every week" for different alcoholic drinks. The measure is identical in both surveys.

Excessive alcohol consumption (drunkenness) is assessed by the question as to whether the adolescent had so much alcohol that they were really drunk in the last 30 days. The constructed variable includes the option "Never" or "1–2 days" vs. the responses, ranging from "3–5 days" to "30 days (or more)". The measure is identical in both surveys.

Cannabis use is recorded only for 15-year-old students by the question on how many days (if any) the student smoked cannabis in the last 30 days. The constructed variable includes response option "Never" and "1–2 days" vs. the response options, ranging from "3–5 days" to "30 days (or more)". The measure is identical in both surveys.

The independent variables, assessed at the individual level, include age recoded in two groups of 11–14- and 15–16-year-old students, gender and ethnicity in the study on adolescents' lives, (mental) health, and wellbeing during the pandemic. In HBSC-2018, age is recoded in the following two groups: 11–13- and 15-year-old students. Ethnic belonging covers the main ethnic groups in the country (Bulgarian, Turkish, and Roma). The category "Other ethnic group" was recoded as missing due to the low number of cases. The question is available only in the study on adolescents' lives, (mental) health, and wellbeing during the pandemic.

The family-related variables include family affluence assessed by the Family Affluence Scale, third revision (FAS III) [30]. The measure combines different material belongings in the family and distinguishes families with low, medium, and high material status. It is available in both surveys.

In HBSC-2018, parental employment status is recorded by the options "[Mother/father is...] In paid work", "Mother/Father does not work", and "I do not know (no mother/father).

In the study on adolescents' lives, (mental) health, and wellbeing during the pandemic, the economic strains of the family are measured by the authors' developed questions related to parental unemployment, temporary lay-offs, and reductions in income caused by the pandemic: "Due to the coronavirus (COVID-19) pandemic, have your mother/father lost their jobs/temporarily stopped working/was paid less?" The response options are "Yes", "No", and "I do not know".

Family dynamics during the pandemic uses the authors' developed scale in measuring the relationships in the family. The following item is used in the present analysis: "In my family, we were more irritable and argued more often than before". The 5-level response options range from "Never" to "All the time". The mean was used as a cut-off point, and two groups were created. The first group includes adolescents who never or sometimes experienced conflicts in the family vs. those who experienced family conflicts more frequently.

The experience of missing face-to-face contact with extended family members during the pandemic is part of the authors' developed scale on social contacts and interactions with significant others during the pandemic. The following item is used in the present analysis: "During the pandemic, I missed face-to-face meetings and the time spent with my grandparents and other elderly or sick relatives". The mean was used as a cut-off point, and two groups were created. The first group includes adolescents who never or sometimes missed contacts with close relatives vs. those who were missing these contacts more frequently.

The communication with parents is assessed separately for mother and father by questions with response options "Easy", "Difficult", and "I do not see mother/father (no mother/father)". The questions are available in both surveys.

3. Results

The distributions in Table 1 show that, in the pre-pandemic period, the most prevalent HRB among adolescents was alcohol consumption (28.9%). Cigarette smoking and cannabis use were reported by 12.4% and 11.6% of the young people. Drunkenness was reported by 6.9%. In the pandemic period, the prevalence of HRBs increased (except for alcohol use and cannabis use). The prevalence of alcohol consumption decreased to 21.5% but drunkenness followed an upward trend, reaching 12.7%. Cigarette smoking increased to 19.2%, and the prevalence of vaping was 22.5%. Cannabis use was reported by 10.8% of the adolescents, remaining close to the prevalence in the pre-pandemic period.

Table 1. Descriptive statistics of the variables used in the analysis of Bulgarian adolescents' HRBs before and during the COVID-19 pandemic.

Variables and Scales	Response Options	2018 N	2018 Percent	2021/2022 N	2021/2022 Percent
Cigarette smoking	Not smoking	3985	87.6	2006	80.8
	Smoking	563	12.4	478	19.2
	Total	4548	100	2484	100
E-cigarette use (vaping)	Not vaping			1856	77.5
	Vaping			539	22.5
	Total			2395	100
Alcohol consumption	Not drinking	3159	71.1	1949	78.5
	Drinking	1283	28.9	535	21.5
	Total	4442	100	2484	100
Excessive alcohol consumption (drunkenness)	Did not get drunk	4235	93.1	2121	87.3
	Got drunk	313	6.9	309	12.7
	Total	4548	100	2430	100
Cannabis use	Did not use cannabis	1341	88.4	914	89.2
	Used cannabis	176	11.6	111	10.8
	Total	1517	100	1025	100
Gender	Girl	2348	51.6	1637	49.6
	Boy	2200	48.4	1667	50.5
	Total	4548	100	3304	100
Age	11–13 years	3031	66.6	2003	59.9
	HBSC—15 years/14–16 years	1517	33.4	1342	40.1
	Total	4548	100	3345	100
Ethnicity	Bulgarian			1976	83.6
	Turkish			147	6.2
	Roma			242	10.2
	Total			2365	100
Family structure	Two parents	3537	78.4	1635	74.5
	One parent/foster care/with Other relatives	974	21.6	559	25.5
	Total	4511	100	2194	100
Family affluence (Material status of the family)	Low	1887	43.6	1272	57.6
	Medium	760	17.6	382	17.3
	High	1680	38.8	555	25.1
	Total	4327	100	2209	100

Table 1. *Cont.*

Variables and Scales		2018		2021/2022	
	Response Options	**N**	**Percent**	**N**	**Percent**
Mother's employment status	In paid work	3935	89.7		
	Mother does not work	358	8.2		
	I do not know/no mother	93	2.1		
	Total	4386	100		
Father's employment status	In paid work	4138	94.3		
	Father does not work	119	2.7		
	I do not know/no father	130	3.0		
	Total	4387	100		
Mother lost job due to the pandemic	No			2419	84.6
	Yes			117	4.1
	I do not know/no mother			324	11.3
	Total			2860	100
Father lost job due to the pandemic	No			2467	84.8
	Yes			113	3.9
	I do not know/no father			329	11.3
	Total			2909	100
Mother temporarily stopped working due to the pandemic	No			1851	63.9
	Yes			589	20.3
	I do not know/no mother			459	15.8
	Total			2899	100
Father temporarily stopped working due to the pandemic	No			1830	61.9
	Yes			569	19.3
	I do not know/no father			556	18.8
	Total			2955	100
Mother paid less due to the pandemic	No			1719	60.0
	Yes			406	14.2
	I do not know/no mother			741	25.9
	Total			2866	100
Father paid less due to the pandemic	No			1615	55.4
	Yes			482	16.5
	I do not know/no father			820	28.1
	Total			2917	100
Family conflicts during the pandemic	No			1115	38.3
	Yes			1800	61.8
	Total			2915	100
Missing close relatives during the pandemic	No			2636	89.9
	Yes			296	10.1
	Total			2932	100
Communication with mother	Easy	3775	84.3	1846	81.0
	Difficult	546	12.2	372	16.3
	Do not see her/no mother	155	3.5	62	2.7
	Total	4476	100	2280	100

Table 1. *Cont.*

Variables and Scales	Response Options	2018 N	2018 Percent	2021/2022 N	2021/2022 Percent
Communication with father	Easy	3285	73.42	1639	71.5
	Difficult	935	20.9	499	21.8
	Do not see him/no father	254	5.68	156	6.8
	Total	4474	100	2294	100

Notes: In the HBSC-2018 and the study on adolescents' lives, (mental) health, and wellbeing during the pandemic, only 15-year-old students responded to the question about cannabis use. Age groups slightly differ in both surveys. The age groups in HBSC-2018 include 11–13- and 15-year-old adolescents. The study on adolescents' lives, (mental) health, and wellbeing during the pandemic includes young people at ages 11–13 and 14–16 years. In HBSC-2018, parental employment status is measured in three categories: "In paid work", "Mother/father does not work", and "I do not know/no mother/father". In the study on adolescents' lives, (mental) health and wellbeing during the pandemic parents' employment status is measured by joblessness, temporary lay-offs, and decreases in income caused by the pandemic.

In the pre-pandemic period, father's unemployment/economic inactivity was reported by 2.7% of the adolescents, while mother's unemployment/economic inactivity was somewhat higher, comprising 8.2% of the families. Of all adolescents, 3.9% reported that their father became unemployed due to the pandemic, and 4.1% reported the same for their mother. Temporary lay-offs due to the pandemic occurred more frequently in adolescents' families. Father temporarily stopped working in 19.3% of the young people's families, while mother's temporary joblessness was 20.3%. A decrease in family income occurred in 16.5% of the families due to the father's reduction in income caused by the pandemic and in 14.2% of the families due to the reduction in the mother's income.

In both periods, students were found to experience more difficulties in the communication with father compared to the communication with mother. Difficulties in communication with mothers were reported by 12.2% of the young people in the pre-pandemic period. The percentage increased to 16.3% during the pandemic. Difficulties in communication with father were reported by 20.9% of the adolescents in the pre-pandemic period. During the pandemic, the same response was given by an almost equal share of the young people—21.8%.

3.1. Multivariate Analysis of Cigarette Smoking among Bulgarian Adolescents

The results from the models of cigarette smoking show that, before the pandemic, boys had significantly lower odds of cigarette smoking compared to girls (reference group) (Table 2, Model 1a). During the pandemic, gender differences ceased to be significant (Table 2, Models 1b and 1c). In both periods, higher age was significantly associated with higher odds of cigarette smoking. During the pandemic period, Roma adolescents were significantly more likely to smoke cigarettes compared to young people with Bulgarian ethnicity (reference group). In both periods, the risk of cigarette smoking significantly increased among students from single-parent families or living in foster care/with other relatives (reference group—students living with both parents). Family affluence was not in a significant relationship with cigarette smoking in the period before the pandemic. During the pandemic, adolescents from high-affluence families had significantly higher odds of cigarette smoking compared to students from medium-status families (reference group).

Table 2. Logistic regression models of cigarette smoking among Bulgarian adolescents before and during the COVID-19 pandemic.

	Model 1a (Baseline) OR	Model 1b OR	Model 1c OR
Gender			
Girl (ref.)	1	1	1
Boy	0.79 (0.65–0.95) **	1.01 (0.80–1.28)	1.01 (0.80–1.27)
Age			
11–13 years (ref.)	1	1	1
HBSC—15 years/14–16 years	5.68 (4.65–6.95) ***	3.91 (3.08–4.97) ***	3.96 (3.11–5.03) ***
Ethnicity			
Bulgarian (ref.)		1	1
Turkish		1.28 (0.80–2.06)	1.26 (0.78–2.02)
Roma		2.53 (1.71–3.75) ***	2.70 (1.82–4.01) ***
Family structure			
Two parents (ref.)	1	1	1
One parent/foster care/with other relatives	1.80 (1.43–2.26) ***	1.99 (1.52–2.61) ***	1.95 (1.48–2.55) ***
Family affluence (FAS III)			
Low	0.85 (0.62–1.15)	0.78 (0.54–1.11)	
Medium (ref.)	1	1	
High	0.98 (0.76–1.26)	1.35 (1.02–1.80) ***	
Mother's employment status			
In paid work (ref.)	1		
Mother does not work	1.06 (0.74–1.54)		
I do not know/no mother	4.33 (2.50–7.51) ***		
Father's employment status			
In paid work (ref.)	1		
Father does not work	2.64 (1.64–4.25) ***		
I do not know/no father	1.07 (0.62–1.84)		
Mother lost job due to the pandemic			
No (ref.)		1	1
Yes		1.81 (1.02–3.21) **	1.80 (1.01–3.21) **
I do not know		1.51 (0.86–2.64)	1.48 (0.84–2.58)
Father lost job due to the pandemic			
No (ref.)		1	1
Yes		2.90 (1.64–5.12) ***	2.90 (1.64–5.14) ***
I do not know		2.44 (1.50–3.97) ***	2.49 (1.53–4.06) ***
Mother temporarily stopped working due to the pandemic			
No (ref.)		1	1
Yes		1.24 (0.88–1.74)	1.23 (0.88–1.73)
I do not know		0.62 (0.37–1.06) *	0.63 (0.37–1.07) *
Father temporarily stopped working due to the pandemic			
No (ref.)		1	1
Yes		0.96 (0.67–1.37)	0.97 (0.68–1.38)
I do not know		1.07 (0.69–1.67)	1.09 (0.70–1.70)

Table 2. *Cont.*

	Model 1a (Baseline) OR	Model 1b OR	Model 1c OR
Mother paid less due to the pandemic			
No (ref.)		1	1
Yes		0.72 (0.47–1.10)	0.74 (0.48–1.12)
I do not know		0.85 (0.56–1.27)	0.86 (0.57–1.29)
Father paid less due to the pandemic			
No (ref.)		1	1
Yes		0.85 (0.56–1.27)	0.88 (0.58–1.32)
I do not know		0.63 (0.42–0.94) **	0.63 (0.42–0.95) **
Family conflicts during the pandemic			
No (ref.)		1	
Yes		1.65 (1.26–2.15) ***	
Missing close relatives during the pandemic			
No (ref.)		1	1
Yes		1.05 (0.72–1.51)	0.98 (0.68–1.42)
Communication with mother			
Easy (ref.)	1	1	1
Difficult	1.27 (0.97–1.65) *	2.70 (1.99–3.66) ***	2.72 (2.00–3.69) ***
Do not see her/no mother	0.91 (0.56–1.48)	2.99 (1.57–5.69) **	2.82 (1.47–5.37) **
Communication with father			
Easy (ref.)	1	1	1
Difficult	1.09 (0.87–1.37)	1.07 (0.79–1.44)	1.07 (0.80–1.45)
Do not see him/no father	0.96 (0.65–1.42)	1.01 (0.64–1.61)	1.04 (0.65–1.66)
Family affluence (FAS III) * Family conflicts during the pandemic			
Low FAS * No family conflicts			1.52 (0.76–3.04)
Medium FAS * No family conflicts (ref.)			1
High FAS * No family conflicts			1.55 (0.91–2.64)
Low FAS * Family conflicts			1.81 (1.24–2.63) **
Medium FAS * Family conflicts			1.09 (0.66–1.78)
High FAS * Family conflicts			2.41 (1.57–3.70) **
Constant	0.05 (0.04–0.07) ***	0.04 (0.03–0.06) ***	0.04 (0.02–0.06) ***
N	4548	2484	2484
Log likelihood	−1474.49	−997.74	−997.14
Pseudo R2	0.13	0.18	0.18

Notes: (1) Missing values included as a separate category in the models. Results are not reported in this table. (2) OR—odds ratio. (3) Sig: ***: $p < 0.001$, **: $p < 0.01$, *: $p < 0.05$.

Before the pandemic, father's unemployment/economic inactivity was associated with higher odds of cigarette smoking (reference category—fathers in paid work). The likelihood of smoking was significantly higher also among students who did not know if mother worked or had no mother (reference group—mother in paid work). Adolescents whose mother or father became unemployed due to the pandemic had a significantly higher risk of cigarette smoking (Table 2, Models 1b and 1c). The risk was higher also among students who did not know if father lost a job due to the pandemic (reference group—father did not become unemployed due to the pandemic). Students who did not know if their mother temporarily stopped working due to the pandemic and those whose fathers experienced a reduction in income had significantly lower odds of cigarette smoking.

Increased family conflicts during the pandemic are associated with higher odds of cigarette smoking. In both periods, young people who experienced difficulties in communication with mother had significantly higher odds of cigarette smoking (reference group—students who easily communicate with mother). The communication with father was not significant in the models on cigarette smoking.

In Model 2c, we include an interaction between family dynamics (conflicts in family during the pandemic) and family affluence. The results show that young people from low and high material status families who frequently experienced conflicts in family during the pandemic had significantly higher odds of cigarette smoking (reference group—students from medium-status families who did not or rarely experienced family conflicts during the pandemic).

3.2. Multivariate Analysis of E-Cigarette Use (Vaping) among Bulgarian Adolescents

The analysis of the factors related to e-cigarette use (vaping) is based on data from the period of the COVID-19 pandemic. The results presented in Table 3 Model 2a show that boys are significantly less likely to vape compared to girls (reference group). The increase in age is significantly associated with a higher risk of vaping. Young people from the Roma ethnic group have significantly higher odds of vaping compared to adolescents with Bulgarian ethnicity (reference group). Young people from single-parent families/living in foster care or with other relatives are significantly more likely to use e-cigarettes (reference group—students living with both parents). The odds of vaping are significantly higher among young people from well-off families compared to young people from medium-status families (reference group). Young people from families with low material status are significantly less likely to vape.

Table 3. Logistic regression models of e-cigarette use (vaping) among Bulgarian adolescents during the COVID-19 pandemic.

	Model 2a **OR**	**Model 2b** **OR**
Gender		
Girl (ref.)	1	1
Boy	0.78 (0.63–0.97) **	0.77 (0.62–0.96) **
Age		
11–13 years (ref.)	1	1
HBSC—15 years/14–16 years	2.59 (2.09–3.21) ***	2.60 (2.10–3.23) ***
Ethnicity		
Bulgarian (ref.)	1	1
Turkish	1.36 (0.87–2.12)	1.34 (0.86–2.09)
Roma	2.28 (1.52–3.40) ***	2.29 (1.54–3.42) ***
Family structure		
Two parents (ref.)	1	1
One parent/foster care/with other relatives	1.96 (1.52–2.53) ***	1.93 (1.49–2.49) ***
Family affluence (FAS III)		
Low	0.44 (0.30–0.65) ***	
Medium (ref.)	1	
High	1.25 (0.97–1.63) *	
Mother lost job due to the pandemic		
No (ref.)	1	1
Yes	1.24 (0.69–2.20)	1.27 (0.71–2.25)
I do not know	1.16 (0.69–1.95)	1.15 (0.68–1.93)

Table 3. *Cont.*

	Model 2a OR	Model 2b OR
Father lost job due to the pandemic		
No (ref.)	1	1
Yes	2.06 (1.16–3.67) **	2.01 (1.13–3.57) **
I do not know	1.81 (1.13–2.90) **	1.84 (1.15–2.94) **
Mother temporarily stopped working due to the pandemic		
No (ref.)	1	1
Yes	1.15 (0.84–1.58)	1.14 (0.83–1.56)
I do not know	1.01 (0.63–1.61)	1.00 (0.63–1.61)
Father temporarily stopped working due to the pandemic		
No (ref.)	1	1
Yes	1.09 (0.79–1.50)	1.10 (0.80–1.51)
I do not know	0.64 (0.42–0.98) **	0.65 (0.43–0.99) **
Mother paid less due to the pandemic		
No (ref.)	1	1
Yes	0.92 (0.63–1.36)	0.94 (0.64–1.38)
I do not know	0.95 (0.66–1.38)	0.97 (0.67–1.40)
Father paid less due to the pandemic		
No (ref.)	1	1
Yes	0.80 (0.55–1.18)	0.81 (0.56–1.19)
I do not know	0.75 (0.52–1.07)	0.74 (0.52–1.07)
Family conflicts during the pandemic		
No (ref.)	1	
Yes	1.42 (1.13–1.80) **	
Missing close relatives during the pandemic		
No (ref.)	1	1
Yes	0.92 (0.64–1.32)	0.87 (0.61–1.25)
Communication with mother		
Easy (ref.)	1	1
Difficult	2.20 (1.64–2.95) ***	2.21 (1.65–2.96) ***
Do not see her/no mother	4.57 (2.50–8.37) ***	4.46 (2.43–8.18) ***
Communication with father		
Easy (ref.)	1	1
Difficult	1.19 (0.90–1.58)	1.20 (0.90–1.58)
Do not see him/no father	0.97 (0.61–1.52)	0.98 (0.63–1.55)
Family affluence (FAS III) * Family conflicts during the pandemic		
Low FAS * No family conflicts		0.67 (0.32–1.39)
Medium FAS * No family conflicts (ref.)		1
High FAS * No family conflicts		1.32 (0.84–2.07)
Low FAS * Family conflicts		1.45 (1.05–2.01) **
Medium FAS * Family conflicts		0.59 (0.36–0.95) **
High FAS * Family conflicts		1.83 (1.26–2.67) **
Constant	0.10 (0.07–0.13) ***	0.09 (0.07–0.13) ***
N	2395	2395
Log likelihood	−1119.13	1120.60
Pseudo R2	0.12	0.12

Notes: (1) The question of e-cigarette use is available only in the study on adolescents' (mental) health and wellbeing during the pandemic. (2) Missing values included as a separate category in the models. Results are not reported in this table. (3) OR—odds ratio. (4) Sig: ***: $p < 0.001$, **: $p < 0.01$, *: $p < 0.05$.

Students whose fathers became unemployed due to the pandemic and those who did not know about this had significantly higher risk of vaping (reference group—students whose fathers did not become unemployed due to the pandemic). Young people who did not know if their father temporarily stopped working due to the pandemic had significantly lower odds of vaping (reference group—students whose fathers temporarily stopped working due to the pandemic).

The risk of vaping is significantly higher among students who experienced frequent family conflicts during the pandemic. Young people who experienced difficulties in communication with mother or did not see her/have no mother have significantly higher odds of vaping (reference group—students who easily communicate with mother). The communication with fathers had no significant effect on the risk of vaping.

The interaction between family dynamics during the pandemic and family affluence presented in Model 2b shows that frequent family conflicts are associated with a higher risk of vaping among young people from less and high-affluent families (reference group—adolescents from medium-status families who did not or rarely experience family conflicts during the pandemic).

3.3. Multivariate Analysis of Alcohol Use among Bulgarian Adolescents

The results from the models on alcohol use presented in Table 4 show that, in both periods, before and during the pandemic, boys were more likely to report that they drunk alcohol compared to girls (reference group). The likelihood of alcohol consumption significantly increased with age. Adolescents from the Roma ethnic group had significantly higher odds of alcohol use compared to young people with Bulgarian ethnicity (reference group). In both periods, students from single-parent families and those living in foster care or with other relatives had significantly higher odds of alcohol use compared to young people living with a mother and father (reference group). In the pre-pandemic period, family affluence was not significantly associated with the risk of alcohol consumption (Model 3a). During the pandemic, students from low-status families had significantly lower odds of alcohol use, while those from affluent families had a significantly higher risk of alcohol use (reference group—adolescents from medium-status families).

Table 4. Logistic regression models of alcohol use among Bulgarian adolescents before and during the COVID-19 pandemic.

	Model 3a (Baseline) OR	Model 3b OR	Model 3c OR
Gender			
Girl (ref.)	1	1	1
Boy	1.50 (1.31–1.72) ***	1.51 (1.22–1.87) ***	1.51 (1.22–1.87) ***
Age			
11–13 years (ref.)	1	1	1
HBSC—15 years/14–16 years	2.45 (2.13–2.82) ***	1.81 (1.47–2.24) ***	1.82 (1.47–2.25) ***
Ethnicity			
Bulgarian (ref.)		1	1
Turkish		1.04 (0.66–1.63)	1.02 (0.65–1.61)
Roma		1.99 (1.37–2.90) ***	2.11 (1.44–3.09) ***
Family structure			
Two parents (ref.)	1	1	1
One parent/foster care/with other relatives	1.43 (1.21–1.70) ***	1.89 (1.47–2.44) ***	1.83 (1.42–2.37) ***

Table 4. *Cont.*

	Model 3a (Baseline) OR	Model 3b OR	Model 3c OR
Family affluence (FAS III)			
Low	0.96 (0.77–1.19)	0.63 (0.44–0.89) *	
Medium (ref.)	1	1	
High	1.08 (0.90–1.29)	1.27 (0.98–1.66) *	
Mother's employment status			
In paid work (ref.)	1		
Mother does not work	0.93 (0.72–1.20)		
I do not know/no mother	2.33 (1.45–3.77) **		
Father's employment status			
In paid work (ref.)	1		
Father does not work	1.60 (1.07–2.39) **		
I do not know/no father	1.14 (0.74–1.75)		
Mother lost job due to the pandemic			
No (ref.)		1	1
Yes		2.38 (1.40–4.05) **	2.39 (1.40–4.07) **
I do not know		1.18 (0.71–1.95)	1.18 (0.72–1.96)
Father lost job due to the pandemic			
No (ref.)		1	1
Yes		1.32 (0.76–2.29)	1.32 (0.76–2.30)
I do not know		1.53 (0.95–2.44) *	1.56 (0.97–2.50) *
Mother temporarily stopped working due to the pandemic			
No (ref.)		1	1
Yes		1.35 (0.99–1.84) *	1.33 (0.98–1.82) *
I do not know		1.11 (0.70–1.76)	1.09 (0.69–1.73)
Father temporarily stopped working due to the pandemic			
No (ref.)		1	1
Yes		1.19 (0.87–1.63)	1.19 (0.87–1.63)
I do not know		0.77 (0.51–1.16)	0.78 (0.52–1.18)
Mother paid less due to the pandemic			
No (ref.)		1	1
Yes		0.62 (0.42–0.92) **	0.63 (0.42–0.93) **
I do not know		1.29 (0.89–1.87)	1.29 (0.89–1.87)
Father paid less due to the pandemic			
No (ref.)		1	1
Yes		1.18 (0.82–1.70)	1.23 (0.85–1.77)
I do not know		0.50 (0.34–0.72) ***	0.49 (0.34–0.72) ***
Family conflicts during the pandemic			
No (ref.)		1	
Yes		1.31 (1.03–1.65) **	
Missing close relatives during the pandemic			
No (ref.)		1	1
Yes		1.09 (0.77–1.54)	1.04 (0.74–1.47)
Communication with mother			
Easy (ref.)	1	1	1
Difficult	1.36 (1.11–1.66) **	2.09 (1.55–2.82) ***	2.09 (1.55–2.82) ***
Do not see her/no mother	0.95 (0.65–1.38)	3.73 (2.04–6.83) ***	3.52 (1.91–6.48) ***

Table 4. *Cont.*

	Model 3a (Baseline) OR	Model 3b OR	Model 3c OR
Communication with father			
Easy (ref.)	1	1	1
Difficult	0.83 (0.70–0.99) **	0.95 (0.71–1.27)	0.96 (0.72–1.28)
Do not see him/no father	0.82 (0.60–1.11)	0.71 (0.44–1.15)	0.74 (0.46–1.19)
Family affluence (FAS III) * Family conflicts during the pandemic			
Low FAS * No family conflicts			1.22 (0.66–2.25)
Medium FAS * No family conflicts (ref.)			1
High FAS * No family conflicts			1.06 (0.67–1.68)
Low FAS * Family conflicts			1.31 (0.94–1.81)
Medium FAS * Family conflicts			0.62 (0.38–0.99) **
High FAS * Family conflicts			1.82 (1.25–2.66) **
Constant	0.21 (0.18–0.24) ***	0.08 (0.06–0.11) ***	0.08 (0.06–0.12) ***
N	4442	2484	2484
Log likelihood	−2537.74	−1149.08	−1144.66
Pseudo R2	0.05	0.11	0.12

Notes: (1) Missing values included as a separate category in the models. Results are not reported in this table. (2) OR—odds ratio. (3) Sig: ***: $p < 0.001$, **: $p < 0.01$, *: $p < 0.05$.

In the pre-pandemic period, students who did not know if their mother works/have no mother were significantly more likely to drink alcohol compared to young people whose mothers were employed (reference group) (Model 3a). Students whose fathers were unemployed/economically inactive also had a significantly higher risk of alcohol use (reference group—adolescents whose fathers are employed).

Young people whose mothers became unemployed due to the pandemic had significantly higher odds of alcohol use (reference group—students whose mothers did not become unemployed due to the pandemic). Father's unemployment caused by the pandemic is significantly associated with a higher risk of alcohol consumption among young people. Students whose mothers temporarily stopped working due to the pandemic showed significantly higher likelihood of alcohol use. Young people whose mothers were paid less due to the pandemic also had lower odds of alcohol use. The same relationship is found also among students who did not know if father experienced income reduction due to the pandemic.

Frequent family conflicts during the pandemic are related to significantly higher odds of alcohol use among young people. In both periods, before and during the pandemic, difficulties in communication with mother are associated with significantly higher likelihood of alcohol consumption (reference group—young people who easily communicate with mother). In the pre-pandemic period, young people who experienced difficulties in communication with father had significantly lower risk of alcohol use (reference group—students who easily communicate with father). In Models 3b and 3c about the pandemic period, the difference was not statistically significant.

In Model 3c, we test the interaction between conflicts in the family during the pandemic and the material status of the family. The results show that students from medium-status families who frequently experienced family conflicts were significantly less likely to use alcohol, while young people from affluent families who frequently experienced conflicts and tensions in the family had a significantly higher risk of alcohol use.

3.4. Multivariate Analysis of Excessive Alcohol Use (Drunkenness) among Bulgarian Adolescents

The results from the logistic regression models of excessive alcohol use (drunkenness) among Bulgarian students before and during the pandemic are presented in Table 5, Models 4a–c. In both periods, boys were found to have a significantly higher risk of drunkenness compared to girls (reference group). The association between age and excessive alcohol use is significant and positive. Roma adolescents have significantly higher odds of excessive alcohol use compared to young people with Bulgarian ethnicity (reference group). In the pre-pandemic period, family stricture was not significantly associated with the risk of drunkenness (Model 4a). During the pandemic, students from single-parent families and those living in foster care or with other relatives had significantly higher odds of excessive alcohol use.

Table 5. Logistic regression models of excessive alcohol use (drunkenness) among Bulgarian adolescents before and during the COVID-19 pandemic.

	Model 4a (Baseline) OR	Model 4b OR	Model 4c OR
Gender			
Girl (ref.)	1	1	1
Boy	1.37 (1.08–1.74) **	1.85 (1.39–2.46) ***	1.84 (1.38–2.44) ***
Age			
11–13 years (ref.)	1	1	1
HBSC—15 years/14–16 years	2.68 (2.10–3.41) ***	2.18 (1.65–2.88) ***	2.18 (1.66–2.88) ***
Ethnicity			
Bulgarian (ref.)		1	1
Turkish		0.96 (0.52–1.77)	0.95 (0.52–1.74)
Roma		2.05 (1.28–3.28) **	2.01 (1.26–3.22) **
Family structure			
Two parents (ref.)	1	1	1
One parent/foster care/with other relatives	1.23 (0.92–1.65)	2.88 (2.10–3.94) ***	2.81 (1.26–3.22) ***
Family affluence (FAS III)			
Low	0.96 (0.65–1.42)	0.55 (0.34–0.88) **	
Medium (ref.)	1	1	
High	1.30 (0.96–1.75) *	1.63 (1.16–2.29) **	
Mother's employment status			
In paid work (ref.)	1		
Mother does not work	0.64 (0.38–1.10)		
I do not know/no mother	2.95 (1.59–5.47) **		
Father's employment status			
In paid work (ref.)	1		
Father does not work	1.68 (0.90–3.12)		
I do not know/no father	1.37 (0.73–2.54)		
Mother lost job due to the pandemic			
No (ref.)		1	1
Yes		1.86 (0.97–3.56) *	1.90(1.00–3.6) **
I do not know		1.46 (0.80–2.67)	1.41 (0.77–2.56)
Father lost job due to the pandemic			
No (ref.)		1	1
Yes		2.70 (1.43–5.07) **	2.66 (1.42–5.01) **
I do not know		1.50 (0.87–2.59)	1.54 (0.89–2.66)

Table 5. *Cont.*

	Model 4a (Baseline) OR	Model 4b OR	Model 4c OR
Mother temporarily stopped working due to the pandemic			
No (ref.)		1	1
Yes		1.00 (0.66–1.50)	0.99 (0.66–1.49)
I do not know		0.84 (0.47–1.50)	0.86 (0.48–1.53)
Father temporarily stopped working due to the pandemic			
No (ref.)		1	1
Yes		1.32 (0.89–1.98)	1.31 (0.88–1.95)
I do not know		0.83 (0.49–1.40)	0.82 (0.49–1.39)
Mother paid less due to the pandemic			
No (ref.)		1	1
Yes		0.72 (0.44–1.18)	0.74 (0.45–1.22)
I do not know		1.00 (0.63–1.60)	1.02 (0.64–1.63)
Father paid less due to the pandemic			
No (ref.)		1	1
Yes		0.84 (0.52–1.35)	0.86 (0.53–1.38)
I do not know		0.67 (0.42–1.08) *	0.67 (0.42–1.07) *
Family conflicts during the pandemic			
No (ref.)		1	
Yes		1.52 (1.12–2.07) **	
Missing close relatives during the pandemic			
No (ref.)		1	1
Yes		1.84 (1.23–2.76) **	1.74 (1.17–2.61) **
Communication with mother			
Easy (ref.)	1	1	1
Difficult	1.46 (1.06–2.01) **	2.50 (1.74–3.59) ***	2.52 (1.76–3.61) ***
Do not see her/no mother	0.94 (0.51–1.72)	4.09 (2.11–7.90) ***	3.93 (2.03–7.63) ***
Communication with father			
Easy (ref.)	1	1	1
Difficult	0.90 (0.67–1.21)	0.97 (0.67–1.41)	0.98 (0.68–1.43)
Do not see him/no father	1.28 (0.81–2.02)	1.52 (0.92–2.52) *	1.54 (0.93–2.55) *
Family affluence (FAS III) * Family conflicts during the pandemic			
Low FAS * No family conflicts			0.65 (0.26–1.62)
Medium FAS * No family conflicts (ref.)			1
High FAS * No family conflicts			1.28 (0.69–2.38)
Low FAS * Family conflicts			1.26 (0.81–1.96)
Medium FAS * Family conflicts			0.70 (0.38–1.30)
High FAS * Family conflicts			2.29 (1.41–3.72) **
Constant	0.03 (0.03–0.04) ***	0.02(0.01–0.03) ***	0.02 (0.01–0.03) ***
N	4548	2430	2430
Log likelihood	−1076.34	−750.09	−753.68
Pseudo R2	0.06	0.19	0.19

Notes: (1) Missing values included as a separate category in the models. Results are not reported in this table. (2) OR—odds ratio. (3) Sig: ***: $p < 0.001$, **: $p < 0.01$, *: $p < 0.05$.

In both periods, before and during the pandemic, students from high-affluent families were more likely to report excessive alcohol use (reference group—students from medium-status families). During the pandemic period, students from low-material-status families were significantly less likely to report excessive alcohol use (no statistical difference in the pre-pandemic period).

During the pre-pandemic, students who did not know if their mother works/have no mother had a significantly higher probability of excessive alcohol use (reference group—mother in paid work). Young people whose mothers became jobless due to the pandemic had significantly higher odds of drunkenness (reference group—students whose mothers did not become jobless due to the pandemic). The same relationship is found with respect to father's unemployment caused by the pandemic. Students who did not know if father experienced income reduction due to the pandemic were less likely to report that they became drunk (reference group—students whose fathers did not experience income reduction due to the pandemic).

Family conflicts during the pandemic were significantly related to a higher risk of excessive alcohol consumption among young people. Adolescents who frequently missed contacts with close relatives also had a significantly higher likelihood of reporting excessive alcohol use. In both periods, young people who experienced difficulties in communication with their mothers were significantly more likely to report that they became drunk. In the case of communication with father, young people who did not see father/have no father were more likely to report excessive alcohol use (Models 4b and 4c).

The results from Model 4c, which includes interaction between family dynamics (conflicts in the family during the pandemic) and family affluence, show that students from affluent families who experienced frequent family conflicts during the pandemic had significantly higher odds of excessive alcohol use.

3.5. Multivariate Analysis of Cannabis Use among Bulgarian Adolescents

In Models 5a–c presented in Table 6, we explore the factors associated with cannabis use among 15-year-old students before and during the pandemic. In both periods, boys showed significantly higher odds of cannabis use compared to girls (reference group). Minority status (Turkish or Roma) is related to significantly higher risk of cannabis use (reference group—students with Bulgarian ethnicity). Family structure is seen to have a significant effect only in the period before the pandemic, showing that adolescents who lived in single-parent families or in foster care/with other relatives were more likely to smoke cannabis (reference group—students living with both parents). In the period before the pandemic, young people whose mothers did not work were significantly less likely to report that they used cannabis, while those in the category "I do not know/have no mother" had significantly higher risk (reference group—students whose mothers were in paid work).

Table 6. Results from logistic regression models of cannabis use among Bulgarian adolescents during the COVID-19 pandemic.

	Model 5a (Baseline) OR	Model 5b OR	Model 5c OR
Gender			
Girl (ref.)	1	1	1
Boy	1.35 (0.98–1.86) *	1.89 (1.11–3.21) **	1.82 (1.07–3.08) **
Ethnicity			
Bulgarian (ref.)		1	1
Turkish		3.87 (1.71–8.79) **	3.68 (1.63–8.33) **
Roma		2.82 (1.22–6.50) **	2.94 (1.29–6.71) **
Family structure			
Two parents (ref.)	1	1	1
One parent/foster care/with other relatives	1.60 (1.05–2.41) **	1.52 (0.85–2.70)	1.48 (0.83–2.64)

Table 6. *Cont.*

	Model 5a (Baseline) OR	Model 5b OR	Model 5c OR
Family affluence (FAS III)			
Low	0.80 (0.45–1.40)	0.63 (0.29–1.40)	
Medium (ref.)	1	1	
High	1.26 (0.84–1.88)	1.48 (0.82–2.68)	
Mother's employment status			
In paid work (ref.)	1		
Mother does not work	0.32 (0.11–0.92) **		
I do not know/no mother	3.05 (1.14–8.15) **		
Father's employment status			
In paid work (ref.)	1		
Father does not work	1.31 (0.45–3.79)		
I do not know/no father	1.68 (0.62–4.56)		
Mother lost job due to the pandemic			
No (ref.)		1	1
Yes		4.13 (1.57–10.87) **	4.32 (1.66–11.22) **
I do not know		3.55 (1.25–10.07) **	3.73 (1.33–10.47) **
Father lost job due to the pandemic			
No (ref.)		1	1
Yes		5.31 (1.89–14.90) **	5.09 (1.81–14.30) **
I do not know		1.87 (0.72–4.84)	1.86 (0.72–4.81)
Mother temporarily stopped working due to the pandemic			
No (ref.)		1	1
Yes		1.14 (0.54–2.40)	1.19 (0.57–2.50)
I do not know		0.47 (0.15–1.53)	0.46 (0.14–1.48)
Father temporarily stopped working due to the pandemic			
No (ref.)		1	1
Yes		0.92 (0.44–1.90)	0.87 (0.42–1.81)
I do not know		1.38 (0.51–3.72)	1.31 (0.49–3.55)
Mother paid less due to the pandemic			
No (ref.)		1	1
Yes		0.57 (0.23–1.45)	0.58 (0.23–1.48)
I do not know		0.83 (0.34–1.99)	0.85 (0.35–2.07)
Father paid less due to the pandemic			
No (ref.)		1	1
Yes		1.06 (0.46–2.46)	1.05 (0.45–2.45)
I do not know		0.39 (0.15–1.02) *	0.39 (0.15–1.01) *
Family conflicts during the pandemic			
No (ref.)		1	
Yes		1.25 (0.71–2.21)	
Missing close relatives during the pandemic			
No (ref.)		1	1
Yes		2.35 (1.21–4.57) **	2.26 (1.16–4.43) **
Communication with mother			
Easy (ref.)	1	1	1
Difficult	1.75 (1.16–2.64) **	4.32 (2.39–7.81) ***	4.31 (2.38–7.80) ***
Do not see her/no mother	1.04 (0.47–2.31)	8.92 (2.90–27.42) ***	9.09 (2.94–28.12) ***

Table 6. *Cont.*

	Model 5a (Baseline) OR	Model 5b OR	Model 5c OR
Communication with father			
Easy (ref.)	1	1	1
Difficult	0.90 (0.62–1.30)	0.62 (0.32–1.23)	0.62 (0.31–1.23)
Do not see him/no father	0.56 (0.27–1.16)	0.84 (0.35–2.03)	0.84 (0.35–2.02)
Family affluence (FAS III) * Family conflicts during the pandemic			
Low FAS * No family conflicts			0.54 (0.10–2.83)
Medium FAS * No family conflicts (ref.)			1
High FAS * No family conflicts			2.04 (0.70–5.93)
Low FAS * Family conflicts			1.35 (0.60–3.02)
Medium FAS * Family conflicts			0.86 (0.29–2.51)
High FAS * Family conflicts			1.38 (0.54–3.49)
Constant	0.09 (0.07–0.13) ***	0.02 (0.01–0.04) ***	0.02 (0.01–0.05) ***
N	1517	1025	1025
Log likelihood	−520.43	−256.97	−257.29
Pseudo R2	0.04	0.27	0.27

Notes: (1) Missing values included as a separate category in the models. Results are not reported in this table. (2) OR—odds ratio. (3) Sig: ***: $p < 0.001$, **: $p < 0.01$, *: $p < 0.05$.

Students reporting that mother became unemployed due to the pandemic or did not know about this had significantly higher risk of cannabis use (reference group—students whose mothers did not become unemployed due to the pandemic). Adolescents who did not know if father experienced income reduction due to the pandemic were less likely to report that they used cannabis (reference group—students whose fathers did not experience income reduction due to the pandemic).

Young people who frequently missed contact with close family members during the pandemic were significantly more likely to use cannabis. In both periods, before and during the pandemic, students who experienced difficulties in the communication with mother were significantly more likely to report that they used cannabis (reference group—students who easily communicate with mother). The variable about the communication with father was not statistically significant.

Model 5c shows that the interaction between family conflicts during the pandemic and family affluence is not significantly associated with cannabis use.

4. Discussion

This study aimed to explore family dynamics and socioeconomic hardships during the COVID-19 pandemic and their associations with substance use (cigarette smoking, vaping, alcohol use, drunkenness, and cannabis use) among young people in Bulgaria. Data from HBSC 2018 were used for comparisons with the pre-pandemic period. We selected factors at the persona and family level, including young people's sociodemographic characteristics and family-related variables such as structure and material status of the family, parental unemployment, lay-offs, and reductions in income due to the pandemic, conflicts in the family, limited social interactions with close family members during the pandemic, and communication with parents. We explored also the interdependence between family dynamics (family conflicts during the pandemic) and family affluence.

The results from the multivariate analysis uncover strong differentials by gender, age, and ethnicity in substance use among young people in Bulgaria and changes in the effect of some of the sociodemographic dependencies during the pandemic. At that period, boys showed a higher risk of alcohol consumption, drunkenness, and cannabis use and a lower risk of vaping compared to girls. The difference between boys and girls was not statistically significant in cigarette smoking. In the pre-pandemic period, the risk of smoking was significantly higher among girls, and the gender difference in cannabis use was not significant. These results suggest changes in HRBs of boys and girls in Bulgaria that have occurred during the pandemic [2,31]. In a broader perspective, studies focused on substance use among young people reveal also diverging and inconsistent effects of gender in different contexts. Studies show that, rather, gender differences in coping with adverse experiences caused by the pandemic were differentiating factors in the disproportionate risk of substance use among boys and girls [8,32].

Similarly to the pre-pandemic period, substance use was prevalent among older adolescents in Bulgaria. This result shows that, despite the restrictions and the imposed social isolation, the older adolescents remained more susceptible to substance use [33,34]. In the pandemic period, substance use remained part of young people's recreational and socialising activity and featured adolescents' pathways to adulthood [35,36].

The present study uncovers a strong differentiating effect of ethnicity, with Roma adolescents having a higher likelihood of cigarette smoking, vaping, alcohol consumption, drunkenness, and cannabis use. Strong socioeconomic deprivation and social exclusion of Roma ethnic minority in Bulgaria was exacerbated during the pandemic as a consequence of the unfolding economic crisis, which increased the vulnerability of young people from this ethnic group, negatively affecting also young people's health behaviours [37,38].

Family structure shows a consistent effect on adolescents' HRBs in both periods, before and during the pandemic. Young people living with one of the parents/in foster care, or with other relatives were found to have a higher likelihood of cigarette smoking, vaping, alcohol consumption, drunkenness, and cannabis use. Studies show that increased difficulties experienced by single parents in combining different tasks during the pandemic had negative implications on parental and adolescents' (mental) health and family relationships [39–41], emphasising also the need for family-focused help and support during the pandemic [42].

Bulgarian adolescents who frequently experienced family conflicts during the pandemic were found to have a higher risk of substance use (cigarette smoking, vaping, alcohol use, drunkenness). Young people who were frequently missing contact with close family members were more likely to use cannabis. Difficulties in communication with mother are associated with significantly higher risk of substance use among young people in both periods, before and during the pandemic. Difficulties in communication with father are in a significant relationship with the use of alcohol in the period before the pandemic and with drunkenness during the pandemic. The correlation between communication with mother and father may influence the significance of ease of communication with father. Monitoring and involvement of mothers in the daily routines and activities of adolescents may explain the significant effect of the communication with the mother on young people's HRBs [43–45]. In countries with more traditional family culture, like Bulgaria, the father's authority is built on perceptions of discipline, decision-making, material support, and provision for the family, while the mother is the person who is more involved in the daily routines of the family and care for children and adolescents [46–48]. These findings confirm our first hypothesis about the importance of family dynamics for young people's HRBs during the pandemic.

Research shows that poverty and prolonged parental unemployment have a harmful effect on adolescent development, including also long-term negative consequences on health at later stages in life [49–51]. The results from the multivariate analysis reveal that, in the period before the pandemic, parental unemployment/economic inactivity was significantly associated with higher engagement of young people in cigarette smoking, vaping, alcohol consumption, drunkenness, and cannabis use. The economic hardships experienced by the families during the COVID-19 pandemic, related to parental joblessness, temporary lay-offs, and decreases in income caused by the pandemic, were associated with a heightened risk of cigarette smoking, vaping, alcohol consumption, drunkenness, and cannabis use among young people. The results reveal also increased differences in HRBs of students from different material status families during the pandemic. In the pre-pandemic period, the material status of the family had a significant effect on drunkenness, with students from affluent families having a higher risk for excessive alcohol use. During the period of the global health crisis, the risk of vaping, alcohol use, and drunkenness was significantly lower among students from less affluent families, and the effect was not significant in cigarette smoking and cannabis use. Heightened risk of substance use (cigarette smoking, vaping, alcohol use, and drunkenness) was observed among students from affluent families, and a non-significant effect was found for cannabis use. These results partly confirm our second hypothesis, revealing a disproportional effect of family affluence during the pandemic with an increased risk of substance use observed among young people from affluent families and a decrease in the risk among adolescents from materially disadvantaged families.

In order to test the interrelatedness between family dynamics (family conflicts) during the pandemic, family affluence, and adolescents' HRBs, we applied additional models with interaction between family conflicts and the material status of the family during the pandemic. The results show that conflictual family relationships are associated with a higher likelihood of smoking, vaping, alcohol use, and drunkenness among young people from affluent families, while among students from low-material-status families the association is positive and significant only for cigarette smoking and vaping. These results partly confirm our third hypothesis. Conflictual family relationships among young people from less affluent families may strengthen the negative effect of economic hardships on young people's HRBs. Among adolescents from high-material-status families, worsened family relationships and the availability of resources may increase young people's engagement in substance use as a response to financial problems and conflicts in the family [52,53]. Studies show that economic difficulties leading to worsened parental mental health and increased tensions and conflicts in families during the pandemic were associated with heterogeneous responses in young people, including also maladaptive coping strategies of increased substance use [54–58]. In the case of Bulgarian adolescents, the economic hardships experienced by the families during the pandemic may affect young people's behavioural health through increased anxiety and depression, provoking higher engagement in substance use [29,59].

5. Conclusions

The COVID-19 pandemic challenged the protective function of the family and reshaped young people's lives in multiple directions. The health crisis created a specific environment of distress and strengthened socioeconomic difficulties for families, increasing the vulnerability of young people. The present study affirms that the economic hardships caused by parental unemployment, temporary lay-offs, and reductions in income are associated with a higher susceptibility to substance use as a maladaptive coping mechanism, especially among young people who experienced worsened family dynamics and increased conflictual relationships in the family during the COVID-19 pandemic.

5.1. Limitations of This Study

In the present analysis, we used cross-sectional surveys, which allows us to focus only on the associations between young people's substance use, family dynamics (relationships in the family during the pandemic, missing contacts with extended family members, communication with parents), and the socioeconomic hardships experienced by the families during the pandemic. Both surveys include self-reported data that are subjected to response biases. The age groups of students in the surveys are slightly different, but the similarities in the design and in the measures used in the analyses allow for group-level comparisons. In HBSC-2018, parental unemployment and economic inactivity are combined in one category. In the study on adolescents' (mental) health and wellbeing during the pandemic, parental unemployment, temporary lay-offs, and decreases in income caused by the pandemic are assessed for the whole period, which does not allow for a more differentiated look into the dynamics of parental economic status changes and their effect on adolescents' HRBs.

Ease of communication with parents is measured by a single question asked separately for mother and father. More complex measures are needed in order to outline more precisely the effect of openness and ease of communication with parents on adolescents' HRBs.

5.2. Implications for Practice

The present analysis reveals that the socioeconomic hardships experienced by the families during the pandemic and worsened family relationships are related to higher engagement of young people in substance use (cigarette smoking, vaping, alcohol use, drunkenness, and cannabis use). These findings highlight the need for special interventions focused on different types of families in terms of material status, parental employment status, family dynamics, and parent-adolescent relationships. The results from this study can serve for the development of prevention programmes targeting the health behaviours of young people from families experiencing economic hardships and worsened family dynamics.

Author Contributions: Conceptualisation, E.D. and A.A.-K.; methodology, E.D. and A.A.-K.; software, E.D.; validation, E.D. and A.A.-K.; formal analysis, E.D.; investigation, E.D. and A.A.-K.; resources, A.A.-K. and E.D.; data curation, A.A.-K. and E.D.; writing—original draft preparation, E.D. and A.A.-K.; writing—review and editing, E.D. and A.A.-K.; visualisation, E.D.; supervision, A.A.-K.; project administration, A.A.-K.; funding acquisition, A.A.-K. and E.D. All authors have read and agreed to the published version of the manuscript.

Funding: This research was funded by the Bulgarian National Science Fund, Project No. КП-06-Н55/7, within Competition for financial support of basic research projects–2021.

Institutional Review Board Statement: The study was conducted in accordance with the Declaration of Helsinki and approved by the Ethics Committee of the Institute for Population and Human Studies at the Bulgarian Academy of Sciences (protocol code RD-5-90/05.05.2022).

Informed Consent Statement: Informed consent was obtained from the adolescents involved in the study and from their parents.

Data Availability Statement: The data presented in this study are available upon request from the corresponding author. The data are not publicly available due to ethical restrictions (data contain sensitive personal information).

Conflicts of Interest: The authors declare no conflicts of interest.

References

1. Inchley, J.; Currie, D.; Budisavljevic, S.; Torsheim, T.; Jåstad, A.; Cosma, A.; Kelly, C.; Arnarsson, Á.M.; Samdal, O. (Eds.) *Spotlight on Adolescent Health and Well-Being. Findings from the 2017/2018 Health Behaviour in School-Aged Children (HBSC) Survey in Europe and Canada*; International Report. Key Data; WHO Regional Office for Europe: Copenhagen, Denmark, 2020; Volume 2.
2. Kotzeva, T.; Dimitrova, E. Risky Behaviours: Tracking Youth Health and Well-being in Bulgaria 2006–2008. In *Wohlbefinden und Gesundheit im Jugendalter. Theoretische Perspektiven, Empirische Befunde und Praxisansätze*; Heinen, A., Samuel, R., Vögele, C., Willems, H., Eds.; Springer-VSL: Wiesbaden, Germany, 2022; pp. 665–668. Available online: https://link.springer.com/chapter/10.1007/978-3-658-35744-3_30 (accessed on 14 April 2024).
3. Bozzini, A.B.; Bauer, A.; Maruyama, J.; Simões, R.; Matijasevich, A. Factors associated with risk behaviors in adolescence: A systematic review. *Braz. J. Psychiatry* **2021**, *2*, 210–221. [CrossRef]
4. Rangachev, A.; Marinov, G.K.; Mladenov, M. The Impact and Progression of the COVID-19 Pandemic in Bulgaria in its First Two Years. *Vaccines* **2022**, *11*, 1901. [CrossRef] [PubMed]
5. Sobczak, M.; Pawliczak, R. COVID-19 Mortality Rate Determinants in Selected Eastern European Countries. *BMC Public Health* **2022**, *22*, 2088. [CrossRef] [PubMed]
6. Sterev, N. Economic Impact of COVID-19 Pandemic: Case of Bulgaria. *SHS Web Conf.* **2021**, *120*, 02005. [CrossRef]
7. Maeva, M. Family Well-Being During the COVID-19 Pandemic in Bulgaria. *Psychol. Res.* **2022**, *25*, 128–137. [CrossRef]
8. Magson, N.R.; Freeman, J.Y.A.; Rapee, R.M.; Richardson, C.E.; Oar, E.L.; Fardouly, J. Risk and Protective Factors for Prospective Changes in Adolescent Mental Health during the COVID-19 Pandemic. *J. Youth Adolesc.* **2021**, *50*, 44–57. [CrossRef]
9. Temple, J.R.; Baumler, E.; Wood, L.; Guillot-Wright, S.; Torres, E.; Thiel, M. The Impact of the COVID-19 Pandemic on Adolescent Mental Health and Substance Use. *J. Adolesc. Health* **2022**, *71*, 277–284. [CrossRef] [PubMed]
10. Pourghazi, F.; Eslami, M.; Ehsani, A.; Ejtahed, H.S.; Qorbani, M. Eating Habits of Children and Adolescents during the COVID-19 Era: A Systematic Review. *Front. Nutr.* **2022**, *9*, 1004953. [CrossRef]

11. Lua, V.Y.Q.; Chua, T.B.K.; Chia, M.Y.H. A Narrative Review of Screen Time and Wellbeing among Adolescents before and during the COVID-19 Pandemic: Implications for the Future. *Sports* **2023**, *11*, 38. [CrossRef]
12. Prime, H.; Wade, M.; Browne, D.T. Risk and Resilience in Family Well-Being during the COVID-19 Pandemic. *Am. Psychol.* **2020**, *75*, 631–643. [CrossRef]
13. Martin-Storey, A.; Dirks, M.; Holfeld, B.; Dryburgh, N.S.J.; Craig, W. Family Relationship Quality during the COVID-19 Pandemic: The Value of Adolescent Perceptions of Change. *J. Adolesc.* **2021**, *93*, 190–201. [CrossRef]
14. Argabright, S.T.; Tran, K.T.; Visoki, E.; DiDomenico, G.E.; Moore, T.M.; Barzilay, R. COVID-19-related Financial Strain and Adolescent Mental Health. *Lancet Reg. Health—Am.* **2022**, *16*, 100391. [CrossRef] [PubMed]
15. Donker, M.H.; Mastrotheodoros, S.; Branje, S. Development of Parent-Adolescent Relationships during the COVID-19 Pandemic: The Role of Stress and Coping. *Dev. Psychol.* **2021**, *10*, 1611–1622. [CrossRef]
16. Pauly, T.; Lüscher, J.; Berli, C.; Scholz, U. Dynamic Associations between Stress and Relationship Functioning in the Wake of COVID-19: Longitudinal Data from the German Family Panel (Pairfam). *J. Soc. Pers. Relat.* **2022**, *39*, 3183–3203. [CrossRef]
17. Kim, C.; Lee, H.; Jung-Choi, K.; Park, H. Changes in Adolescent Health Behavior and the Exacerbation of Economic Hardship During the COVID-19 Pandemic: A Cross-sectional Study From the Korea Youth Risk Behavior Survey. *J. Prev. Med. Public Health* **2024**, *57*, 18–27. [CrossRef] [PubMed]
18. Richard, V.; Dumont, R.; Lorthe, E.; Loizeau, A.; Baysson, H.; Zaballa, M.E.; Pennacchio, F.; Barbe, R.P.; Posfay-Barbe, K.M.; Guessous, I.; et al. Impact of the COVID-19 Pandemic on Children and Adolescents: Determinants and Association with Quality of Life and Mental Health—A Cross-Sectional Study. *J. Child Psychol. Psychiatry* **2023**, *17*, 17. [CrossRef]
19. Holloway, K.; Murray, S.; Buhociu, M.; Arthur, A.; Molinaro, R.; Chicken, S.; Thomas, E.; Courtney, S.; Spencer, A.; Wood, R.; et al. Lessons from the COVID-19 Pandemic for Substance Misuse Services: Findings from a Peer-Led Study. *Harm. Reduct. J.* **2022**, *19*, 140. [CrossRef]
20. Richter, L. The Effects of the COVID-19 Pandemic on the Risk of Youth Substance Use. *J. Adolesc. Health* **2020**, *4*, 467–468. [CrossRef] [PubMed]
21. Calihan, J.B.; Levy, S. Coronavirus Disease Pandemic and Adolescent Substance Use. *Curr. Opin. Pediatr.* **2022**, *4*, 334–340. [CrossRef]
22. Layman, H.M.; Thorisdottir, I.E.; Halldorsdottir, T.; Sigfusdottir, I.D.; Allegrante, J.P.; Kristjansson, A.L. Substance Use among Youth during the COVID-19 Pandemic: A Systematic Review. *Curr. Psychiatry Rep.* **2022**, *24*, 307–324. [CrossRef]
23. Pelham, W.E., 3rd; Tapert, S.F.; Zúñiga, M.L.; Thompson, W.K.; Wade, N.E.; Gonzalez, M.R.; Patel, H.; Baker, F.C.; Dowling, G.J.; Van Rinsveld, A.M.; et al. Pandemic-Related Changes in the Prevalence of Early Adolescent Alcohol and Drug Use, 2020-2021: Data from a Multisite Cohort Study. *J. Adolesc. Health* **2023**, *73*, 338–346. [CrossRef]
24. Rosenthal, S.R.; Noel, J.K.; Skierkowski-Foster, D.; Gately, K.A.; Borden, S.K. Perceived Parent and Peer Substance Use Disapproval and Perceptions of Harm among Youth Before and After COVID-19 Lockdowns. *J. Subst. Use* **2024**, 1–6. [CrossRef]
25. Branquinho, C.; Paiva, T.; Guedes, F.; Gaspar, T.; Tomé, G.; Gaspar de Matos, M. Health Risk Behaviors before and during COVID-19 and Gender Differences. *J. Community Psychol.* **2022**, *2*, 1102–1110. [CrossRef]
26. Bowen, M. The use of family theory in clinical practice. *Compr. Psychiatry* **1966**, *7*, 345–374. [CrossRef] [PubMed]
27. Bowen, M. *Family Therapy in Clinical Practice*; Jason Aronson: New York, NY, USA, 1978.
28. Inchley, J.; Currie, D.; Samdal, O.; Jåstad, A.; Cosma, A.; Nic Gabhainn, S. (Eds.) *Health Behaviour in School-Aged Children (HBSC) Study Protocol: Background, Methodology and Mandatory Items for the 2021/22 Survey*; MRC/CSO Social and Public Health Sciences Unit, University of Glasgow: Glasgow, UK, 2023.
29. Dimitrova, E.; Alexandrova-Karamanova, A. Biopsychosocial Factors of Adolescent Health Risk Behaviours during the COVID-19 Pandemic—Insights from an Empirical Study. *Societies* **2023**, *13*, 169. [CrossRef]
30. Torsheim, T.; Cavallo, F.; Levin, K.A.; Schnohr, C.; Mazur, J.; Niclasen, B.; Currie, C. Psychometric Validation of the Revised Family Affluence Scale: A Latent Variable Approach. *Child. Indic. Res.* **2016**, *9*, 771–784. [CrossRef]
31. Vasileva, L.; Alexandrova, B.; Bogdanova, E. Relationship Satisfaction with Family Relationships among Students 7th and 9th grade. In *Young People in European Bulgaria*; Mitev, P.-E., Kotzeva, T., Mihova, G., Eds.; CPS-BAS: Sofia, Bulgaria, 2007; pp. 490–500.
32. Romano, I.; Patte, K.A.; de Groh, M.; Jiang, Y.; Wade, T.J.; Bélanger, R.E.; Leatherdale, S.T. Substance-related Coping Behaviours among Youth during the Early Months of the COVID-19 Pandemic. *Addict. Behav. Rep.* **2021**, *14*, 100392. [CrossRef] [PubMed]
33. Rodríguez-Cano, R.; Kypriotakis, G.; Cortés-García, L.; Bakken, A.; von Soest, T. Polysubstance Use And Its Correlation With Psychosocial And Health Risk Behaviours among more than 95,000 Norwegian Adolescents during the COVID-19 Pandemic (January to May 2021): A Latent Profile Analysis. *Lancet Reg. Eur.* **2023**, *28*, 100603. [CrossRef] [PubMed]
34. Noel, J.K.; Rosenthal, S.R.; Skierkowski-Foster, D.; Borden, S.K. Effect of COVID-19 Lockdown on Substance Use Among Middle School and High School Students: A Natural Experiment. *Public Health Rep.* **2023**, *138*, 349–356. [CrossRef]
35. Schulenberg, J.; Maslowsky, J.; Jager, J. Substance Use and Abuse during Adolescence and the Transition to Adulthood are Developmental Phenomena: Conceptual and Empirical Considerations. In *Alcohol Use Disorders: A Developmental Science Approach to Etiology*; Fitzgerald, H.E., Puttler, L.I., Eds.; Oxford University Press: New York, NY, USA, 2018; pp. 199–222. [CrossRef]
36. Adalbjarnardottir, S.; Rafnsson, F.D. Adolescent Antisocial Behavior and Substance Use: Longitudinal Analyses. *Addict. Behav.* **2022**, *27*, 227–240. [CrossRef]

37. Children and COVID-19. The Impact of the Crisis on the Rights and Interests of Children in the Republic of Bulgaria. Special Report of the Ombudsman of the Republic of Bulgaria. 2021. Available online: https://www.ombudsman.bg/storage/pub/files/20220729171046_ANNUAL%20REPORT%202021_OMBUDSMAN%20OF%20BULGARIA.pdf (accessed on 18 August 2024).
38. UNICEF Europe and Central Asia Regional Office. *Un/Equal Childhood: Deep Dive in Child Poverty and Social Exclusion in Bulgaria*; UNICEF-Bulgaria Report; UNICEF: UNICEF Europe and Central Asia Regional Office: Geneva, Switzerland, 2021.
39. Dawes, J.; May, T.; McKinlay, A.; Fancourt, D.; Burton, A. Impact of the COVID-19 Pandemic on the Mental Health and Wellbeing of Parents with Young Children: A Qualitative Interview Study. *BMC Psychol.* **2021**, *9*, 194. [CrossRef]
40. Hoffmann, J.P. Family Structure, Unstructured Socializing, and Heavy Substance Use among Adolescents. *Int. J. Environ. Res. Public Health* **2022**, *19*, 8818. [CrossRef] [PubMed]
41. Spina, G.; Giordano, F.; Cristofolini, F.; Landoni, M.; Grazioli, S.; Viggiani, C.; Gnagnarella, C.; Simione, L. Mental Health of Mothers and Children during the COVID-19 Lockdown: A Cross-sectional Study on a Large Sample of Italian Families. *J. Child Fam. Stud.* **2023**, *32*, 3666–3680. [CrossRef]
42. Baldus, C.; Franz, S.; Thomasius, R. Help Needs among Parents and Families in Times of the COVID-19 Pandemic Lockdown in Germany. *Int. J. Environ. Res. Public Health* **2022**, *19*, 14159. [CrossRef]
43. Levin, K.A.; Currie, C. Family Structure, Mother-Child Communication, Father-Child Communication, and Adolescent Life Satisfaction: A Cross-Sectional Multilevel Analysis. *Health Educ.* **2010**, *110*, 152–168. [CrossRef]
44. Moore, G.F.; Cox, R.; Evans, R.E.; Hallingberg, B.; Hawkins, J.; Littlecott, H.J.; Long, S.J.; Murphy, S. School, Peer and Family Relationships and Adolescent Substance Use, Subjective Wellbeing and Mental Health Symptoms in Wales: A Cross Sectional Study. *Child Indic. Res.* **2018**, *11*, 1951–1965. [CrossRef] [PubMed]
45. Zaborskis, A.; Kavaliauskienė, A.; Eriksson, C.; Dimitrova, E.; Makari, J. Family Structure through the Adolescent Eyes: A Comparative Study of Current Status and Time Trends over Three Decades of HBSC Study. *Societies* **2022**, *12*, 88. [CrossRef]
46. Novianti, R.; Suarman, S.; Nur, I. Parenting in Cultural Perspective: A Systematic Review of Paternal Role across Cultures. *J. Ethn. Cult. Stud.* **2023**, *10*, 22–44. [CrossRef]
47. Heaton, K.G.; Camacho, N.L.; Gaffrey, M.S. Associations between Pre-Pandemic Authoritative Parenting, Pandemic Stressors, and Children's Depression and Anxiety at the Initial Stage of the COVID-19 Pandemic. *Sci. Rep.* **2023**, *13*, 15592. [CrossRef]
48. Williams, O.C.; Prasad, S.; Khan, A.A.; Ayisire, O.E.; Naseer, H.; Abdullah, M.; Nadeem, M.; Ashraf, N.; Zeeshan, M. Tailoring parenting styles and family-based interventions cross-culturally as an effective prevention strategy for youth substance use: A scoping review. *Ann. Med. Surg.* **2023**, *86*, 257–270. [CrossRef]
49. Mooi-Reci, I.; Wooden, M. Jobless Parents, unhealthy children? How Past Exposure to Parental Joblessness Influences Children's Future Health. *SSM Popul. Health* **2022**, *19*, 101144. [CrossRef]
50. Judd, N.; Hughes, K.; Bellis, M.A.; Hardcastle, K.; Amos, R. Is Parental Unemployment Associated with Increased Risk of Adverse Childhood Experiences? A Systematic Review and Meta-analysis. *J. Public Health* **2023**, *4*, 829–839. [CrossRef] [PubMed]
51. Drydakis, N. Economic Recession, Parental Unemployment and Adolescents' Health-Related Quality of Life and Mental Health Outcomes in Greece. *Southeast Eur. Black Sea Stud.* **2023**, *2*, 275–298. [CrossRef]
52. Plenty, S. Too Much or Too Little? A short-term Longitudinal Study of Youth's Own Economic Resources and Risk Behaviour. *J. Adolesc.* **2018**, *66*, 21–30. [CrossRef]
53. Foley, S.; Badinlou, F.; Brocki, K.; Frick, M.; Ronchi, L.; Hughes, C. Family Function and Child Adjustment Difficulties in the COVID-19 Pandemic: An International Study. *Int. J. Environ. Res. Public Health* **2021**, *18*, 11136. [CrossRef]
54. Shroff, A.; Fassler, J.; Fox, K.R.; Schleider, J.L. The Impact of COVID-19 on U.S. Adolescents: Loss of Basic Needs and Engagement in Health Risk Behaviors. *Curr. Psychol.* **2022**, *43*, 12023–12033. [CrossRef]
55. Morgan, D.D.; Higgins, C.D.; Ingram, P.B.; Rogers, C.R. Predicting Parental Mental Health during COVID-19: Economic Pressure, COVID-19 Stress, and Coping Strategies. *Front. Psychol.* **2022**, *13*, 909978. [CrossRef]
56. Wang, Z.; Li, C.; Ai, K. Family Economic Strain and Adolescent Aggression during the COVID-19 Pandemic: Roles of Interparental Conflict and Parent–Child Conflict. *Appl. Res. Qual. Life* **2022**, *17*, 2369–2385. [CrossRef]
57. Lee, J.B.; Ross, K.M.; Ntanda, H.; Fiest, K.M.; Letourneau, N.; The APrON Study Team. Mothers' and Children's Mental Distress and Family Strain during the COVID-19 Pandemic: A Prospective Cohort Study. *Children* **2023**, *11*, 1725. [CrossRef]
58. Campione-Barr, N.; Skinner, A.; Moeller, K.; Cui, L.; Kealy, C.; Cookston, J. The Role of Family Relationships on Adolescents' Development and Adjustment during the COVID-19 Pandemic: A Systematic Review. *J. Res. Adolesc.* 2024; *early view*. [CrossRef]
59. Alexandrova-Karamanova, A.; Kotzeva, T.; Paunova-Markova, E.; Mineva, K.; Dimitrova, E.; Yordanova, T. COVID-19 Exposure and COVID-19 Disease in the Family: Effects on Adolescent Mental Health. *Bulg. J. Psychol.* **2023**, *1*, 279–296.

children

Systematic Review

Systematic Review of Psychosocial Risk and Protective Factors in Children Reported from Developmental Criminology

Daniela Zúñiga [1,*], Francesco Carretta [2], Macarena Contreras [3], Erica Cornejo [3], Constanza Gallardo [3], Isidora Guichapani [3] and Constansa Muñoz [3]

1 Institute of Psychological Studies, Faculty of Medicine, Universidad Austral de Chile, Isla Teja Campus, Valdivia 5110566, Chile
2 Faculty of Law, Pontificia Universidad Católica de Valparaíso, Valparaíso Campus, Valparaíso 2340025, Chile; francesco.carretta@pucv.cl
3 School of Psychology, Faculty of Medicine, Universidad Austral de Chile, Isla Teja Campus, Valdivia 5110566, Chile; macarena.contreras01@alumnos.uach.cl (M.C.); erica.cornejo@alumnos.uach.cl (E.C.); contanza.gallardo@alumnos.uach.cl (C.G.); isidora.guichapani@alumnos.uach.cl (I.G.); constansa.munoz@alumnos.uach.cl (C.M.)
* Correspondence: daniela.zuniga@uach.cl; Tel.: +56-998-485-649

Abstract: Background/Objectives: Evidence indicates that persistent transgressive behaviors often begin early in development and increase around age twelve, and warns that children who exhibit transgressive behaviors in childhood or early adolescence tend to develop criminal behaviors in adulthood which makes childhood a critical unit of analysis for timely intervention. The study examines risk and protective factors in childhood related to illegal behavior, through the perspective of developmental criminology. The observation of risk and protective factors in early stages allows us to design interventions that prevent social adjustment problems in children from becoming more complex by maintaining the transgression of social norms over time. Factors identified by developmental criminology can be organized according to ecological systems theory and discussed in relation to previous criminological studies. Methods: Using a systematic review based on the PRISMA method, the study identifies 24 updated developmental criminology articles that study early protective factors between birth and age twelve. Result: Risk factors at the individual level include biological, socioemotional, behavioral, symptomatic aspects and adverse life experiences. Individual protective factors include cognitive, socioemotional, and personality development aspects. Risk factors at an interpersonal and contextual level are related to family, school, peers, socioeconomic situation and governance. Conclusions: This review highlights the importance of recognizing risk and protective factors in child development, contemplating interventions at multiple levels where an articulation between the various institutions involved in child care is possible.

Keywords: developmental criminology; childhood; children; protective factors; risk factors; criminality; crime; life course; systematic review

1. Introduction

Understanding criminal behavior involves examining multiple factors related to antisocial, delinquent, and criminal activities, considering their duration, frequency, intensity, and severity [1,2]. Comprehensive approaches from a specialized field enable the prevention, prediction, and detection of antisocial behavior and personality [3].

Numerous theories have contributed to explaining criminal behavior in adolescence, and it is possible to organize them into three groups: the classic theories of crime that try to explain crime from different biological, psychological, and sociological approaches; the critical or criminalization theories; and the integrative theories that are built by incorporating previous theoretical proposals, which allow us to visualize the problem of crime from a broad comprehensive framework and reflecting its complexity [4].

One theoretical integrative framework is developmental criminology, a branch built on evidence from various disciplines [5,6]; it has been considered one of the most accurate theories to understand delinquency in the juvenile stage since developmental criminology encompasses crime throughout the life course, in contrast to traditional or classic criminological theories that do not consider the passage of time, focusing particularly on childhood and adolescence [7–11]. From this perspective, law-breaking is viewed as part of a life trajectory that can begin early in childhood and continue into adolescence, with desistance or intensification of criminal behavior being common [12]. This approach seeks to explain the development of delinquency through an age-graded framework based on empirical observations from prospective longitudinal studies [6]. Research consistently views delinquency as part of a broader social phenomenon encompassing antisocial behavior that persists throughout the life cycle and across generations [13]. Consequently, the challenge lies in preventing and disrupting its persistence.

The literature delimits two lines of research that have in common observing life history and social development, differing in their emphases. Developmental theories, rooted in psychology, emphasize psychosocial factors, the appearance of delinquency, and the role of psychological factors. early protective and risk factors [13]. In contrast, life course theories, with a sociological orientation, focus on social structure and life events, investigating desistance and turning points [13]—for example, the research of Sampson and Laub [14] emphasizes the desistance of antisocial behavior. Both approaches, life course and developmental criminology, provide insights into various aspects of criminality that had not been previously considered and allow design preventive strategies [14].

In recent years, various reviews of the theoretical body that underpins developmental criminology have been developed [13,15,16]. McGee and Farrington [6] reviewed and compared six of the most relevant theories: the integrated cognitive antisocial potential theory [17]; the social development model [18]; antisocial behavior persistent throughout life and limited in adolescence [9,19]; the theory of informal social control by age [14,20]; the situational action theory of crime causation [21,22]; and interactional theory [23,24].

Currently, the most important theories, Farrington, Loeber, and Catalano and Hawkins, base their developments on several classic theories, such as those of social learning, social control, opportunities, differential association, and labeling, and test them through longitudinal and experimental studies [25]. Farrington, Wikström, Hawkins, and Catalano work from early socialization, postulating that children learn practices from their parents and the community during childhood [6]. Moffitt, another important theory, explores the early neuropsychological factors that result in two types of criminality: persistent and adolescent-limited [6].

In summary, current developmental criminology has managed to focus on three perspectives of analysis: (1) the development of criminal and antisocial behaviors, (2) risk and protective factors at different stages of life, and (3) the effects of certain life events in development [26]. These studies have contributed significantly to criminology, allowing preventive interventions to be designed based on evidence [25]. In relation to risk factors, it is important to point out the work of Bonta and Andrews [27], who, based on general personality and cognitive social learning theory of criminal behavior, determine psycho-social–biological factors that initiate and maintain these behaviors that are called the eight risk/need factors that are identified in meta-analysis studies; these are criminal history, procriminal attitudes, procriminal associates, antisocial personality patterns, family/marital, school/work, substance misuse, leisure/recreation. These factors are associated with the decision to engage in criminal conduct (rewards/cost favorable to crime), mediated by four factors (called the big four) that come from family, neighborhood, gender, age, and ethnicity [27].

Within developmental criminology, there has been a priority in the study of risk and protective factors in adolescents, possibly due to the minimum age of juvenile criminal responsibility that, in most countries, coincides with this stage of the life cycle. Childhood is receiving less attention in research, which, from a life course perspective, spans from birth to 12 years of age [28]; however, evidence indicates that persistent transgressive behaviors often begin early and increase at age 12. Farrington [29] warns that children exhibiting transgressive behaviors in childhood or adolescence tend to develop criminal behaviors in adulthood, making childhood a critical unit of analysis for timely intervention.

Children are not criminally responsible until the minimum age of criminal responsibility established in each country, and they require different treatment than adults focused on protection [30], but few studies describe the factors involved when illicit behavior begins at early ages (between four and seven years), the period in which these behaviors tend to begin [26]. Identifying early biopsychosocial mechanisms could help prevent children from starting a trajectory of chronic antisocial behavior that continues into adulthood [31].

Therefore, it is crucial to understand the risk and protective factors underlying children's social behaviors, as these could predict and antisocial or prosocial behavior. These factors include individual characteristics and the social environment in which children develop, with the family being the primary reference, along with friends, school, and society [25,32].

Risk factors include a conflicting and disorganized bond between the child and caregivers, discipline techniques applied by caregivers, having friends involved in delinquency, and certain individual psychological and moral factors acquired and developed in childhood that may relate to social adaptation [25,33]. However, despite exposure to the same risk factors, some children do not develop criminal behavior due to individual and environmental variables that function as protective factors against severe cumulative events and stressful situations. These protective factors refer to individual characteristics and the family or community context that can mitigate the effect of risk factors, increasing resilience and preventing the development or persistence of such behaviors [25]. One such factor is guilt related to morality, which reinforces self-control in high-criminal temptation scenarios [33].

Taking the above into account, focusing on children is crucial due to their greater capacity for change and flexibility. Most individuals with persistent criminal behavior began their activities at an early age, closely related to developmental contexts [25]. Observing risk and protective factors allows us to design interventions that prevent social adjustment problems in children from becoming more complex by maintaining the transgression of social norms [9,34].

The factors identified by developmental criminology can be organized according to the theory of ecological systems [35], which proposes that human behavior is understood in a dynamic relationship with other systems, distinguishing from the close ones (microsystem) to the most distant ones (macrosystem, exosystem) [36]; classifying them from this point of view could contribute to understanding the criminal behavior of children and adolescents considering the contexts, situation, and social position. In addition, it is possible to consider individual resources, community, and social needs and the articulations between systems. Behavioral changes require a collaborative effort between different systems of which children, adolescents, and adults responsible for care and interventions will have less or more control, so it is possible to assess which elements are under the one domain of children and those who accompany their development (family, school, health, and justice systems, among other systems), as well as factors that cannot be addressed immediately and that require long-term structural change. Classifying the risk and protective factors described in the updated literature from the perspective of developmental criminology and considering the person and transactions with the context (Person-Process-Context-Time Model of Development) or what Sheldon calls "Develecology," such as "the study of the processes of development of organisms and their changing relations with their environments, employing a combination of systemic and longitudinal perspectives that include the mutual and reciprocal transactions of organism and context" [37], could lead to reflection about when to intervene, the social systems involved, and how they are articulated. If the models proposed from criminology dialogue with the current systemic health and educational models, it would be possible to advance in multisystemic, comprehensive, and collaborative interventions between different agents, since the justice system by itself will not be able to solve the social problem of crime in childhood and youth [35].

Given the complexity of addressing crime in childhood, the objective of this study arises: to analyze the existing updated empirical studies on psychosocial factors in developmental, risk, and protection criminology in relation to crime in childhood and then classify them according to the ecological model. The specific objectives are: 1. Describe the articles found by country, year of publication, and methodology; 2. Identify the protective and risk factors in the analyzed texts; 3. Categorize protective and risk factors at systemic levels: individual, interpersonal, and contextual; 4. Identify early behavioral factors, from birth to 7 years, reporting on updated literature.

2. Materials and Methods

This research is a systematic review, which involves summarizing evidence by one or more experts on a specific topic, identifying, evaluating, and synthesizing it to answer a particular question and draw conclusions from the collected data [38]. In this study, an analysis is conducted on psychosocial factors related to criminality in children, selected under predefined inclusion and exclusion criteria.

To ensure the validity and quality of the systematic review, the PRISMA methodology was used (Preferred Reporting Items for Systematic Reviews and Meta-Analyses). Yepes-Núñez et al. [39] in "PRISMA 2020 Statement: An Updated Guideline for Reporting Systematic Reviews" indicated that the PRISMA Statement has been developed for systematic reviews to assess the effects of health interventions regardless of the design of the selected studies. It is noteworthy that PRISMA 2020 can be applied to original, updated, or continuously updated systematic reviews.

2.1. Study Selection

A bibliographic search was conducted during October and November 2023, selecting empirical quantitative and qualitative scientific articles from indexed journals that indicate psychosocial factors in children, as reported in the literature from 2017 to 2023. For the systematic review, the following elements were included:

("Developmental criminology" OR "life course criminology") AND ("risk factors" OR "protect factor" OR "protective factors").

And for EBSCOhost:

Developmental criminology OR life course criminology AND protective factors OR risk factors.

2.2. Inclusion and Exclusion Criteria

This systematic review includes articles published in popular science journals. Articles from the following databases are considered: SCIELO, SCOPUS, Web of Science, PubMed, and EBSCOhost, from those open access repositories in English, Portuguese, and Spanish. Articles were included whose study subjects belonged to the age group of 1 to 12 years. Empirical methodology articles related to the topic and published between 2017 and 2023 were included due to the need for updated information on psychosocial factors. The exclusion criteria exclude articles not related to the topic, articles that are not open access in languages other than English, Portuguese, and Spanish, as well as books, press articles, essays, theses, reports, opinion columns, and conference papers. The filters applied in the search databases are empirical studies, the year range from 2017 to 2023, language as indicated in the inclusion criteria, and open access articles. The selection and data collection process conforms to the PRISMA model and is organized in the following steps: 1. A search for articles is carried out in SCIELO, SCOPUS, Web of Science, PubMed, and EBSCOhost. 2. One researcher reviewed the articles from each database, totaling five researchers, one for each database. 3. All researchers use the same ad hoc instrument, an Excel database, where each sheet corresponds to an inclusion criterion. In a systematic and sequential manner, it is possible to reach the results. This standardized procedure helps reduce bias in the results and ensures reliability.

3. Results

The systematic review results can be seen in Figure 1. After applying the exclusion criteria, 24 articles were reviewed, allowing us to respond to our objectives.

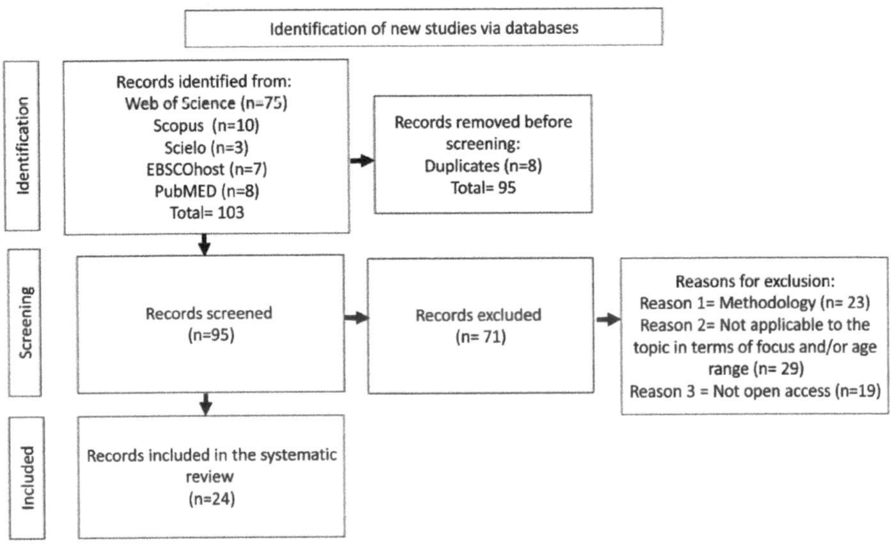

Figure 1. Search identification flow diagram. Based on the PRISMA Statement.

3.1. Article Characterization

Regarding the methodology, 23 of the selected articles have a quantitative approach, and one article employs a mixed-method approach. Concerning the design, 22 articles are longitudinal, and two are cross-sectional. Among the analyzed articles, 50% use a database of male participants, 42% are mixed, and 8% are female only.

The geographical distribution of the reviewed studies shows that 13 are from North America, with 11 from the USA and 2 from Canada. Only one study is from Latin America (Brazil).

In terms of publication years, the distribution is as follows: seven articles from 2021; five from 2020; four from 2019; four from 2017; and one each from 2018, 2022, and 2023.

3.2. Contents of the Selected Articles

To address the proposed objectives, the 24 selected articles are organized into content trees for each systemic level of analysis: individual, interpersonal, and contextual. Bronfenbrenner's ecological theory is used as a basis for categorization, with the individual level being everything related to the child's characteristics (Figure 2), while the interpersonal and contextual (Figure 3) encompass the microsystem and mesosystem (family, peers/school), in addition to the exosystem and macrosystem (community/wider environment). Each tree includes protective and risk factors in childhood with respect to delinquency according to updated literature on developmental criminology.

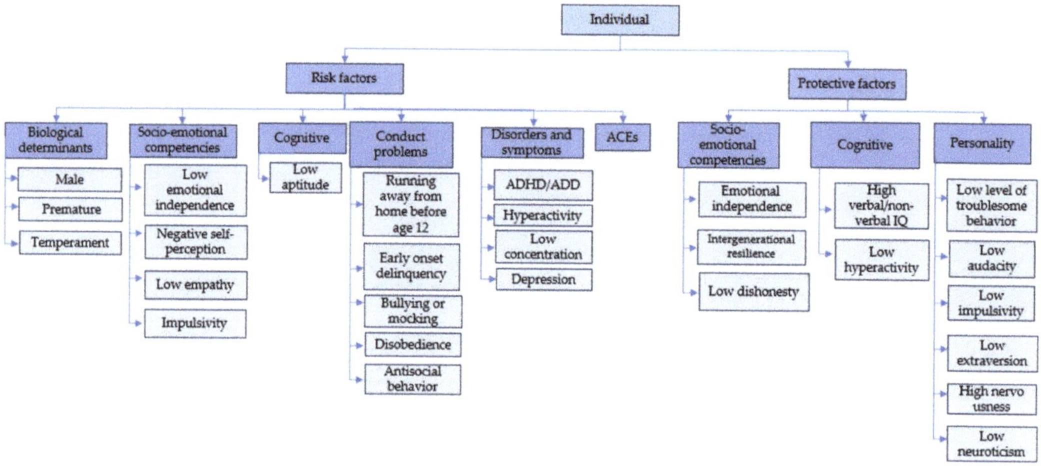

Figure 2. Individual-level content.

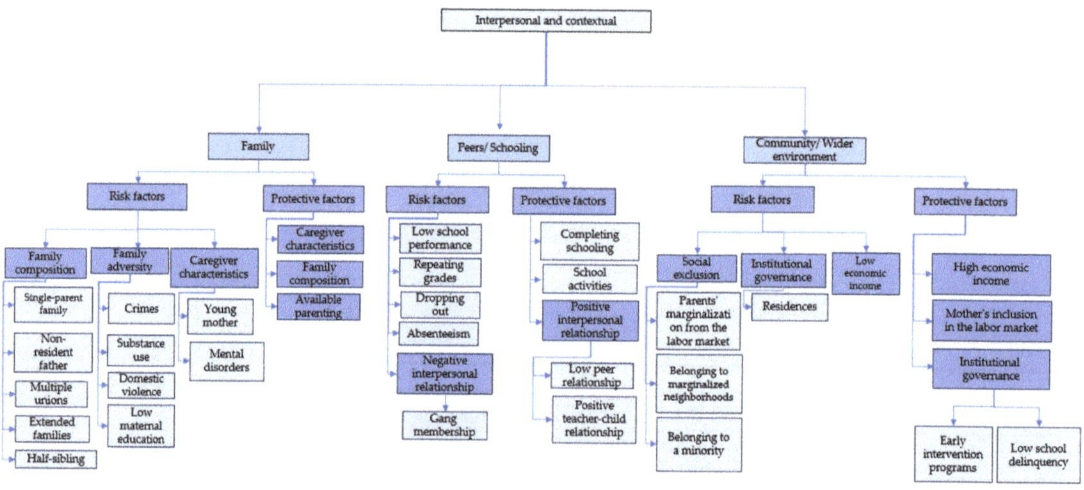

Figure 3. Interpersonal and contextual-level content.

3.2.1. Individual Risk Factors

The individual risk factors reported in the literature include biological determinants, socio-emotional competencies, cognitive factors, conduct problems, psychopathological disorders and symptoms, and adverse childhood experiences (see Figure 2).

In the category of biological determinants, Van Hazebroek et al. [40] mention that being male is associated with antisocial behaviors and higher recidivism in serious violent and chronic (SVC) crimes [41]. Herrera and Stuewig [42] also note that being male is a risk factor, especially when interrelated with other components such as witnessing spousal violence (for adolescent delinquency) or living in violent contexts with substance use. Regarding preterm birth, Givens and Reid [43] link it to early-onset delinquency. Additionally, temperament, specifically "hyperreactivity" and a "short temper," increases the likelihood of SVC infractions in adulthood [41]. Neuroticism is also identified as a risk factor for the development of chronic persistent delinquency, characterized by younger age at first conviction and longer criminal careers [44].

The socio-emotional competencies category highlights low emotional independence from an incarcerated father and negative self-perception as risk factors. The former facilitates intergenerational continuities in crime [41], while the latter increases the likelihood of developing RORD and slow-rising chronic (SRC) delinquent trajectories [45]. Impulsivity, referring to low self-control, can lead to antisocial behaviors [46,47]. Low empathy is linked to sexual crimes in adolescence [48].

Cognitive factors include low aptitude, referring to low verbal and non-verbal IQ, which is an early risk characteristic for delinquency [44,46,49].

Conduct problems refer to early behaviors that are indicators of the possible development of the disorder in its entirety [50]. Gushue et al. [45] mention that running away from home before age 12 increases the likelihood of quickly engaging in and desisting from delinquency (Rapid Onset Rapid Desistance, RORD).

Early-onset delinquency is another critical factor. Authors such as Han and Park [51] and Wolff [41] indicate that delinquent behaviors in childhood increase the risk of lifelong delinquency. Solomon et al. [52] identify bullying, mocking others, and disobedience as factors that can lead to antisocial behaviors in adulthood. Koegl et al. [53] and Solomon et al. [52] also mention that such behaviors in children are related to delinquency in adolescence and adulthood.

The category of disorders and symptoms refers to psychopathological indicators. Rosa et al. [48] mention that attention deficit hyperactivity disorder (ADHD) is linked to nonsexual crimes. Solomon et al. [52] and Whitten et al. [44] indicate that low concentration levels and hyperactivity are predictors of persistent delinquency, understood as those with older age at first conviction but longer criminal careers. Depression also influences serious crimes in both women and men [42].

Finally, adverse childhood experiences (ACEs) can act as risk factors according to Craig et al. [54]. The study indicates that the more ACEs a child has, the more likely they are to commit crimes in late adulthood. However, the number of ACEs was not predictive in women with SVC crimes [41].

3.2.2. Individual Protective Factors

The factors are divided into socio-emotional competencies. Socio-emotional competencies include high emotional independence from incarcerated parents [41], low dishonesty [53], and intergenerational resilience in children. Intergenerational resilience refers to a reduction in crime across generations within the same family, mediated by various protective elements that manifest in each age group. However, since it is a recent concept, it lacks detailed factors mediating its appearance [55].

Concerning cognitive factors, Craig et al. [54] and Capaldi et al. [56] indicate that high verbal IQ (vocabulary and reading) significantly reduces the likelihood of delinquency in males. This factor, along with low hyperactivity, also protects against ACEs [56].

Finally, in terms of personality, Craig et al. [54] identify low troublesome behavior, described as "being unproblematic", as a protective factor against delinquency. Additional elements that significantly reduce the risk of committing a crime include low audacity, low impulsivity, low extraversion, high nervousness, and low neuroticism [54].

3.2.3. Family Risk Factors

Family composition factors identified as risk factors include single-parent families, non-resident fathers, having half-siblings, and multiple maternal unions before childbirth, with the most prevalent factor being a non-resident father [52]. Criminality increases with the number of these components in the family [52]. Basto-Pereira and Farrington [49] identify that extended family, along with other factors, can predict the criminal behaviors of the "serious and persistent versatile" group, characterized mainly by committing violent and, to a lesser extent, minor crimes. Finally, Whitten et al. [44] indicate that this risk element, along with high audacity, predicts chronic criminal behaviors.

The authors report a set of situations related to family adversity (see Figure 3). Having a convicted father influences the appearance of chronic persistent delinquency [44]. Similarly, Han and Park [51] indicate that substance use by caregivers is a risk component related to early alcohol and drug use in children.

Family violence and spousal violence are significant factors. Herrera and Stuewig [42] indicate that both are related to delinquency in adolescence, as minors are socialized to imitate behaviors that transgress social limits. Low maternal education (less than nine years of completed schooling) [52], child maltreatment as corporal punishment [57,58], severe or authoritarian parenting, and discipline [58] are predictors of delinquency from childhood to adolescence. Farrington [58] also mentions that caregiver neglect, understood as low parental involvement in their children's education, is an indicator for persistent delinquency. Similarly, Whitten et al. [44] indicate that low supervision over children's whereabouts and actions predicts longer criminal careers. Martins et al. [59] report that low stimulation in children under four correlates with the manifestation of violent crimes.

Regarding sexual abuse, Rosa et al. [48] link childhood sexual abuse to the early onset of sexual delinquency.

Regarding caregiver characteristics, Solomon et al. [52] and Basto-Pereira and Farrington [46] identify young mothers as a risk component, predicting minor crimes. Martins et al. [59] indicate that mothers with mental disorders influence the appearance of violent crimes.

3.2.4. Family Protective Factors

Family protective factors include caregiver characteristics, such as the older age of the mother; family composition, which refers to reduced family sizes; and available parenting, which points to high parental interest in education. Craig et al. [54] indicate that these elements are associated with a lower prevalence of committing crimes between the ages of 10 and 56. Reduced family sizes and/or older parents significantly reduce criminal behaviors [54].

3.2.5. Peers/Schooling Risk Factors

Regarding schooling, studies such as Koegl et al. [53] indicate that low academic performance is related to future antisocial behavior. Similarly, Basto-Pereira and Farrington [49] identify low academic achievement as a predictor. Whitten et al. [44] also highlight low performance and interrupted schooling trajectories, which are linked to chronic delinquency characterized by shorter criminal careers but with a higher number of crimes and convictions. Additionally, youths who repeated grades three times and/or dropped out of school were twice as likely to commit violent crimes [59]. School absenteeism in women also constitutes a risk factor [45].

Educational environments with high crime rates and the development of links with delinquent peers are mentioned [51], representing a short-term risk for criminal behavior.

Peer risk factors include negative interpersonal relationships—for example, gang membership is linked to delinquent trajectories in incarcerated youth [60] and women in juvenile residences with SVC delinquency [41].

3.2.6. Peers/Schooling Protective Factors

Regarding schooling, completing education, even with grade repetition, serves as a protective element by preventing the development of violent and nonviolent criminal careers [59], predominantly in males [54]. School activities are also protective against substance use in children [51].

Peer protective factors include positive interpersonal relationships, such as low peer relationships [54]. A positive relationship between teacher and child is also significant, allowing for the development of positive affection and the construction of healthy interactions with peers [57].

3.2.7. Community Risk Factors

Community risk factors include social exclusion, comprising three aspects (see Figure 3): exclusion from the labor market for both parents [52], belonging to marginalized neighborhoods, and minorities that may be racial, ethnic, or gender-based [40].

Regarding institutional governance, authors such as Yang et al. [60] and Valdivia-Devia et al. [61] indicate that attending residences reduces the possibility of experiencing positive turning points. Finally, low economic income, defined as situations where none of the child's parents or caregivers receive a work income [52].

3.2.8. Community Protective Factors

Community protective factors including high economic income, which includes the mother's inclusion in the labor market, is another protective factor [54].

Children exposed to higher risk factors who do not engage in delinquency tend to have few friends. In terms of governance and institutionalization, early multicomponent intervention programs [18] promote prosocial behaviors and prevent problematic behaviors. Finally, Craig et al. [54] identify a low school crime rate as a protective factor.

The last specific objective raises the need to identify factors before the age of 7. Few studies have been found, with the following being noted: antisocial behaviors, physical aggression, noncompliance with rules, low child responsiveness, high hyperactivity, and impulsiveness.

4. Discussion

This study aimed to analyze existing empirical studies on psychosocial factors in the field of developmental criminology, such as risk and protective factors related to crime in children, incorporating an ecological perspective. As a result of the review, 24 updated articles were identified. The factors in each of the reviewed texts are categorized into different levels: individual, interpersonal, and contextual. These are visualized in Figures 2 and 3.

The review shows that crime in childhood is a complex phenomenon, influenced by several factors throughout the life cycle [13]. Developmental criminology studies highlight this complexity by providing a longitudinal view of various areas of child development, allowing individual, relational, and contextual aspects to be considered to understand criminal behavior. From this perspective, children who exhibit delinquent behavior in childhood or adolescence are more likely to engage in delinquency in adulthood [29], making childhood an opportune time to intervene.

Risk factors usually act early, and some disruptive behaviors manifest before the age of seven, such as antisocial behavior, physical aggression, noncompliance with rules, low child responsiveness, high hyperactivity, and impulsivity [43,44,53,61]. Various studies highlight childhood and its care context as critical points for the possible development of criminal behavior in adolescence and/or adulthood [62–67].

Proposing interventions involves establishing conducive care and attention environments for children that promptly and adequately address behavioral problems in childhood. However, the child's context is socially conditioned by a culture that does not emphasize care [68]. Given that young people who exhibit criminal behavior often come from vulnerable contexts and experience childhood victimization, it is understood that the cycle of violence does not occur in a vacuum [69–72].

A systematic analysis of the updated literature reveals a dynamic link between several factors identified in the development of criminal behavior. At the community level, risk factors such as labor market exclusion and low income indicate material deprivation and vulnerability [52]. This is connected to the family level, where parental crime [44] and family violence are primary elements within a context of vulnerability. However, this vulnerability is not static, reflecting the possibility of intervention and prevention through economic, labor, and social opportunities that promote contexts of early development and inclusion for children and their families.

Schooling constitutes both a protective and risk factor at individual and community levels. Situations of schooling at the individual level, such as repeating grades [59] and high school crime rates at the community level, relate to developing delinquent behaviors in children [51]. However, schooling can be a significant protective factor when individuals participate in school activities [57] and when there is a low school crime rate [54], as well as when children form meaningful bonds with their teachers. This reflects the importance of strengthening the individual educational experience from an early age while also promoting communication and inclusion of families in the school community.

From this perspective, protective and risk factors at different levels are dynamic conditions in the life history that can become more complex or resolved. To prevent early antisocial behaviors, it is essential to observe the available evidence, generate research from an evolutionary and systemic approach, and consider the experiences, learnings, and contexts in which children develop. It is also crucial for justice actors to prevent actions reported in the literature that could result in victimization and risk factors, such as institutionalization as a protection measure. Its application should be exceptional and not preferred, as living in residences or foster homes constitutes a significant risk factor for chronic crimes despite exposure to other risk factors [60].

The literature indicates that an important protective factor is working from early childhood to promote prosocial actions through activities that include the entire family unit. Parenting styles significantly influence the socio-emotional and moral development of children and, consequently, the behaviors they will exhibit throughout their lives [33,51]. Intervention and prevention strategies should focus on reducing risk and promoting factors that promote resilience. We believe that an appropriate strategy that is consistent with developmental criminology and evidence is a multisystemic intervention since factors are observed at different levels related to each other and change over time [47].

Although preventive efforts focus on adolescence, they could be more effective if it is recognized that the complexity of crime has its roots in childhood [73] and that it is crucial to address children's adverse experiences in their early stages, as they are related to criminal behavior at later stages of development [74]. This is consistent with Bonta and Andrews [27], who emphasize understanding criminal behavior as the result of a series of factors that require attention and that influence the cost–benefit evaluation that people make when starting and maintaining crime. In the case of childhood, decision-making has its limitations due to the characteristics of children's development and their life contexts, which possibly has a greater influence in the early stages of development due to its relationship with learning. Unlike the eight risk/need factors, this study, by focusing on childhood, allows us to observe other recent elements of importance for children: the presence of adverse childhood experiences, the early appearance of behavioral problems in close environments, and cognitive and affective difficulties. Substance consumption is not yet relevant at this stage; even so, it is logical to think that as children begin and maintain transgressive behaviors, substance consumption can begin constituting a risk factor.

According to the characterization of the articles, there is a lack of research on this approach in Latin America [59]. It is necessary to investigate the nuances for Latin America, considering that studies carried out on adolescents in Brazil [59] and Chile establish a more active role of family risk factors than in Anglo-Saxon studies [75–77]. Furthermore, the samples focus mainly on men, although social factors may act differently in girls and boys; this requires further studies [41,42].

Focusing on childhood when studying crime from a complex or integrative and multilevel perspective is essential. Addressing it requires evidence-based actions and a collective commitment from various institutions and social actors to build a society that cares for and respects the rights of children and their families. This study makes it clear that family, school, justice, and health systems should work collaboratively with children and their families when some of the individual, relational, and contextual factors occur, implementing strategies with families to support them socially, if required, so that it is possible to exercise their care functions, without neglecting structural aspects such as poverty, prejudice, stigmatization of minority social groups, neighborhood conditions, and the relationship that families and children build with justice actors.

The results allow us to reflect on the relevance of legislative proposals that aim to reduce the age of criminal responsibility of children in an attempt to prevent criminal behavior; evidence suggests that increasing the severity of penalties is not an effective method to prevent crimes, and if the crime rate committed by adolescents increases, the severity of sanctions will also increase, causing a downward spiral phenomenon. Studies have shown that incentives can work better than punitive measures. Therefore, timely detection of risk factors that facilitate children's criminal behavior is essential for effective prevention [41]. Solutions to juvenile delinquency should focus on promoting research to deepen the understanding of this phenomenon and implementing preventive mechanisms based on such research findings, rather than toughening sanctions.

This systematic review covers studies from a limited time period, reviewing only articles from 2017 to 2023, consideredupdated evidence in the population of children involved in criminal behavior. However, this may leave out relevant evidence prior to 2017. Additionally, certain languages are included in this review, excluding studies that do not meet the inclusion criteria. This is a limitation of our study because research in other languages and other age groups, older than 12 years, may be left out of this review. Future systematic review studies could address gender differences, articles from previous years, and incorporating other languages and theoretical perspectives.

Author Contributions: Conceptualization, D.Z.; methodology, D.Z.; validation, D.Z., M.C., E.C., C.G., I.G. and C.M.; formal analysis, D.Z. and F.C.; investigation, D.Z., F.C., M.C., E.C., C.G., I.G. and C.M.; writing—original draft preparation, D.Z., F.C., M.C., E.C., C.G., I.G. and C.M.; writing—review and editing, D.Z. and F.C. All authors have read and agreed to the published version of the manuscript.

Funding: This research was funded by the Agencia Nacional de Investigación y Desarrollo (ANID) of the Chilean government, FONDECYT Project N° 11240951 "factores criminológicos y victimológicos vinculados al comportamiento delictivo en la infancia y su relación con las prácticas del tribunal de familia", with director Daniela Zúñiga Silva; and by FONDECYT Project N° 1221075 "Estudio histórico-jurídico sobre la ejecución de las pensiones de alimentos para niños, niñas y adolescentes, de cara a su adecuada compresión, aplicación y reforma en la justicia de familia chilena", director Francesco Carretta Muñoz.

Institutional Review Board Statement: Not applicable.

Informed Consent Statement: Not applicable.

Data Availability Statement: All data are included in the article or in the tables.

Conflicts of Interest: The authors declare no conflicts of interest.

References

1. De la Peña, M.; Gómez, J. Agresión y conducta antisocial en la adolescencia: Una integración conceptual. *Psicopatología Clínica Leg. Y Forense* **2006**, *6*, 9–24.
2. Milano, W. Entre la psicología criminal, la psicología forense y la psicología penitenciaria. *Cienc. Digit.* **2019**, *3*, 23–39. [CrossRef]
3. Verde, M.; Roca, D. *Psicología Criminal*; Cañizal, A., Bazaco, E., Eds.; Pearson Prentice Hall. Madrid, Spain, 2006; ISBN 978-84-8322-306-2.
4. Vázquez, C. *Delincuencia Juvenil. Consideraciones Penales y Criminologías*; Colex: Madrid, Spain, 2003.
5. Carreón, W. Criminología del Desarrollo: Estudio del Desarrollo en la Formación de la Conducta Criminal. *Ratio Juris UNAULA* **2023**, *18*, 3–22. [CrossRef]
6. McGee, T.; Farrington, D. Developmental and Life-Course Explanations of Offending. *Psychol. Crime Law* **2018**, *25*, 609–625. [CrossRef]
7. Farrington, D.; Ttofi, M.; Piquero, A. Risk, promotive, and protective factors in youth offending: Results from the Cambridge study in delinquent development. *J. Crim. Justice* **2016**, *45*, 63–70. [CrossRef]
8. Loeber, R.; Farrington, D.; Waschbusch, D. *Serious and Violent Juvenile Offenders: Risk Factors and Successful Interventions*; Loeber, R., Farrington, D., Eds.; Thousand Oaks: Washington, DC, USA, 1998; pp. 313–345, ISBN 978-14-5224-374-0.
9. Moffitt, T. Adolescence limited and life-course-persistent antisocial behavior: A developmental taxonomy. *Psychol. Rev.* **1993**, *100*, 674–701. [CrossRef] [PubMed]

10. Farrington, D. *The School Years: Current Issues in the Socialization of Young People Chapter 6: Juvenile Delinquency*, 2nd ed.; Coleman, J., Ed.; Routledge: London, UK, 1992; pp. 123–163, ISBN 9780415061704.
11. Farrington, D. Criminal career research in the United Kingdom. *Br. J. Criminol.* **1992**, *32*, 521–536. [CrossRef]
12. Le Blanc, M.; Trudeau Le Blanc, P. La Réadaptation de l'Adolescent Antisocial: Un Programme Cognitivo-Emotivo-Comportemental. Presses de l'Université de Montréal: Montreal, QC, Canada, 2014; ISBN 9782760633537.
13. Farrington, D.; Kazemian, L.; Piquero, A. *The Oxford Handbook of Developmental and Life-Course Criminology*; Oxford University Press: Oxford, UK, 2019; ISBN 9780190201388.
14. Sampson, R.; Laub, J. Life-Course and Developmental Criminology: Looking back, moving forward. ASC Division of Developmental and Life-Course Criminology inaugural David P. Farrington lecture, 2017. *J. Dev. Life-Course Criminol.* **2020**, *6*, 158–171. [CrossRef]
15. McAra, L.; McVie, S. *Developmental and Life-Course Criminology: Innovations, Impacts, and Applications, 6th ed*; Liebling, A., Maruna, S., McAra, L., Eds.; Oxford University Press: Oxford, UK, 2017; ISBN 9780190201371.
16. McGee, T.; Farrington, D. *Handbook of Criminological Theory*; Piquero, A., Ed.; Wiley-Blackwell: Chinchester, UK, 2016; pp. 336–354, ISBN 978-0190201371.
17. Farrington, D. *Integrated Developmental and Life-Course Theories of Offending: Advances in Criminological Theory*; Farrington, D., Ed.; Transaction Publisher: New York, NY, USA, 2005; Volume 4, pp. 73–92, ISBN 9871412807999.
18. Catalano, R.; Hawkins, J.; Kosterman, R.; Bailey, J.; Oesterle, S.; Cambron, C.; Farrington, D. Applying the social development model in middle childhood to promote healthy development: Effects from primary school through the 30s and across generations. *J. Dev. Life-Course Criminol.* **2021**, *7*, 66–86. [CrossRef]
19. Moffitt, T. Life-course persistent versus adolescence limited antisocial behavior. In *Developmental Psychopathology*; Cicchetti, D., Cohen, D., Eds.; Wiley: Hoboken, NJ, USA, 2006; pp. 570–598. [CrossRef]
20. Sampson, R.; Laub, J. Desistance from crime over the life course. In *Handbook of the Life Course*; Springer: Boston, MA, USA, 2003; pp. 295–309. [CrossRef]
21. Wikström, P.; Treiber, K. What drives persistent offending? The neglected and unexplored role of the social environment. In *The Development of Persistent Criminality*; Savage, J., Ed.; Oxford University Press: Oxford, UK, 2009; pp. 389–420, ISBN 9780190295004.
22. Wikström, P.; Treiber, K. The Dynamics of Change: Criminogenic Interactions and Life-Course Patterns in Crime. In *The Oxford Handbook of Developmental and Life-Course Criminology*; Farrington, D., Kazemian, L., Piquero, A., Eds.; Oxford University Press: Oxford, UK, 2019; pp. 272–294.
23. Thornberry, T.; Krohn, M. Applying Interactional Theory to the explanation of continuity and change in antisocial behaviour. In *Integrated Developmental and Life-Course Theories of Offending*; Farrington, D., Ed.; Transaction Publishers: Piscataway, NJ, USA, 2005; pp. 183–209.
24. Thornberry, T.; Krohn, M. Interactional Theory. In *The Oxford Handbook of Developmental and Life-Course Criminology*; Farrington, D., Kazemian, L., Piquero, A., Eds.; Oxford University Press: Oxford, UK, 2019; pp. 248–271.
25. Vásquez, C. Predicción y prevención de la delincuencia juvenil según las teorías del desarrollo social (social development theories). *Rev. Derecho* **2003**, *14*, 135–158.
26. Requena, L. *Principios Generales de Criminología del Desarrollo y las Carreras Criminales*; JM Bosch: Cataluna, Spain, 2014; pp. 11–104.
27. Bonta, J.; Andrews, D.A. *The Psychology of Criminal Conduct*; Routledge: New York, NY, USA, 2016.
28. Faas, A.E. *Psicología del Desarrollo de la Niñez*; Editorial Brujas: Córdoba, Argentina, 2018; pp. 13–417.
29. Farrington, D. The Development of Offending and Antisocial Behavior from Childhood: Key Findings from the Cambridge Study in Delinquent Development. *J. Child Psychol Psychiat* **1995**, *360*, 929–964. [CrossRef]
30. Schneider, F. Measuring the Size and Development of the Shadow Economy. Can the Causes be Found and the Obstacles be Overcome? In *Essays on Economic Psychology*; Brandstätter, H., Güth, W., Eds.; Springer: Berlin/Heidelberg, Germany, 1994; pp. 193–212.
31. Tremblay, R. Early development of physical aggression and early risk factors for chronic physical aggression in humans. In *Neuroscience of Aggression*; Miczek, K., Meyer-Lindenberg, A.A., Eds.; Springer Publishing: New York, NY, USA, 2014; pp. 315–327.
32. Molinedo-Quílez, M. Factores de riesgo psicosociales en menores infractores. *Rev. Española Sanid. Penit.* **2020**, *22*, 110–118.
33. Maggi, S.; Zaccaria, V.; Breda, M.; Romani, M.; Aceti, F.; Giacchetti, N.; Ardizzone, I.; Sogos, C. A Narrative Review about Prosocial and Antisocial Behavior in Childhood: The Relationship with Shame and Moral Development. *Children* **2022**, *9*, 1556. [CrossRef] [PubMed]
34. Morizot, J. The contribution of temperament and personality traits to criminal and antisocial behavior development and desistance. In *The Development of Criminal and Antisocial Behavior*; Morizot, J., Kazemian, L., Eds.; Springer International Publishing: New York, NY, USA, 2015; pp. 137–165. [CrossRef]
35. Bronfenbrenner, U. Ecological systems theory. In *Six Theories of Child Development: Revised Formulations and Current Issues*; Vasta, R., Ed.; Jessica Kingsley: London, UK, 1992; pp. 187–249.
36. April, K.; Schrader, S.W.; Walker, T.E.; Francis, R.M.; Glynn, H.; Gordon, D.M. Conceptualizing juvenile justice reform: Integrating the public health, social ecological, and restorative justice models. *Child. Youth Serv. Rev.* **2023**, *148*, 106–887. [CrossRef]
37. Shelton, L. *The Bronfenbrenner Primer: A Guide to Develecology*; Routledge: New York, NY, USA, 2018.
38. Adolf, S. Utilidad y revisión de literatura. *Rev. Enfermería* **2015**, *9*, 2–13. [CrossRef]

39. Yepes-Nuñez, J.; Urrutia, G.; Romero-García, M.; Alonso-Fernández, S. The PRISMA 2020 statement: An updated guideline for reporting systematic reviews. *Rev. Esp. Cardiol.* **2021**, *74*, 790–799. [CrossRef]
40. Van Hazebroek, B.; Blokland, A.; Wermink, H.; De Keijser, J.; Popma, A.; Van Domburgh, L. Delinquent development among early-onset offenders: Identifying and characterizing trajectories based on frequency across types of offending. *Crim. Justice Behav.* **2019**, *46*, 1542–1565. [CrossRef]
41. Wolff, K.; Baglivio, M.; Vaughn, M.; DeLisi, M.; Piquero, A. For males only? The search for serious, violent, and chronic female juvenile offenders. *J. Dev. Life-Course Criminol.* **2017**, *3*, 168–195. [CrossRef]
42. Herrera, V.; Stuewig, J. Gender differences in pathways to delinquency: The impact of family relationships and adolescent depression. *J. Dev. Life-Course Criminol.* **2017**, *3*, 221–240. [CrossRef]
43. Givens, E.; Reid, J. Developmental Trajectories of Physical Aggression and Nonaggressive Rule-Breaking During Late Childhood and Early Adolescence. *Crim. Justice Behav.* **2019**, *46*, 395–414. [CrossRef]
44. Whitten, T.; McGee, T.; Homel, R.; Farrington, D.; Ttofi, M. Comparing the Criminal Careers and Childhood Risk Factors of Persistent, Chronic, and Persistent- Chronic Offenders. *Aust. N. Z. J. Criminol.* **2019**, *52*, 151–173. [CrossRef]
45. Gushue, K.; Mccuish, E.; Corrado, R. Developmental Offending Patterns: Female Offending Beyond the Reference Category. *Crim. Justice Behav.* **2021**, *48*, 139–156. [CrossRef]
46. Basto-Pereira, M.; Farrington, D. Lifelong conviction pathways and self-reported offending: Towards a Deeper comprehension of criminal career development. *Br. J. Criminol.* **2020**, *60*, 285–302. [CrossRef]
47. Fox, B.; Kortright, K.; Gill, L.; Oramas, D.; Moule, R.; Verona, E. Heterogeneity in the Continuity and Change of Early and Adult Risk factor Profiles of Incarcerated Individuals: A latent Transition Analysis. *Youth Violence Juv. Justice* **2021**, *19*, 68–93. [CrossRef]
48. Rosa, M.; Fox, B.; Jennings, W. Do Developmental and Life-Course Theory Risk Factors Equally Predict Age of Onset Among Juvenile Sexual and Nonsexual Offenders? *Sex. Abus.* **2020**, *32*, 55–78. [CrossRef] [PubMed]
49. Basto-Pereira, M.; Farrington, D. Advancing knowledge about lifelong crime sequences. *Br. J. Criminol.* **2019**, *59*, 354–377. [CrossRef]
50. Asociación Americana de Psiquiatría. *Manual Diagnóstico y Estadístico de los Trastornos Mentales (DSM-5®)*, 5th ed.; Asociación Americana de Psiquiatría: Arlington, VA, USA; Madrid, España, 2014.
51. Han, S.; Park, Y. Which risk factors plays the most critical role for delinquent behavior? Examining integrated cognitive antisocial potencial theory. *Crime Delinq.* **2023**, *69*, 1947–1972. [CrossRef]
52. Solomon, S.; Savolainen, J.; Mason, W.; Miettunen, J.; January, S.; Järvelin, M. Does educational marginalization mediate the path from childhood cumulative risk to criminal offending? *J. Dev. Life-Course Criminol.* **2017**, *3*, 326–346. [CrossRef] [PubMed]
53. Koegl, C.; Farrington, D.; Augimeri, L. Predicting Future Criminal Convictions of Children Under Age 12 Using the Early Assessment Risk Lists. *J. Dev. Life-Course Criminol.* **2021**, *7*, 17–40. [CrossRef]
54. Craig, J.; Piquero, A.; Farrington, D.; Ttofi, M. A little early risk goes a long bad way: Adverse childhood experiences and life-course offending in the Cambridge study. *J. Crim. Justice* **2017**, *53*, 34–45. [CrossRef]
55. Thornberry, T. Intergenerational Patterns in Offending: Lessons from the Rochester Intergenerational study-ASC Division of Developmental and Life Course Criminology David P. Farrington Lecture, 2019. *J. Dev. Life-Course Criminol.* **2020**, *6*, 381–397. [CrossRef] [PubMed]
56. Capaldi, D.; Wiesner, M.; Kerr, D.; Owen, L.; Tiberio, S. Intergenerational associations in crime for an at-risk sample of US men: Factors that may mitigate or exacerbate transmission. *J. Dev. Life-Course Criminol.* **2021**, *7*, 331–358. [CrossRef]
57. Neaverson, A.; Murray, A.; Ribeaud, D.; Eisner, M. Disrupting the Link Between Corporal Punishment Exposure and Adolescent Aggression: The Role of Teacher- child Relationships. *J. Youth Adolesc.* **2022**, *51*, 2265–2280. [CrossRef] [PubMed]
58. Farrington, D. Childhood Risk Factors for Criminal Career Duration: Comparisons with Prevalence, Onset, Frequency and Recidivism. *Crim. Behav. Ment. Health* **2020**, *30*, 159–171. [CrossRef] [PubMed]
59. Martins, R.; Gonçalves, H.; Blumenberg, C.; Könsgen, B.; Houvèssou, G.; Carone, C.; Murray, J. School performance and young adult crime in a Brazilian birth cohort. *J. Dev. Life-Course Criminol.* **2022**, *8*, 647–668. [CrossRef]
60. Yang, J.; McCuish, E.; Corrado, R. Is the Foster Care-Crime Relationship a Consequence of Exposure? Examining Potential Moderating Factors. *Youth Violence Juv. Justice* **2021**, *19*, 94–112. [CrossRef]
61. Valdivia-Devia, M.; Oyanedel, J.; Andrés-Pueyo, A. Trayectoria y reincidencia criminal. *Rev. Crim.* **2018**, *60*, 251–267.
62. Andolfi, M. El niño consultante. *Cah. Crit. Ther. Fam. Prat. Réseaux* **2001**, *2*, 99–116.
63. Barudy, J. *Dolor Invisible de la Infancia*; Paidós: Barcelona, Spain, 1998.
64. Ortega, B.; Jimeno, M.V.; Topino, E.; Latorre, J.M. Direct and indirect childhood victimization and their influence on the development of adolescents antisocial behaviors. *Psychol. Trauma Theory Res. Pract. Policy* **2023**, *16*, 72–80. [CrossRef]
65. Chopin, J.; Fortin, F.; Paquette, S. Childhood victimization and poly-victimization of online sexual offenders: A developmental psychopathology perspective. *Child Abus. Negl.* **2022**, *129*, 105–659. [CrossRef]
66. Wolff, K.T.; Cuevas, C.; Intravia, J.; Baglivio, M.T.; Epps, N. The effects of neighborhood context on exposure to adverse childhood experiences (ACE) among adolescents involved in the juvenile justice system: Latent classes and contextual effects. *J. Youth Adolesc.* **2018**, *47*, 2279–2300. [CrossRef] [PubMed]
67. Miley, L.; Fox, B.; Muniz, C.; Perkins, R.; DeLisi, M. Does childhood victimization predict specific adolescent offending? An analysis of generality versus specificity in the victim-offender overlap. *Child Abus. Negl.* **2020**, *101*, 2–12. [CrossRef] [PubMed]

68. Hein, A. Factores de riesgo y delincuencia juvenil: Revisión de la literatura nacional e internacional. *Fund. Paz Ciudad.* **2004**, 1–21. Available online: https://pazciudadana.cl/biblioteca/documentos/factores-de-riesgo-y-delincuencia-juvenil-revision-de-la-literatura-nacional-e-internacional/ (accessed on 7 August 2024).
69. Berg, M.; Mulford, C. Reappraising and redirecting research on the victim-offender overlap. *Trauma Violence Abuse.* **2020**, *21*, 16–30. [CrossRef] [PubMed]
70. Kushner, M.; Botchkovar, E.; Antonaccio, O.; Hughes, L. Exploring vulnerability to deviant coping among victims of crime in two Post-Soviet cities. *Justice Q.* **2020**, *38*, 1182–1209. [CrossRef]
71. Kushner, M. Betrayal Trauma and Gender: An Examination of the Victim-Offender Overlap. *J. Interpers. Violence.* **2022**, *37*, NP3750–NP3778. [CrossRef]
72. Da Costa, E.; Faúndes, A.; Nunes, R. The association between victim-offender relationship and the age of children and adolescents who suffer sexual violence: A cross-sectional study. *J. De Pediatr.* **2022**, *98*, 310–315. [CrossRef]
73. Beckley, A.; Caspi, A.; Arseneault, L.; Barnes, J.; Fisher, H.; Harrington, H.; Moffitt, T. The Developmental Nature of the Victim-Offender Overlap. *J. Dev. Life-Course Criminol.* **2017**, *4*, 24–49. [CrossRef]
74. Silva, C.; Moreira, P.; Moreira, D.; Rafael, F.; Rodrigues, A.; Leite, A.; Lopes, S.; Moreira, D. Impact of adverse Childhood Experiences in Young Adults and Adults: A Systematic Literature Review. *Pediatr. Rep.* **2024**, *16*, 461–481. [CrossRef]
75. Alarcón, P.; Luco, R.; Chesta, S.; Wenger, L. Examinando factores de riesgo y recursos para la intervención con adolescentes infractores. In *Psicología Jurídica, Conocimiento y Práctica*; Bringas, C., Novo, M., Eds.; Sociedad Española de Psicología Jurídica y Forense: Sevilla, Spain, 2017; pp. 425–442, ISBN 978-84-8408-326-9.
76. Zambrano, V.; Gemignani, M.; Fernández-Pacheco, G.; Ergas, L. Resiliencia en adolescentes infractores con trayectorias en los sistemas chilenos de bienestar infantil y de justicia adolescente. *Rev. De Estud. Soc.* **2024**, *88*, 59–78. [CrossRef]
77. Maldonado, J.; Garrido, Á.; Henríquez, S. Trayectorias de vida de jóvenes infractores de ley internados y respuesta educativa en el servicio nacional de menores de Chile. *Interciencia* **2022**, *47*, 191–198.

children

MDPI

Article

Parenting in the Face of Trauma: Music Therapy to Support Parent–Child Dyads Affected by War and Displacement

Tamar Hadar

School of Creative Arts Therapies, Faculty of Social Welfare and Health Sciences, University of Haifa, Haifa 3498838, Israel; thadar1@staff.haifa.ac.il

Abstract: Background: The literature highlights the profound psychological impact of war on children, families, and communities, emphasizing the prevalence of Post-Traumatic Stress Disorder (PTSD), anxiety, and other symptoms among affected individuals. Interventions, such as Child-Parent Psychotherapy (CPP) and music therapy, show promise in mitigating trauma effects, underscoring the need for holistic approaches that address familial and community dynamics alongside individual well-being. Methods: Aiming to explore the influences of dyadic music therapy sessions on parents' capacity to support their children, this study involved four families displaced from their home-kibbutz as result of a terrorist attack. All dyads participated in music therapy sessions with a focus on parent–child interactions and trauma processing (CPP informed). Embedded in a qualitative, phenomenological approach, the research utilized interpretative phenomenological analysis (IPA) and micro-analytic methods to explore meaningful moments in the music therapy sessions. Results: Findings identified four central categories: (1) Discovering the child's grounding song: identifying resources; (2) Musical improvisation sets the grounds for parent–child mutual recognition of the child's traumatic experience; (3) Musical performance empowers child and parent; (4) A sense of agency is gained through controlling the musical environment. Conclusions: The significance of restoring the children's freedom of play, the parents' sense of competency, and of enhancing families' capacity to connect to their traumatic experiences through the musical environment is discussed.

Keywords: music therapy; Child-Parent Psychotherapy (CPP); dyadic therapy; trauma; interpretative phenomenology

1. Introduction

1.1. Children Experiencing War and Displacement

A significant body of literature highlights the psychological trauma and post-traumatic stress experienced by children who have been exposed to war [1–5]. Children living in chronic war zones display high rates of Post-Traumatic Stress Disorder (PTSD), anxiety, and other psychological symptoms due to continual exposure to violence and distressing events [6–8]. According to Sagi-Schwartz [7], the impact of war on children is mediated by a combination of risk and protective factors. Factors such as the availability of social support systems, familial relationships, and community cohesiveness play crucial roles in determining the extent of war's debilitating effects on children. The research underscores the importance of understanding these dynamics for creating interventions that foster resilience among children [7].

Pat-Horenczyk et al. [9] found high levels of post-traumatic stress among both children and mothers in Sderot, Israel, due to frequent missile attacks, showcasing the wide-reaching psychological impact of constant conflict exposure on family units. The authors presented an integrative model focusing on clinical services, resilience-building workshops, and enhancing local resources in the community. The model was implemented effectively to address the symptoms and enhance resilience among affected families and educators. Preliminary results showed positive outcomes in reducing symptoms of distress in children and improving coping skills among parents and teachers, highlighting the potential of community and clinical efforts in fostering resilience in conflict-affected populations.

Moreover, the psychosocial consequences of war seem to extend beyond the individual level, to affect family and community systems [9,10]. Studies from Afghanistan and Sri Lanka [3] have established correlations between exposure to war and increased incidents of domestic violence. This interaction suggests the necessity for family- and community-based programs tailored to address the multifaceted impacts of mass trauma. Despite the profound adversities faced, some children develop resilience and find ways to cope with the horrifying experiences.

Bryant et al. [10] revealed the high rates of PTSD among refugee caregivers and its impact on child mental health. The researchers found that 38% of 411 adult caregivers who participated in their study had probable PTSD, which is consistent with other research on refugee populations. The study showed that caregiver PTSD persisted over time and was linked to harsh parenting, which negatively affected children's mental health. This effect was stronger than the direct impact of PTSD on children's emotional problems. The study also highlighted that previous trauma and post-migration stressors contributed to ongoing PTSD and harsh parenting, leading to various psychological issues in children. Understanding the impact of early and overwhelming stress on individuals is crucial because childhood trauma can predispose them to being overwhelmed by stress later in life and may lead to misdiagnosis of stress-related behaviors as conditions like ADHD [11,12]. The influence of trauma and war-induced trauma on parenting practices has been of growing interest in the past decade [10,13,14] and will be explored next.

1.2. Parenting, War and Intergenerational Trauma

The significance of parenting practices as either mitigating or exacerbating the impact of mass trauma on child adjustment was highlighted by different studies [9,10,13–17]. Khamis [18] showed how parental psychological distress served as a mediator in the impact of war on children's emotional and behavioral disorders. Using hierarchal regression analyses, the study demonstrated how trauma exposure and parents' psychological distress predicted the occurrence of disorders in children. In a study focusing on the long-term effect of the 9/11 attacks [19], the authors highlighted not only its influence on parents but the severe psychological effects on their children. In an attempt to mitigate the intergenerational transmission of trauma effects, the authors underscored the child's risk of psychological distress when exposed to a combination of maternal depression and PTSD. This research contributes to the understanding of how very young children, given their developmental stage, are particularly vulnerable to the effects of maternal psychological conditions triggered by extremely stressful events. Additionally, it highlights the necessity of considering the mother–child dyad in the context of trauma exposure and treatment.

An important consequence of war relates not only to parental psychological distress and post-traumatic reactions but to its impact on their parenting practices [14]. Drawing from a wide range of studies, Murphy et al. [14] explored the complex dynamics of family relationships amidst the backdrop of war and explored how war related experiences impacts not only the mental health of parents but also affects their parenting styles, which in turn, influences the psychological and emotional well-being of children. The authors argued that parents exposed to war experiences may undergo significant shifts in their behavior and parenting styles. Such experiences can lead to increased authoritarianism, hesitancy, and withdrawal in how parents interact with their children. Conversely, some mothers, upon facing horrifying events, may become less strict and exercise lower control, thereby affecting the dynamics of mother–child interaction. Ultimately, this study emphasizes the intricate link between war events, parenting, and children's mental health. It advocates for a holistic approach to intervention that considers the entire family system, aiming to mitigate the adverse effects of war trauma across generations. One such holistic, evidence-based and integrative approach to treatment of trauma-induced symptoms is Child-Parent Psychotherapy (CPP).

1.3. Child-Parent Psychotherapy

Child-Parent Psychotherapy is a trauma-informed dyadic intervention model for young children. This model is highlighted as an evidence-based intervention suited for the experiences of children, aiming to restore the child's healthy developmental trajectory following traumatic experiences [20]. In a study examining the efficacy of Child-Parent Psychotherapy (CPP) in reducing symptoms of trauma in both children and their parents who have experienced trauma [21], the authors found a decrease in post-traumatic stress symptomatology (PTSS), indicating that CPP effectively ameliorates trauma symptoms in both population groups. Recent years gave rise to the integration of various art therapy approaches, among them music therapy, within trauma-informed practices [22,23]. We will now examine the distinctive aspects of music therapy that make it an appropriate clinical practice for clients who have experienced traumatic and post-traumatic symptoms.

1.4. Music Therapy in the Context of Trauma

A growing amount of literature delves into the multifaceted role of music therapy in addressing the complex needs of individuals experiencing trauma [2,24,25], including those bearing the weight of transgenerational trauma [26]. Abrams delineates an intimate exploration into how analytical music therapy (AMT) can be harnessed as a therapeutic conduit to navigate and alleviate the deeply ingrained scars of transgenerational trauma. Through reflective vignettes, the paper underscores AMT's potency in facilitating a unique therapeutic space, enabling individuals to confront and therapeutically engage with transgenerational trauma. Several mechanisms underlying musical experiences are associated with the therapeutic effect of music therapy, and are pertinent to trauma-informed practice: relationality in music [24,27]; music-related emotional regulation [25–31]; and communicative musicality [32]. Bensimon [24] expands on the realms of relational needs (RNs) of trauma victims—within a spectrum encompassing recognition, acceptance, emotional witnessing, responsiveness, safety, trust, and outreach, the author elucidates how these pivotal psycho-emotional requirements can be efficaciously addressed within the music therapy milieu. Employing a constructivist methodology, the paper articulates the observed therapeutic mechanism whereby music validates, witnesses, and tactfully engages with the emotional states of trauma victims. Through music therapy, a profound space of emotional safety and understanding is crafted.

Several researchers advocate for the possible role of music intervention in supporting emotional regulation (ER) among clients [29–31]. Sena-Moore and Hanson-Abromeit [31] provide a theoretical rationale for the Therapeutic Function of Music (TFM) Plan, applied to a music-based emotional regulation intervention for preschoolers, known as the Musical Contour Regulation Facilitation (MCRF) intervention. The study suggests that music can effectively address limitations in current verbal and behavioral ER treatments by offering real-time, adult-child interactions that support stress management and emotional regulation through alternating arousal states. As trauma and post-trauma are highly associated with difficulties in emotional regulation [33,34], music-based interventions may be of particular interest when establishing parent–child, trauma-informed protocols.

Another aspect of the music therapy relevant to trauma processing is its non-verbal nature [23,32,35]. As described by Trevarthen and Malloch [32], music can be seen as a basic language that nurtures coordinated interaction and closeness, forming the basis for later verbal communication. When discussing the mechanisms of change underlying music therapy interventions in the treatment of trauma and post-trauma, Bensimon [23] highlights that music, as a sensory stimulus, can bypass linguistic barriers and access unprocessed traumatic memories, allowing clients to express trauma-related super-expressive emotions. Through the process of emotional contagion, the music therapist and client engage in a reciprocal exchange, where the therapist validates the client's emotions, helping to restore empathy and enhance the therapeutic process. The benefit of employing a non-verbal approach for trauma processing becomes even more significant when working with children, as they may find verbal communication difficult or inaccessible as a result of such experiences [36].

1.5. The Current Research

A smaller range of literature deals with the impact of music therapy interventions on childhood and adolescents dealing with the consequences of stressful events (e.g., [2,37]) and even less attention is given to interventions including parents' role in the context of trauma which, when addressed, is predominantly concerned with NICU-induced trauma [38–40]. Music and music therapy approaches have been used to address the needs of adults [25,41] and children [42–44] experiencing war and conflict-induced anxiety and trauma. Inasmuch, there is as yet a dearth of research concerning the significance of including parents in the therapeutic process, in the context of childhood and adolescence trauma. This study aims at shedding some light on the significance of including the child–parent dyad in therapy when dealing with war-induced trauma in a music therapy context. A more integral, holistic approach to childhood trauma, including the role of parents in mediating the traumatic experience and its by-products specifically in the context of war, is missing in the music therapy literature. This study aims at addressing this gap in the literature, by presenting a thematic analysis of four courses of dyadic music therapy provided to families who had experienced displacement for six months, following the deadly attack performed by Hamas on 7 October 2023.

Beyond presenting a music-based approach towards trauma, the current study introduces an ecological and psychobiological approach to therapy, through acknowledging different aspects of the child's being, possibly affected by the distressing experience: the war induced trauma component (i.e., environmental and neural aspect); trauma's possible influence on the child's relations with their care-takers with consideration of child's developmental stage and attachment predisposition [36]; trauma's possible influence on the whole family system; and trauma's influence on the community system as well as on the child's specific peer-group. Throughout the analysis and interpretation of therapy vignettes, the author integrates multiple angles to encompass the various layers of well-being attended through the musical-therapeutic intervention, including the child's changes in the physiological, behavioral, emotional, social, relational, and cognitive realms. Therefore, the author believes that, though originating in a specific, music-based mind-set, this paper can expand clinical thought in new integrative and trans-modal directions when addressing child and youth trauma.

1.6. Research Questions

The research questions guiding this analysis were:

1. What are the salient characteristics of significant moments in parent–child music therapy sessions for dyads who had experienced acute trauma?
2. How can those significant moments be understood in the context of each client's individual course of therapy?
3. How can those significant moments be understood in the context of each client's relationships with their parents?
4. How can those significant moments be understood in light of clients' and families' traumatic narratives?

2. Materials and Methods

2.1. Background and Intervention

The participants in this study included four families who were displaced from their home-kibbutz situated on the Israeli border with Gaza, following Hamas's deadly terror attack on 7 October 2023. The families were relocated to a hosting village in the northern part of Israel. As part of the governmental rehabilitation plan, all families were offered by social services the opportunity to meet with various professionals (e.g., social workers, psychologists and art therapists), to process their traumatic experiences and the consequent displacement, which endured for six months. The author is a music therapist who participated in this plan by initiating a temporary music therapy clinic in the hosting village, offering music therapy sessions for families of young children and adolescents. The author is an experienced music therapist, who also specialized in Child–Parent Psychotherapy.

Most of the families who engaged in the music therapy program were interested in dyadic, i.e., parent–child, meetings, which were encouraged by the therapist, who incorporated a CPP protocol into her approach. However, several families chose to engage only their child in therapy. All families met for parental consultations separately. All the children met for weekly one-hour sessions.

To foster inclusive language and perspectives, the author acknowledges the impact of her cultural background on social science inquiry ([45,46]). As an Israeli, white female studying music and music therapy in Western-oriented institutions, she recognizes the potential for oppressive language and thinking. While this study primarily examines the effects of war and trauma on a specific group affected by a terror attack, the author acknowledges the broader impact of war on all involved parties, hoping that the research findings will benefit anyone experiencing trauma. Throughout the paper, person-first language is used, such as "children who experienced trauma" rather than "traumatized children".

2.2. Participants

Four participants were included in the analysis (see Table 1). The inclusion/exclusion criteria were as follows: (1) families who opted for Child-Parent Therapy instead of individual sessions for the child; (2) the child had no additional diagnoses other than experiencing the traumatic event of the October 7 attack; and (3) the dyad attended a minimum of four therapy sessions.

Table 1. Research Participants.

Name	Gender	Age	# Sessions
Yana	F	13	6
Rani	M	8	16
Sarit	F	10	14
Maya	F	5.5	17

2.3. Research Approach

Embedded in a qualitative, phenomenological school [47,48], this study was informed by both interpretative phenomenological analysis (IPA) approaches in the study of music therapy sessions ([49–51]), as well as micro-analytic methods applied for the analysis of musical and non-musical occurrences within the client–therapist relationship [49,52,53]. Hadar and Amir [50] adapted Forinash and Gonzales's phenomenological method to investigate moments of joint improvisation in music therapy, adapting their multi-stage process into a four-step analysis of meaningful moments. Lee and Mcferran [49] integrated IPA with video micro-analysis, highlighting both the possibility of studying delicate nuances emerging in every session, without leaving out their contextual relationship to the therapy as a whole.

2.4. Procedure

Informed mainly by Hadar and Amir [50] and Lee and McFerran [49], the following steps were applied: (1) Preliminary Data Screening—Congruent with Smith et al. [48], all data included (in this case: the recordings of the sessions) were reviewed thoroughly. The author listened to all recordings of all participants' sessions and indicated moments which revealed themselves as possibly significant to the research foci: parenting and trauma. (2) Understanding the moment—similar to Lee and McFerran [49]'s approach, in this phase, a short narrative was developed around certain moments, which were deemed important and had been marked by the author in the first stage. (3) Understanding the whole—following Lee and McFerran [49], in this stage the moments were contextualized within the bigger picture of the child's course of therapy as unfolded through the author's immersion in the recordings. This step included a first level of meaning induction out of the raw data. (4) Contextualizing the moment in the triadic or dyadic relationships in the room—this part leans on Hadar and Amir [50], who emphasized listening to the relationship in the music in their phenomenological protocol. In this study, the researcher highlighted the possible relational meanings, including both the child–parent relationship, the therapist–child relationship, and the therapist–parent relationship. Although not always present in the room, the role of the parent and their relevance to the moment was highlighted. (5) Contextualizing the moment in the traumatic experience—all moments were revisited in light of the family's traumatic story, and possible interpretations were applied by the therapist-researcher. (6) Integrating parts and whole—following both Hadar and Amir [50] and Lee and McFerran [49], this stage supported the therapist-researcher in consolidating overlapping descriptions from earlier stages into a unified narrative of meaningful dyadic (and triadic) moments. The process of iteratively analyzing parts and wholes directed the therapist-researcher in exploring layers of influences, relating to the trauma as well as to the child–parent relationship, until reaching personal saturation. In this step, the author deployed Corbin and Strauss's (2008) [54] coding method as follows: first, the author used open coding to break down the data into discrete parts, and to examine and compare them for similarities and differences. This phase included developing categories from the narratives created for each client, by assigning labels to chunks of data, such as words, sentences, or paragraphs. These labels represented key concepts or themes emerging from the data. This step was led by the author's research questions, focusing on the possible meanings ascribed to participants' experiences in the sessions, in the context of their traumatic narratives and the relational dynamics. Reoccurring patterns across clients were highlighted, giving rise to codes such as "being in control"; "singing as grounding"; "the child as a director" and "trauma narratives". In the next stage, axial coding was deployed to organize the open codes into more distinct categories and to systematically explore the relationships among them. This permitted the researchers to gather new data while also building on the categories that had already emerged. At this point, following Charmaz's [55] approach, the research focus was further honed, allowing the researchers to formulate their theoretical framework. In this step the author further examined the multi-layered meanings of the emerging categories and continued to consolidate the thematic analysis. In this step, categories such as "grounding songs elevate regulation" and "musical recordings serve as agents of resilience and strength" were articulated. In the final stage of analysis, selective coding was used to develop the core categories explaining the data. In line with Charmaz [56], this step involved an iterative process, in which categories were compared and contrasted to refine them further. The final consolidation of the core categories constructed the findings of this study, presented in Section 3.

2.5. Ethical Considerations

The researcher did not have access to a formal ethics review committee when conducting this study. This study followed the principles of the Declaration of Helsinki. Informed consent was obtained from the research participants prior to their engagement in music therapy sessions. In addition, all names and identifying information were removed from the data. Another important aspect pertinent to the current study relates to the dual role of the music therapist, serving both as a practitioner and a researcher in the study. The advantage of this arrangement is ascribed to the researcher's ability to bring a first-person perspective grounded in extensive clinical experience, which can enhance the depth of reflection, insight, and the meaningful interpretation of findings. In the current study, this dual position enabled the researcher to sound fragile moments of existence for families who had faced horrifying events, and to further make sense of their meeting together, in a different time and space.

However, it also highlights the challenges that come with this dual role, particularly the need to maintain transparency, ensure the research is transferable and accountable, and remain open to different perspectives. The researcher's unique situatedness is also highly germane to the research process itself. It is important to be aware of the potential biases and dilemmas that can arise from this dual role [57]. To address this issue, the short narratives created from each course of therapy, as well as the final thematic analyses, were all sent to the families for their approval. All families approved the materials and felt that they reflected their experiences. One family asked to remove a single quote, which was immediately removed from the data. In addition, the final analysis was sent to four experts in the fields of trauma treatment and qualitative analysis of practice materials for peer debriefing [58], and their comments were integrated to the final manuscript.

3. Results

The analysis of the sessions of four children who came to music therapy with their parents gave rise to four categories: (1) Discovering the child's grounding song: identifying resources; (2) Musical Improvisation sets the grounds for parent–child mutual recognition of the child's traumatic experience; (3) Musical performance empowers child and parent; (4) Gaining a sense of agency through controlling the musical environment.

3.1. Discovering the Child's Grounding Song: Identifying Resources

A major component of all four courses of therapy was manifested in the creation of a grounding-promoting song for each child. In most cases, the grounding song was created in the second or third session, and soon after became a safe base for the child to turn to whenever the meeting became too intense. Mostly, grounding songs were played at the openings and closures of sessions.

Upon her second session, Yana marched in and confessed—"Yesterday I felt free—almost like I felt in music with you, it was when I rode on a horse for the first time". Soon after, Yana and the therapist improvised a song, which included a short melodic dialogue between them:

> Yana—"Yesterday something happened when I rode the horses."
>
> Therapist—"What happened"?
>
> Yana—"I was so happy. . .I was so thrilled."
>
> The refrain "I was so thrilled" was repeated by the therapist and Yana many times, accompanied by Yana's free play on the drum-set, and the therapist's improvising on the piano. Since its first appearance in therapy, the sessions consistently opened and concluded with this song.

In Rani's case, it took several sessions to focus on a certain song. Rani came to most sessions with his dad. After singing through several songs, Rani asked to record one of the Jewish holiday songs. The choice of song, which seemed random at first, revealed itself as touching some basic needs of Rani relating to stability and familiarity. Throughout many sessions, Rani worked on the process of recording the song, adding layers of various instruments to it, for himself as well as his father, enjoying moments of togetherness and synchrony.

Sarit, a young and gentle singer-songwriter, 9 years of age, used music composition extensively, both to connect to areas of strength and resilience, as well as for touching on more turbulent areas of her emotional world. For a considerable part of her therapy time, Sarit started the sessions by playing together with the therapist two–three songs she had learned on her guitar, prior to her sudden leaving of her home due to the terror attack. As her relationship with the therapist developed, Sarit immersed herself in putting new words to the familiar tunes, at first connecting to her dreams and fantasies, and later also revealing her fears and challenges. Through the songs, for example, Sarit expressed her concern for family friends who were being held captive in Gaza by Hamas.

3.2. Musical Improvisation Sets the Grounds for Parent–Child Mutual Recognition of the Child's Traumatic Experience

The analysis revealed that, often after moments of freely exploring the musical instruments or improvising together, the children related spontaneously to a previously unbearable moment, most often revealing a hidden, yet unspoken part of their traumatic story. (Music therapy improvisation is a multifaceted practice, portraying the intentional use of musical expression to address various therapeutic goals. Whether in a medical setting, working with neurological conditions, in social contexts, or delving into psychological and psychodynamic aspects, the therapist guides the improvisational process to tap into the client's needs and experiences. It is this blend of spontaneity, creativity, and therapeutic intentionality that makes music therapy improvisation such a powerful tool for healing and growth ([59,60])) In Yana's third session, she started by singing and improvising musically for several minutes around her grounding song, a song she often turned to at different points of the session to connect to her strengths and resources. At this time, after singing her grounding song, she grabbed the microphone and started narrating a minute-by-minute description of her 17-h experience of hiding in the house-shelter when the terrorists attacked. She was looking at mom in the eye and did not stop talking for about 20 minutes. Mom looked at me intermittently, amazed, somewhat shocked by the unexpected monologue taking place in the room. While I was sharing with her the almost sacred feelings of Yana's words, I also reassured her that this moment was being recorded. One of the salient qualities captured in the recording relates to the "stand-up" tone used by Yana, and her connecting for the first time to details which were out of reach for her for several weeks (as indicated by the family later), while she was navigating between moments of horror...

> "At first, I asked my dad—is this real? Am I only imagining this? But then, another siren came, and we ran to the shelter, and then I opened Tik-Tok and I saw shooting, constant shooting, 24/7."

> and moments which gave her strength in those long hours, for example, her mom going out of the shelter to prepare a feast meal from all the meat she had prepared to cook that day for the unattended family gathering.

Another client, Rani, when asked specifically about the horrifying moments of waiting to be rescued from the terror attack, expressed detached feelings towards the situation, sharing that he could only remember watching a lot of movies. However, several weeks into the therapeutic process, he could share the experience of a traumatic trigger when hearing a siren when playing in the park with his friends (already in the hosting village), his parents being a few hundred meters away, not in sight. The therapy started with Rani's improvisation on the recorder, followed by a joint improvisation between his father, the therapist and Rani, led by his recorder playing. Soon after putting the recorder aside, Rani could connect for the first time to feelings of helplessness, anxiety and fear when remaining alone in a moment of horror, amidst a possible missile attack. "I would rather stay out-side when the missile comes, than to go on my own to the shelter", he added, hence referencing for the first time the levels of panic involved the last time he had to rush to a shelter, on 7 October, a dread he could not imagine going through alone. In the following moments, we could touch for the first time on the more shattered parts of his experience of the 7 October attack.

3.3. Musical Performance Empowers Child and Parent

For all children, moments of listening to their recordings with the parent or performing "live" to the parents were marked as highly significant, and in many cases enabled moments of transformation in the child's well-being, as well as in the child–parent relationship.

It was in the very early stages of therapy that Sarit discovered she could prepare a mini-album in therapy, including a special performance of all the songs to her parents. In our very last session, her parents came to the special concert she had prepared with the therapist. Sarit felt on top of the world. Her parents were in awe and could not stop expressing their amazement at their daughter. Never had they experienced her as such a confident and impressive musician. In their final parental consultation, the parents shared with the therapist their surprise at the level of depth expressed in her songs' lyrics. They had not realized until that moment how deeply her thoughts and emotions were centered around her war experiences.

Rani's grounding song entailed different aspects of his therapeutic growth, addressing various goals. One facet of his work relates to the meticulous attitude he embraced when recording multiple layers for the song, together with dad. Rani's musical requests from dad when recording his song together, across many sessions, reflected in many cases, Rani's basic needs: sometimes, he only wanted to be listened to, and at other times he could engage in an improvised musical dialogue. A special moment emerged when mom visited the session for the first time. Rani immediately wanted to add a recorded layer of her playing and chose for her a very special instrument. Upon listening together to mom's recording, he realized he could not hear her clearly enough and continued to record her part again and again until satisfied. Reflecting together with mom on possible meanings of Rani's request in the session itself and afterwards marked an important milestone in the dyad's relationship.

3.4. Gaining a Sense of Agency through Controlling the Musical Environment

One salient characteristic of the musical behavior among all four children included in this report, relates to their attempt to gain a sense of control through directing the musical activities in the session. For Maya, restoring her sense of control became a central theme in her course of therapy. Already in her first meeting, Maya was preoccupied with directing mom and me in every single step we made in our joint music making. In fact, Maya was very concerned about communicating her detailed instructions about "what happens when", leaving us very little time to actually play together, if at all. Another manifestation of Maya's need for control took place in Maya's recording of "the passing of time". While many children who participate in music therapy enjoy recording their music and listening to it, Maya insisted on recording the silence, while making the therapist and her parent freeze any move (and sometimes breath) while she recorded it and, later, when listening to it. In a slow and delicate process, Maya started to loosen her need to control the situation and direct every step made in therapy and managed to start restoring her ability to play and explore freely.

As mentioned earlier, in his music therapy meetings, Rani created a multi-layered instrumentation for a song. This creative endeavor reflected on many psychological processes Rani was going through. For example, in each layer, Rani added more instruments, changing the musical roles adopted by him and his dad, changing their sounds and their way of relating musically. While, in the first layer, Rani, the therapist and dad were asked by Rani to play and sing the song while adhering strictly to the script (words and music), in the second layer more musical freedom was added, yet dictated closely by Rani. Through articulating the delicate facets of each layer, Rani enabled himself to gain more levels of freedom, in his inner self, as well as within his relationship with his parents.

4. Discussion

The analysis identified four central categories highlighting different aspects of the child–parent relationship in the context of their traumatic experience, as manifested in music therapy. Through integrating different ways in which the war affected the children's sense of safety and attachment, aspects relating to the opportunity music therapy provided for restoring salient child–parent properties will be now explored.

4.1. Reclaiming Security: Children's Growing from Directing to Playfully Exploring

Findings point to the delicate ways children used the therapeutic context to restore their sense of control and feelings of reassurance, as experienced within their relationships with their parents. Most intriguing, all children included in this study utilized the music sessions to gain a sense of safety through deploying the musical experiences, first and foremost, to dictate the minute-by-minute occurrences in the session: whether by giving the parent and therapist specific musical roles, or by directing the adults in the room to hold their breath. Such behaviors reflected not only the children's high levels of anxiety, but, more deeply, it revealed their inability to trust their central attachment figures. Various studies have shown the devastating effect of trauma on children's levels of secure attachment [4,61], as well as on children's extent of freedom and playfulness [62,63].

While CPP was widely proved to decrease traumatic symptoms and restore significant aspects of the child–therapist relationship [36,61,64], this study is the first to show how a CPP-informed approach in music therapy practice may contribute to rebuilding confidence, faith and security among dyads who had experienced war induced trauma.

In addition, and congruent with various acute trauma and post-trauma intervention protocols [65–68], this study emphasized the significance of establishing with clients their inner resources and exercising with them states of grounding and regulation. The current study demonstrated how child–parent and child–therapist joint music making might serve as a regulative activity, supporting clients in visiting their traumatic experiences, as well as in taking a healthy distance from the trauma at the end of an intervention. In this sense, it seems that the musical experience enabled the dyads both to reach a regulative state, which allowed them to touch on traumatic memories, and to further gain additional levels of playfulness and freedom, utilizing the musical environment.

This research's findings conform with additional studies highlighting the significance of embracing a biopsychosocial framework when working with children who had experienced trauma [36,61,64]. The therapist's emphasis on restoring the child's most primary, biological and physiological sense of control, leading to an increase in both parents' and children's regulated state, corresponds to additional perspectives, which urge clinicians to include a comprehensive view of the child's being [69] and on conducting a thorough assessment of the child's history to gain all the required information possibly linked to various developmental symptoms experienced by the child [5,11]. As indicated by additional ecological models for the treatment of childhood trauma [36,61], after reaching a more regulated state, both child and parent were free to explore their environments and relationships more playfully.

4.2. Rehabilitating Parental Sense of Competency

A central component unearthed across various themes relates to the extensive use of the sessions as a means for rebuilding parents' position as being competent and present. In this respect, parents were granted the opportunity to revisit their children's moments of horror by co-creating their war narratives and connecting to parts which were inaccessible for parents and children up until that moment. CPP research advocates for the need to "speak the unspeakable", and for supporting parents in establishing an environment that would allow tapping into the traumatic experiences [21,36,61,64]. This research further highlights different ways whereby musical experiences can assist parents in delving into such horrifying moments and have a chance to witness and acknowledge their child's experiences, especially in situations where they could not fully be present, e.g., when the terror attack occurred. Music, and specifically songwriting, was found to provide a mediating role, allowing both the child to connect to their experience and the parent to be able to contain their child's unbearable experiences. Moreover, engaging in a performance or finalizing a musical recording seemed to provide families with a concrete object to hold on to and relate to, an object representing their sense of healing, reconnecting, and celebrating life, rather than being caught in the deadly, frozen past.

Finally, different approaches to trauma emphasized the devastating effect of trauma on both children's [4,36] and adult's [65] sense of helplessness, inability, failure and passiveness. This study suggests that engaging in joint music making provides a multi-layered experience that might support parent–child dyads in becoming more present and active, and in restoring their sense of agency and competency. Through becoming playful and innovative in the musical space, parents and children were able to attend to each other's musical requests and enjoy regulative moments of joint music making. Therefore, music therapy was found to be an important approach in the context of trauma treatment for this population.

The ongoing state of war and conflict in Israel and Palestine indicated an urgent need for therapists specialized in trauma-informed practice, particularly highlighting its adverse effect on children and adolescence [9,63]. Numerous centers for supporting citizens' resilience (i.e., "Hosen-Centers") are spread throughout Israel. First-aid trauma in Israel is managed by social workers who specialize in trauma informed practice [70]. This study points to possible benefits of integrating music therapy-informed practice within such services: in Israel, Palestine and anywhere that trauma endures. Most importantly, it seems that the music-based intervention was able to touch on different realms of the child's experience: the physiological (regulation), cognitive (trauma-song narrative), emotional (sharing emotions through singing and co-music), relational (interacting musically with parents and therapist), and more. This holistic approach to children who had experienced trauma ratifies the significance of applying an ecological perspective when treating childhood trauma and further suggests the possible contribution of the arts to such models.

4.3. Limitations

The thematic analysis of a music therapy intervention for children and adolescents who had experienced trauma revealed promising possibilities in promoting attachment, regulation and healing. This study serves as a preliminary attempt to outline the key components of a child–parent approach to trauma within the context of music therapy. However, it faces several limitations, including the use of a relatively small sample size. Further research is required to test and consolidate applicable protocols which include music making as a prominent agent. As raised by one of the auditors of this manuscript, the data analysis also failed to capture any contra-indications for using music in therapy with individuals who experienced acute stress symptoms. More research is required to reveal what kinds of clinical music making is suitable when working with this population and what kinds of music might elevate clients' levels of stress and anxiety rather than support them. To advance the field, future research could employ micro-analytic [52] methods to explore the relationship between verbal content in specific session periods and the level and quality of both the child's and parent's musical engagement. As this study was based on a qualitative framework, it lacked outcome measures and a control group. For more comprehensive recommendations on trauma-informed music therapy treatment and to develop reliable protocols, future studies should include a larger sample size and measurable outcomes, enabling generalization. Expanding the sample to include more child–parent dyads would allow for the examination of the intervention's impact on factors such as attachment, anxiety, stress, regulation, and well-being, thereby strengthening the validity and reliability of trauma-informed, music-based interventions.

5. Conclusions

The literature advocates for long-term studies and interventions to mitigate the enduring effects of war on children's development, stressing the importance of evidence-based interventions aimed at preventing and treating trauma, as well as policies that prioritize the mental well-being of children in conflict zones [10,19,36].

This study showed novel evidence for the benefits of using CPP-informed music therapy in the treatment of families who had experienced a terror attack and were displaced from their home-kibbutz for more than six months. Findings revealed that CPP-informed music therapy provided ample opportunities for children and parents to revisit their traumatic experiences, promoted parental responsiveness and supported children's and parents' feelings of competency, agency, coherence and stability. This study underscores the significance of families engaging in musical activities, fostering a sense of safety, acknowledging their children's traumatic experiences, and paving the way toward rehabilitation, resilience, and playfulness.

Funding: This research received no external funding.

Institutional Review Board Statement: Ethical review and approval were waived for this study due to the author being an independent researcher at the time. (There are related laws and regulations). This study followed the principles of the Declaration of Helsinki. Informed consent was obtained from the research participants prior to their engagement in music therapy sessions.

Informed Consent Statement: Informed consent was obtained from all subjects involved in the study.

Data Availability Statement: Data are contained within the article.

Conflicts of Interest: The author declares no conflicts of interest.

References

1. Michalek, J.; Lisi, M.; Binetti, N.; Ozkaya, S.; Hadfield, K.; Dajani, R.; Mareschal, I. War-related Trauma Linked to Increased Sustained Attention to Threat in Children. *Child. Dev.* **2022**, *93*, 900–909. [CrossRef] [PubMed]
2. Beer, B.L.E.; Birnbaum, J.C. *Trauma-Informed Music Therapy: Theory and Practice*; Routledge: London, UK, 2022.
3. Catani, C.; Schauer, E.; Neuner, F. Beyond Individual War Trauma: Domestic Violence against Children in Afghanistan and Sri Lanka. *J. Marital. Fam. Ther.* **2008**, *34*, 165–176. [CrossRef]
4. Masten, A.S.; Narayan, A.J. Child Development in the Context of Disaster, War, and Terrorism: Pathways of Risk and Resilience. *Annu. Rev. Psychol.* **2012**, *63*, 227–257. [CrossRef]
5. Popham, C.M.; McEwen, F.S.; Karam, E.; Fayyad, J.; Karam, G.; Saab, D.; Moghames, P.; Pluess, M. Predictors of Psychological Risk and Resilience among Syrian Refugee Children. *Child. Psychol. Psychiatry* **2023**, *64*, 91–99. [CrossRef]
6. Hazer, L.; Gredebäck, G. The Effects of War, Displacement, and Trauma on Child Development. *Humanit. Soc. Sci. Commun.* **2023**, *10*, 909. [CrossRef]
7. Sagi-Schwartz, A. The Well Being of Children Living in Chronic War Zones: The Palestinian—Israeli Case. *Int. J. Behav. Dev.* **2008**, *32*, 322–336. [CrossRef]
8. Khamis, V. Posttraumatic Stress Disorder and Emotion Dysregulation among Syrian Refugee Children and Adolescents Resettled in Lebanon and Jordan. *Child. Abus. Negl.* **2019**, *89*, 29–39. [CrossRef] [PubMed]
9. Pat-Horenczyk, R.; Achituv, M.; Rubenstein, A.K.; Khodabakhsh, A.; Brom, D.; Chemtob, C. Growing Up Under Fire: Building Resilience in Young Children and Parents Exposed to Ongoing Missile Attacks. *J. Child. Adol Trauma.* **2012**, *5*, 303–314. [CrossRef]
10. Bryant, R.A.; Edwards, B.; Creamer, M.; O'Donnell, M.; Forbes, D.; Felmingham, K.L.; Silove, D.; Steel, Z.; Nickerson, A.; McFarlane, A.C.; et al. The Effect of Post-Traumatic Stress Disorder on Refugees' Parenting and Their Children's Mental Health: A Cohort Study. *Lancet Public. Health* **2018**, *3*, e249–e258. [CrossRef]
11. Perry, B.D. Examining Child Maltreatment Through a Neurodevelopmental Lens: Clinical Applications of the Neurosequential Model of Therapeutics. *J. Loss Trauma* **2009**, *14*, 240–255. [CrossRef]
12. Shapiro, J.R.; Applegate, J.S. Cognitive Neuroscience, Neurobiology and Affect Regulation: Implications for Clinical Social Work. *Clin. Soc. Work. J.* **2000**, *28*, 9–21. [CrossRef]
13. Kapel Lev-ari, R.; Aloni, R.; Ben-ari, A. Understanding the Dyadic Mental Health of Refugee Parents and Children after Fleeing the 2022 Ukraine War. *Psychol. Trauma Theory Res. Pract. Policy* **2024**. [CrossRef] [PubMed]
14. Murphy, K.M.; Rodrigues, K.; Costigan, J.; Annan, J. Raising Children in Conflict: An Integrative Model of Parenting in War. *Peace Confl. J. Peace Psychol.* **2017**, *23*, 46–57. [CrossRef]
15. Gewirtz, A.; Forgatch, M.; Wieling, E. Parenting Practices as Potential Mechanisms for Child Adjustment Following Mass Trauma. *J. Marital. Fam. Ther.* **2008**, *34*, 177–192. [CrossRef] [PubMed]
16. Hoffman, Y.; Shrira, A. Variables Connecting Parental PTSD to Offspring Successful Aging: Parent–Child Role Reversal, Secondary Traumatization, and Depressive Symptoms. *Front. Psychiatry* **2019**, *10*, 718. [CrossRef] [PubMed]
17. Möllerherm, J.; Saile, R.; Wieling, E.; Neuner, F.; Catani, C. Parenting in a Post-Conflict Region: Associations between Observed Maternal Parenting Practices and Maternal, Child, and Contextual Factors in Northern Uganda. *Dev. Psychopathol.* **2024**, 1–12. [CrossRef]
18. Khamis, V. Does Parent's Psychological Distress Mediate the Relationship between War Trauma and Psychosocial Adjustment in Children? *J. Health Psychol.* **2016**, *21*, 1361–1370. [CrossRef]
19. Chemtob, C.M.; Nomura, Y.; Rajendran, K.; Yehuda, R.; Schwartz, D.; Abramovitz, R. Impact of Maternal Posttraumatic Stress Disorder and Depression Following Exposure to the September 11 Attacks on Preschool Children's Behavior. *Child. Dev.* **2010**, *81*, 1129–1141. [CrossRef]
20. Hoffnung-Assouline, A.; Knei-Paz, C. Supervising Contact Visits: A Trauma-Informed Approach Based on Principles of Child-Parent Psychotherapy. *Clin. Soc. Work J.* **2024**, *52*, 136–149. [CrossRef]

21. Hagan, M.J.; Browne, D.T.; Sulik, M.; Ippen, C.G.; Bush, N.; Lieberman, A.F. Parent and Child Trauma Symptoms During Child–Parent Psychotherapy: A Prospective Cohort Study of Dyadic Change. *J. Trauma. Stress* **2017**, *30*, 690–697. [CrossRef] [PubMed]
22. Gordon, J. Longing and Belonging: Making Mobiles in Art Therapy with Young Ukrainian Refugees. *Int. J. Art Ther.* **2024**, *29*, 165–173. [CrossRef]
23. Bensimon, M. Mechanisms of Change in Music Therapy When Treating Adults Coping with Trauma. In *Trauma-Informed Music Therapy*; Routledge: New York, NY, USA, 2022; pp. 150–157. [CrossRef]
24. Bensimon, M. Relational Needs in Music Therapy with Trauma Victims: The Perspective of Music Therapists. *Nord. J. Music. Ther.* **2020**, *29*, 240–254. [CrossRef]
25. Nnanyelugo, C.E.; Iyendo, T.O.; Emmanuel, N.O.; Okwuowulu, C.; Izuchukwu John, E.; Apuke, O.D.; Gever, V.C. Effect of Internet-Mediated Music Therapy Intervention on Reduction in Generalized Anxiety Disorder Symptoms among Displaced Nigerians of the Russia–Ukraine War. *Psychol. Music.* **2023**, *51*, 1149–1159. [CrossRef]
26. Abrams, B. Encountering Transgenerational Trauma through Analytical Music Therapy. *Nord. J. Music Ther.* **2021**, *30*, 197–218. [CrossRef]
27. Wilhelmsen, C.; Fuhr, G. Reflections on Practice. *Voices* **2018**, *18*. [CrossRef]
28. Uhlig, S.; Jansen, E.; Scherder, E. "Being a Bully Isn't Very Cool...": Rap & Sing Music Therapy for Enhanced Emotional Self-Regulation in an Adolescent School Setting—A Randomized Controlled Trial. *Psychol. Music.* **2018**, *46*, 568–587. [CrossRef]
29. Moore, K.S.; Hanson-Abromeit, D. Feasibility of the Musical Contour Regulation Facilitation (MCRF) Intervention to Promote Emotion Regulation for under-Resourced Preschoolers: Examining Intervention Intensity. *Arts Psychother.* **2023**, *82*, 101984. [CrossRef]
30. Zhang, M.; Ding, Y.; Zhang, J.; Jiang, X.; Xu, N.; Zhang, L.; Yu, W. Effect of Group Impromptu Music Therapy on Emotional Regulation and Depressive Symptoms of College Students: A Randomized Controlled Study. *Front. Psychol.* **2022**, *13*, 851526. [CrossRef]
31. Sena Moore, K.; Hanson-Abromeit, D. Theory-Guided Therapeutic Function of Music to Facilitate Emotion Regulation Development in Preschool-Aged Children. *Front. Hum. Neurosci.* **2015**, *9*, 572. [CrossRef]
32. Malloch, S.; Trevarthen, C. *Communicative Musicality: Exploring the Basis of Human Companionship*; Oxford University Press: Oxford, UK, 2009.
33. Chinchaipong, P. Association of Post-Traumatic Stress Disorder (PTSD) in Children and HPA Axis Regulation. *Int. J. Sci. Healthc. Res.* **2022**, *7*, 64–73. [CrossRef]
34. Russo, J.E.; Dhruve, D.M.; Oliveros, A.D. Childhood Trauma and PTSD Symptoms: Disentangling the Roles of Emotion Regulation and Distress Tolerance. *Res. Child. Adolesc. Psychopathol.* **2023**, *51*, 1273–1287. [CrossRef] [PubMed]
35. Malloch, S.N. Mothers and Infants and Communicative Musicality. *Music. Sci.* **1999**, *3* (Suppl. 1), 29–57. [CrossRef]
36. Lieberman, A.F.; Van Horn, P. *Psychotherapy with Infants and Young Children: Repairing the Effects of Stress and Trauma on Early Attachment, Paperback ed.*; Guilford Press: New York, NY, USA, 2011.
37. Colegrove, V.M.; Havighurst, S.S.; Kehoe, C.E. Emotion Regulation during Conflict Interaction after a Systemic Music Intervention: Understanding Changes for Parents with a Trauma History and Their Adolescent. *Nord. J. Music. Ther.* **2019**, *28*, 405–425. [CrossRef]
38. Chifa, M.; Hadar, T.; Politimou, N.; Reynolds, G.; Franco, F. The Soundscape of Neonatal Intensive Care: A Mixed-Methods Study of the Parents' Experience. *Children* **2021**, *8*, 644. [CrossRef] [PubMed]
39. Loewy, J. NICU Music Therapy: Song of Kin as Critical Lullaby in Research and Practice. *Ann. N. Y. Acad. Sci.* **2015**, *1337*, 178–185. [CrossRef]
40. Loewy, J.V.; Rossetti, A.; Telsey, A.; Dassler, A.M. Assessing & Treating Trauma: Music Psychotherapy for Parents of Neonates. *Music. Med.* **2021**, *13*, 138–149. [CrossRef]
41. Saada, B.; Coombes, E. Music Therapy in the Occupied Palestinian Territories: An Overview and Some Perspectives on Dementia and End-of-Life Care. *Approaches Interdiscip. J. Music. Ther.* **2020**, *12*, 280–285. [CrossRef]
42. Enge, K.E.A.; Stige, B. Musical Pathways to the Peer Community: A Collective Case Study of Refugee Children's Use of Music Therapy. *Nord. J. Music. Ther.* **2022**, *31*, 7–24. [CrossRef]
43. Mallon, T.; Hoog Antink, M. The Sound of Lost Homes—Introducing the COVER Model—Theoretical Framework and Practical Insight into Music Therapy with Refugees and Asylum Seekers. *Voices* **2021**, *21*. [CrossRef]
44. Storsve, V.; Westbye, I.A.; Ruud, E. Hope and Recognition: A Music Project among Youth in a Palestinian Refugee Camp. *Voices* **2010**, *10*. [CrossRef]
45. Bottema-Beutel, K.; Kapp, S.K.; Lester, J.N.; Sasson, N.J.; Hand, B.N. Avoiding Ableist Language: Suggestions for Autism Researchers. *Autism Adulthood* **2021**, *3*, 18–29. [CrossRef] [PubMed]
46. Hadar, T. "What Sound Does a Cat Make in Cantonese?": Advocating for Lingual Plurality in Music Therapy Settings. *Voices* **2022**, *22*. [CrossRef]
47. Ferrara, L. Phenomenology as a Tool for Musical Analysis. *Music. Q.* **1984**, *LXX*, 355–373. [CrossRef]
48. Smith, J.A.; Larkin, M.; Flowers, P. *Interpretative Phenomenological Analysis: Theory, Method and Research*; SAGE: London, UK, 2008.
49. Lee, J.; McFerran, K.S. Applying Interpretative Phenomenological Analysis to Video Data in Music Therapy. *Qual. Res. Psychol.* **2015**, *12*, 367–381. [CrossRef]

50. Hadar, T.; Amir, D. Intimacy, Mutuality & Negotiations: Dialogic Moments in Joint Improvisation. *Nord. J. Music. Ther.* **2021**, *30*, 460–484.
51. Hadar, T.; Amir, D. Discovering the Flute's Voice: On the Relation of Flutist Music Therapists to Their Primary Instrument. *Nord. J. Music. Ther.* **2018**, *27*, 381–398. [CrossRef]
52. Wosch, T.; Wigram, T.; Wheeler, B.L. (Eds.) *Microanalysis in Music Therapy: Methods, Techniques and Applications for Clinicians, Researchers, Educators and Students*; Jessica Kingsley: London, UK; Philadelphia, PA, USA, 2007.
53. Hakvoort, L.; Tönjes, D. Music-Mechanisms at the Core of Music Therapy: Towards a Format for a Description of Music Therapy Micro-Interventions. *Nord. J. Music. Ther.* **2023**, *32*, 67–91. [CrossRef]
54. Corbin, J.M.; Strauss, A.L. *Basics of Qualitative Research: Techniques and Procedures for Developing Grounded Theory*, 3rd ed.; Sage Publ: Los Angeles, CA, USA, 2015.
55. Charmaz, K. *Constructing Grounded Theory: A Practical Guide through Qualitative Analysis*; Sage Publications: London, UK, 2006.
56. Charmaz, K. Rethinking Methods in Psychology. In *The Search for Meanings-Grounded Theory*; Sage Publications: New York, NY, USA, 1996.
57. Wheeler, B.L.; Murphy, K.M. (Eds.) *Music Therapy Research*, 3rd ed.; Barcelona Publishers: Dallas, TX, USA, 2016.
58. Denzin, N.K.; Lincoln, Y.S. (Eds.) *The Sage Handbook of Qualitative Research*, 3rd ed.; Sage Publ: Thousand Oaks, CA, USA, 2009.
59. Bruscia, K.E.; Bruscia, K.E. *Improvisational Models of Music Therapy*; ISMEZ: Roma, Italy, 1987.
60. Hadar, T.; Aigen, K. *Music, Time, and Self: A Time Model for Nordoff-Robbins Clinical Improvisation*; Barcelona Publishers: Glen Rock, PA, USA, 2024.
61. Lieberman, A.F.; Ghosh Ippen, C.; Van Horn, P. Child-Parent Psychotherapy: 6-Month Follow-up of a Randomized Controlled Trial. *J. Am. Acad. Child. Adolesc. Psychiatry* **2006**, *45*, 913–918. [CrossRef]
62. Chazan, S.; Cohen, E. Adaptive and Defensive Strategies in Post-Traumatic Play of Young Children Exposed to Violent Attacks. *J. Child Psychother.* **2010**, *36*, 133–151. [CrossRef]
63. Barbanel, L.; Sternberg, R.J. *Psychological Interventions in Times of Crisis*; Springer: New York, NY, USA, 2006.
64. Sullivan, A.D.W.; Merrill, S.M.; Konwar, C.; Coccia, M.; Rivera, L.; MacIsaac, J.L.; Lieberman, A.F.; Kobor, M.S.; Bush, N.R. Intervening after Trauma: Child–Parent Psychotherapy Treatment Is Associated with Lower Pediatric Epigenetic Age Acceleration. *Psychol. Sci.* **2024**, *35*, 1062–1073. [CrossRef]
65. Farchi, M.; Hirsch-Gornemann, M.B.; Whiteson, A.; Gidron, Y. The SIX Cs Model for Immediate Cognitive Psychological First Aid: From Helplessness to Active Efficient Coping. *Int. J. Emerg. Ment. Health* **2018**, *20*, 395. [CrossRef]
66. Shapiro, E.; Laub, B. Early EMDR Intervention Following a Community Critical Incident: A Randomized Clinical Trial. *J. EMDR Prac. Res.* **2015**, *9*, 17–27. [CrossRef]
67. Zemestani, M.; Mohammed, A.F.; Ismail, A.A.; Vujanovic, A.A. A Pilot Randomized Clinical Trial of a Novel, Culturally Adapted, Trauma-Focused Cognitive-Behavioral Intervention for War-Related PTSD in Iraqi Women. *Behav. Ther.* **2022**, *53*, 656–672. [CrossRef] [PubMed]
68. Tissue, A.; Specker, P.; Hoffman, J.; Uppal, S.; Cloitre, M.; Neuner, F.; O'Donnell, M.; Nickerson, A. Skills Training in Affective and Interpersonal Regulation for Refugees Integrated with Narrative Exposure Therapy: A Case Study on the Treatment of PTSD and Emotion Dysregulation for Refugees and Asylum-Seekers. *Clin. Case Stud.* **2023**, *22*, 285–306. [CrossRef]
69. Berzoff, J.; Drisko, J. What Clinical Social Workers Need to Know: Bio-Psycho-Social Knowledge and Skills for the Twenty First Century. *Clin. Soc. Work. J.* **2015**, *43*, 263–273. [CrossRef]
70. Cohen, M.; Gagin, R.; Peled-Avram, M. Multiple Terrorist Attacks: Compassion Fatigue in Israeli Social Workers. *Traumatology* **2006**, *12*, 293–301. [CrossRef]

children

MDPI

Article

Who Benefits Most from the Family Education and Support Program in Cape Verde? A Cluster Analysis

Adriana Correia [1], Cátia Martins [2,3], Rita dos Santos [2], Victoria Hidalgo [4], Saúl Neves de Jesus [1,3] and Cristina Nunes [2,3,*]

1 Research Centre for Tourism, Sustainability and Well-Being (CinTurs), University of Algarve, Campus de Gambelas, 8005-139 Faro, Portugal; a62613@ualg.pt (A.C.); snjesus@ualg.pt (S.N.d.J.)
2 Psychology Research Centre (CIP), University of Algarve, 8005-135 Faro, Portugal; csmartins@ualg.pt (C.M.); rasantos@ualg.pt (R.d.S.)
3 University Research Center in Psychology (CUIP), University of Algarve, Campus de Gambelas, 8005-139 Faro, Portugal
4 Department of Developmental and Educational Psychology, Faculty of Psychology, University of Seville, 41018 Seville, Spain; victoria@us.es
* Correspondence: csnunes@ualg.pt

Abstract: Background/Objectives: Child parenting programs can enhance parental skills, prevent future issues in child development, and improve children's quality of life. The present research aimed to study the changes promoted by the Family Education and Support Program (FAF) implemented in Cape Verde, regarding parental educational practices, perceived parental efficacy, and attitudes and beliefs of Cape Verdean parents. Methods: To this end, 37 participants were evaluated through a pretest-postest design. The evaluated dimensions were perceived parental competence, parenting practices, Parental attitudes and beliefs, mental health and perceived child quality of life. Results: A cluster analysis was conducted, distinguishing two groups. Both groups benefited from the program. Cluster 1 reported more significant gains in dimensions of parental efficacy and satisfaction, inadequate expectations, affection and support, and reactivity, while cluster 2 showed a greater difference in regulation and reactivity. Conclusions: Overall, the FAF intervention contributed to an increase in positive parenting practices. By analyzing potential underlying profiles in the change process, this study suggests that there are participants who benefit more than others from the intervention, and this information may be relevant for professionals and researchers in the field.

Keywords: family education and support program (FAF); parental attitudes and beliefs; parental educational practices; perceived parental efficacy; positive parenting

1. Introduction

Parenting can be defined as the interactions, emotions, beliefs, attitudes, practices, knowledge, and behaviors of parents that are associated with providing comprehensive care to their children. It refers to the ongoing process of promoting and supporting the full development and socialization of the child. Among the many influences that impact child development, parents are essential for the development, protection, empowerment, adaptation, and success throughout the lives of children. Children who are educated with strategies involving attention, care, and stimulation become more cooperative, react more positively to non-punitive approaches, and demonstrate greater flexibility and adaptability [1,2].

Parenting programs, which promote positive interactions between parents and children, can prevent future issues in child development, strengthen emotional bonds, and consequently protect children from violence, as well as promote their overall health [3–6]. The essential components of parenting programs include education and counseling for parents and caregivers on positive parenting practices, such as the use of non-violent discipline, and effective and sensitive communication strategies to deal with children and adolescents [7–10]. By increasing parents' knowledge about child development, improving parenting skills, and encouraging the use of positive strategies in child education, these programs can prevent the use of negative parenting practices and various forms of violence [11–14].

Positive parenting refers to respectful, caring, protective, nurturing, and affectionate parental behaviors that stimulate and promote the satisfaction of children's basic needs. It involves providing guidance and setting boundaries to strengthen the child's full development [15]. In contrast, negative parenting is characterized by rigid and coercive, punitive, and violent practices [16–18].

Parental practices are strategies adopted to suppress inappropriate behaviors and promote appropriate behaviors [19,20]. They guide, teach, and correct children's attitudes and behaviors and can be either positive (e.g., positive discipline and parental involvement in interactions with children) or negative (e.g., physical and psychological abuse, neglect, negative communication) [20,21]. Parents should combine affection and protection while establishing educational boundaries, as opposed to the undesirable use of physical and psychological punishments, which induce feelings of depreciation, fear, behavioral alterations, and emotional dysregulation in children [22].

Many factors influence parenthood, including evolution and history, culture, socioeconomic level, family typology, number of children, children's ages, and parents' mental health and social support [16,23,24]. The choice of a particular parental practice can also be influenced by the individual characteristics of both parents (e.g., developmental history, personality, psychopathology) and children (e.g., temperament), as well as by the sociocultural context in which they are a part [20,25]. According to Belsky [26], it is crucial to highlight the developmental history of the individual, as it influences their personality, and consequently has implications for their parental practices. In many cases, parents who experienced adverse situations in childhood (e.g., physical punishment) often repeat these practices with their children, perpetuating an intergenerational cycle of violence [18]. Another important aspect concerns the use of violent disciplinary practices, which, instead of being a deliberate choice of discipline, result from parents' anger and frustration or lack of knowledge about the harms of violence and the possibility of using non-violent practices [27,28].

The relationship between parental practices and various dimensions of child well-being has also been extensively studied, highlighting the influence of parental attitudes and behaviors on children's psychosocial adjustment, academic performance, and health [29–31]. While psychological control and coercion have been associated with psychosocial maladjustment in children, behavioral control and positive parenting have been related to healthy development [32–34]. A pattern of punitive parental behavior (e.g., hitting, threatening, and scolding) is associated with long-term risk trajectories for both externalizing and internalizing problems [35,36]. In this regard, parents who employ harsh discipline, including physical punishment with low responsiveness and inconsistency, are associated with adolescents experiencing more health problems such as substance abuse, mental health issues, disengagement, and school dropout [37,38]. Conversely, positive involvement between parents and children has reduced the impact of coercion, decreasing children's behavioral problems [39–41].

Parenting has been extensively studied, assessing the relevance of cultural context in the effectiveness of certain parenting behaviors [20]. Some studies have shown that a high level of parental control may have positive effects for African American and Asian American youths [42,43], but not for European American youths. The cultural and socioeconomic aspects of parents (e.g., educational level and professional qualifications) have a moderating effect on parenting practices, affecting children's psychosocial adjustment and well-being. These differences found across cultures suggest that parenting practices have different meanings and implications depending on the sociocultural context [20].

Regarding parental attitudes, they involve a set of beliefs that position parents regarding a particular issue or decision-making process (e.g., being against or in favor of corporal punishment as an educational strategy) [44]. In studies conducted on parental attitudes, especially in abusive parents, it was observed that they tend to have inappropriate expectations about children's abilities, associated with a lack of knowledge about their needs at different developmental stages [45] and a lack of empathy toward the child [46]. Parte superior do formulário On the other hand, abusive parents typically have a negative self-image, based on experiences of exposure to ridicule, disappointment, and failure during their own childhoods, which they tend to replicate, thereby extending this negative view to their children. The behaviors exhibited by children, which abusive parents believe should be eliminated, often mirror those for which they themselves were punished as children, thus imbuing corporal punishment with a sense of approval and tradition. The outcome of such abusive behavior is the development of aggressive behaviors in the child [47].

The parents' perception of self-efficacy—which translates into their expectations regarding the adequacy of their parenting skills in prioritizing the child's needs according to their level of development [48]—is also related to the parenting practices used. Thus, parents with high perceived self-efficacy use more positive parenting practices, while parents with low self-efficacy have limited abilities to effectively deal with challenging children, opting to give up or use punitive and severe strategies [49]. Therefore, the perception of parental competence is even more important in families at psychosocial risk, where the exercise of parenting can be more challenging [1,24,50,51]. Parents' sense of competence consists of the parents' beliefs about their ability to influence the development of their children in a positive way and the satisfaction derived from the parental role [48–51]. Parental satisfaction includes attitudes towards children, the nature of your relationship with them and the attitudes given the responsibilities inherent to the parental role [9,49].

When parental satisfaction and perception of parental self-efficacy are compromised, high levels of parental stress may arise, resulting in symptomatic consequences at cognitive, emotional, and behavioral levels (e.g., anxiety, depression, post-traumatic stress, obsessive-compulsive thoughts, and somatic complaints) [52]. Therefore, parental stress influences parental well-being, which arises from the conflict between demands and available resources, generating negative feelings about oneself and the child and influencing how parents act. The higher the level of parental stress, the worse the environment provided for the children, as they become more vulnerable to anxiety and externalizing problems [50,53,54]. Parental stress can thus result in low parental satisfaction, especially when there is weak family and social support, a low perceived quality of life, and psychological problems [50,54].

Regarding the influence of parenting practices on parental mental health, results have shown that engaging in positive parenting (i.e., more practices of emotional support and fewer practices of rejection and control) is associated with higher levels of perceived psychological quality of life in adults [55]. This finding underscores that more positive relationships are associated with higher levels of life satisfaction, particularly in the family context, influencing the family environment and contributing to individual well-being [1]. In this sense, there is a need to address not only the needs of children but also the needs of parents, as their psychological well-being is crucial for good parenting practices [56].

Strategies for dealing with stress primarily focus on valuing interpersonal relationships, balancing work and leisure, and maintaining healthcare, so participating in parental intervention programs can be a useful tool because parents can find and increase the necessary social support in this context [24,50]. Thus, the implementation of intervention programs based on positive parenting becomes even more important, especially in contexts that are inherently more likely to generate parental stress, such as in developing countries, where economic difficulties, overcrowding, and low qualifications and literacy lead to environments of greater problems in terms of family functioning, including conflict situations and negative parenting practices [57], as is the case of Cape Verde [58].

In Cape Verde, and more specifically on Boa Vista Island (where the FAF took place), data on living conditions demonstrate very precarious situations, with few resources, overcrowding and poverty, which contribute to the increase in situations of hostility and of conflicting interactions between the couple and their children. Children are exposed to child labor, sexual abuse and mistreatment, with 57% of children aged zero to six being physically punished by caregivers for disobedience. Parents' working conditions are very demanding, which can make it difficult to organize and structure activities with their children, which can result in emotional distance and a lack of parental support [58]. Study of the implementation of positive parenting programs in Africa has been rare, and non-existent in Cape Verde [58]. Several programs promote positive parenting (e.g., Triple P; Sanders [59]; Incredible Years; Gardner et al. [60]; Learning Together, Growing With Family; Amorós-Martí et al. [61]), some of which have been implemented in African contexts [62], albeit in English. The Family Education and Support Program (FAF) [63–65] is an evidence-based program that focuses on positive parenting with a psychoeducational and community-based approach, employing participatory and experiential methodology to enhance parenting skills. This program has been implemented in various countries, particularly low- and middle-income (LMI) countries, with different cultural and socioeconomic backgrounds, with a special emphasis on families at psychosocial risk (e.g., Correia et al. [12]; Hidalgo et al. [66]; Maya and Hidalgo [67]). The main objectives of this program are: (a) to improve parenting practices used by parents; (b) to strengthen feelings of security in their role as parents, enhancing parental competence; (c) to promote community integration of families; and (d) to improve the quality of life for parents and children [64].

The topics covered and the activities carried out were those contained in the FAF program manual (Hidalgo et al., [64]), selected according to the characteristics of the participants and the identified intervention needs, including child development, adolescent development, adult development, family system, educational styles (norms and discipline; affection and communication), conflict resolution, risky sexual behaviors and substance use. The FAF was applied in 12 sessions (on a weekly basis, 2 h per session) by two psychologists, with specific training for this program.

Considering that the FAF intervention had already been translated and adapted for the Portuguese context [68], it was decided to implement the program in the African context, specifically in Cape Verde. Most of the research conducted in African contexts has focused more on the effectiveness of programs [12,69–72], although some investigations in the field of positive parenting promotion had already focused more on participant profiles and underlying characteristics of the change processes [73,74]. Thus, the present research aimed to study the changes promoted by the FAF in parenting practices, perceived parental efficacy, and parents' attitudes and beliefs. Namely, we intend to identify which parents of this group most benefit from the intervention and their characteristics.

2. Methods

2.1. Participants

A total of 35 mothers (94.6%) and 2 fathers (5.4%) participated in this study, ranging in age from 25 to 56 years ($M = 35.62$; $SD = 7.23$). Regarding their educational qualifications, 45.9% had incomplete primary education, 29.7% had incomplete secondary education, and 16.2% had a higher education degree. Overall, most participants were professionally active (91.9%), engaged in low-skilled (56.8%) or medium-skilled jobs (27%), with job stability (86.5%) and incomes ranging from 4.000 to 75.000 Cape Verdean escudos ($M = 30{,}366.67$; $SD = 17{,}991.35$). Regarding family structure, 70.3% were biparental families and 21.6% were monoparental families, with 54.1% being nuclear families and 37.8% being reconstituted families, with 69.4% reporting family stability. Regarding the children, 45.9% of the families had female children and 51.1% had male children with ages ranging from 6 to 12 years ($M = 8.68$; $SD = 2.27$). In terms of past psychosocial risk, 51.4% had no risk, 32.4% had level 1 risk, 10.8% had level 2 risk, and 5.4% had level 3 risk; for current risk, 56.8% had no risk, 24.3% indicated level 1, and 10.8% indicated level 3.

2.2. Measures

Sociodemographic data. Participants responded to an interview-format questionnaire consisting of 13 items that assessed individual indicators (age, origin, level of education, and professional status) and family indicators (family type and size, family stability, number of children, and income).

Level of psychosocial risk. The Inventory of Stressful and Risk Life Events (Hidalgo et al. [75]; translated by Nunes et al. [76]) was used to assess the level of psychosocial risk, consisting of a list of stressful and negative events (e.g., "Conflictual relationship with children" or "Being a victim of abuse"), which can characterize both past life trajectories (i.e., 7 items: "Childhood maltreatment") and the present situation of the individual (i.e., 15 items: "Being a victim of maltreatment"). Higher scores indicate a higher level of associated risk.

Perceived parental competencies. The Portuguese version of the Parental Sense of Competence (PSOC) (Johnston and Mash [77]; adapted by Nunes et al. [5]) consists of 16 items that evaluate parental competence perceived by parents across two dimensions: efficacy (i.e., 7 items: e.g., "Even though it is difficult, I already know how to influence my children"; $\alpha = 0.70$) and satisfaction with the parental role (i.e., 9 items: e.g., "Being a mother makes me feel nervous and anxious"; $\alpha = 0.72$), measured on a scale from 1 to 6 (1 = "No, I totally disagree" and 6 = "Yes, I totally agree"). Higher scores indicate higher levels of efficacy or satisfaction. According to the extensive review of Jones & Prinz [49], the PSOC scale is the most frequently used tool in assessing parenting self-evaluations.

Mental health. The General Health Questionnaire (GHQ-28; Goldberg and Williams [78]; Portuguese adaptation by Pais-Ribeiro and Antunes [79]) was used to assess non-psychotic psychiatric disorders. The GHQ-28 is self-report screening. measure used to detect possible psychological disorder and identifies two main concerns: the inability to carry out normal functions; and the appearance of new and distressing phenomena [78]. It consists of 28 items (e.g., "Have you been feeling perfectly well?"), answered on a Likert-type scale from 0 to 3 (0 = "Not at all" and 3 = "Much"). The total score of the questionnaire varies between 0 and 84, with higher values indicating poorer mental health ($\alpha = 0.91$).

Perceived child quality of life. This was measured using the Kidscreen-10 (The European Kidscreen Group [80]; Portuguese version by Gaspar and Matos [81]), a scale composed of 10 items (e.g., "Think about the last week ... did your child feel lonely?") that assesses the well-being and subjective health of the child on a 5-point scale, ranging from 1 = "Not at all" to 5 = "Completely". Higher values correspond to a better perceived quality of life ($\alpha = 0.74$). The KIDSCREEN-10 is recommended by the International Consortium for Health Outcomes Measurement as part of their standard set of outcome measures for anxiety disorders, depression, obsessive-compulsive behavior disorders, and post-traumatic stress disorder in children and adolescents [80].

Parenting practices. This was an instrument composed of a compilation of subscales from various instruments that assess different aspects related to parental behavior: affection and support, reasoning/induction, democratic participation, permissiveness, excessive reactivity, and intrusion. The Affection and Support (AP), Regulation (RE), and Autonomy (AU) scales are specific subscales of the short version of the Parenting Styles and Dimensions Questionnaire-13 (Robinson et al. [82]; Portuguese adaptation by Martins et al. [19]). For each item, participants indicate the frequency with which they perform the presented behaviors using a 5-point Likert scale (1 = "Never" to 5 = "Always"). The democratic style includes subscales of Support and Affection (5 items; e.g., "I praise my child when they behave or do something well"; $\alpha = 0.69$), Regulation (5 items; e.g., "I emphasize the reasons for the rules I establish"; $\alpha = 0.77$), and Autonomy/Cedence of Autonomy/Democratic Participation (5 items; e.g., "I encourage my child to express themselves freely, even when they disagree with me"; $\alpha = 0.68$). Responses are given using a 5-point Likert scale (1 = "Never" to 5 = "Always"), and higher scores on each scale reflect more frequent use of each practice. Excessive Reactivity (ER; 5 items; e.g., "When my child misbehaves,

I raise my voice or shout"; $\alpha = 0.68$) evaluates the tendency to respond impulsively to children's misbehavior (ER), and Permissiveness evaluates the lack of parental control (5 items; "I let my child do whatever they want"; $\alpha = 0.57$); both are subscales of the reduced version of the Parenting Scale-15 [83]. Items are responded to using a 7-point Likert scale (1 = "Never" to 7 = "Always"). Low scores indicate good parenting. Intrusion is a subscale of the Psychological Control Scale (Barber [84]; Portuguese version by Nunes et al. [20]), composed of 8 items (e.g., "My father/mother tries to make me change my mind"; $\alpha = 0.57$), which assesses the extent to which parents try to intrusively control their children. Items are responded to on a 6-point scale (1 = "Strongly disagree" to 6 = "Strongly agree"), and higher scores reflect more frequent use of this practice.

Parental attitudes and beliefs. We used two subscales from the Adult Adolescent Parenting Inventory (AAPI; Bavolek and Keene [47]; Portuguese version by Lopes and Brandão [85]) to assess parental educational attitudes. The Inappropriate Expectations subscale (7 items: e.g., "Good children always obey their parents"; $\alpha = 0.77$) evaluates the extent to which parents have a realistic perception of children's development, abilities, and limitations. The Physical Punishment subscale (11 items: e.g., "Spanking children when they misbehave teaches them how to behave"; $\alpha = 0.78$) assesses the extent to which parents value or do not value physical punishment as a means of disciplining and educating their children. Higher scores indicate favorable parental attitudes and behaviors, while lower scores indicate a greater potential for abuse or neglect.

2.3. Analysis Plan

The data were entered into SPSS 29.0.1.0 (IBM Corp., Chicago, IL, USA) and cluster analysis was conducted based on the on clValid [86] an *R* package for cluster validation [87]. This package contains several methods for validating the results from a cluster analysis. Multiple clustering algorithms, validation measures, and numbers of clusters were used simultaneously, to determine the most appropriate method and an optimal number of clusters for the dataset. The optimal scores, along with the corresponding cluster method and number of clusters, were extract for the clustering results of a particular algorithm. The validation measures used included internal measures [88], namely, the Dunn Index [89], Silhouette Width [90] and the connectivity (where scores near 0 are preferable), and included stability measures, namely, the average proportion of non-overlap (APN), the average distance (AD), the average distance between means (ADM), and the figure of merit (FOM) [91]. The Silhouette value measures the degree of confidence in the clustering assignment of a particular observation, with well-clustered observations having values near 1 and poorly clustered observations having values near −1. Together with the Dunn Index (the ratio of the smallest distance between observations not in the same cluster to the largest intra-cluster distance), are examples of non-linear combinations of the compactness and separation. Connectivity is another internal measure available in clValid and refers to the more related and nearby observations [91].

The order of clustering algorithms on each validation measure is rarely the same; therefore, to select the cluster algorithm, a rank aggregation was used as it ranks all the clustering algorithms based on their performance, determined by all the validation measures simultaneously, and also determines the overall winner. The rank aggregation was performed using the *R* package RankAggreg.

The internal consistency levels of the measures used were calculated using Cronbach's alpha, with values between 0.60 and 0.70 considered satisfactory, above 0.70 as adequate, and above 0.90 as excellent [92]. To analyze the characteristics of the participants in each cluster, descriptive statistics (mean, standard deviation, minimum and maximum values), as well as frequencies (f) and percentages (%) for categorical variables, were used. Considering the characteristics of the clusters, the non-parametric Mann-Whitney test was used to compare mean values between the two groups, with differences considered significant when $p < 0.05$ ($\alpha = 5\%$). Effect sizes were calculated using the r value, with values between 0.20 and 0.40 considered of low magnitude, between 0.40 and 0.60 of moderate magnitude, between 0.60 and 0.80 high, and above 0.80 as very high [93].

3. Results

The choice for the best performing algorithm was not straightforward in this case because the order of the clustering on each validation measure is not the same (Table 1). Therefore, a rank aggregation was performed using the default cross-entropy method with weighted Spearman's footrule to produce a 4-optimal order (i.e., hierarchical–2, sota-3, diana-3, diana-2; Spearman = 4.309), pointing that an hierarchical solution with 2 clusters was the best performing algorithm for this case (Figure 1).

Table 1. Optimal scores.

Validation Measures		Optimal Score	Method	Clusters
Internal	Connectivity	6.691	Diana	2
	Dunn Index	0.439	Diana	3
	Silhouette	0.525	Diana	2
Stability	APN	0.007	Hierarchical	2
	AD	1.389	Sota	3
	ADM	0.023	Hierarchical	2
	FOM	0.400	Sota	3

Notes. APN = Average proportion of non-overlap; AD = Average distance; ADM = Average distance between means; FOM = Figure of merit.

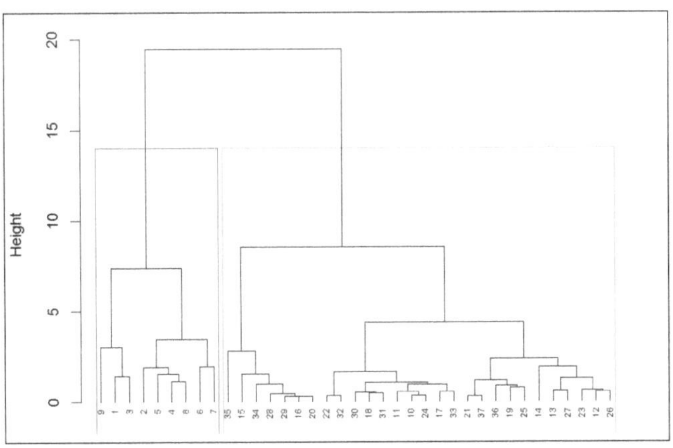

Figure 1. Dendrogram with the 8 variables under analysis.

According to Table 2, cluster 1 (C1) consisted of 9 participants, all mothers (100% female) aged between 26 and 56 years (M_{C1} = 36.78; SD_{C1} = 8.01), predominantly attending group 3 (88.90%). Cluster 2 (C2) showed greater heterogeneity, consisting of 29 participants, mostly mothers (85.70%), followed by fathers (7.10%) and grandparents (7.10%), with 85.70% being female, aged between 25 and 54 years (M_{C2} = 35.25; SD_{C2} = 7.74), distributed across assistance groups 2 (35.70%), 3 (28.60%), and 4 (32.10%).

Per the participants' educational level, in C1, 44.40% reported incomplete primary education and 33.30% had completed secondary education. In C2, 46.40% had incomplete primary education, 28.60% had secondary education, and 17.90% had higher education. Regarding employment, in C1, 100% were active but did not demonstrate stability (88.90%) and performed low/no qualification (55.60%) or medium qualification jobs (33.30%). In C2, 89.30% were active, with stability (85.70%), and performed low/no qualification (57.10%) or medium qualification jobs (25.00%).

Table 2. Sociodemographic and psychosocial characteristics of participants by cluster.

Domains	Categories	Cluster 1 (n = 9)				Cluster 2 (n = 28)			
		f		%		*f*		%	
Assistance Group	1	0		0		1		3.60	
	2	1		11.10		10		35.70	
	3	8		88.90		8		28.60	
	4	0		0		9		32.10	
Education Level	Primary	5		55.50		53		53.50	
	Secondary	3		33.30		8		28.60	
	Higher education	1		11.10		5		17.90	
Family Type	Monoparental	3		33.30		5		17.90	
	Biparental	6		66.70		20		71.40	
Sex of the child	Female	3		33.30		14		50.00	
	Male	6		66.70		14		50.00	
		M	*SD*	*Min*	*Max*	*M*	*SD*	*Min*	*Max*
	Age of the child	8.33	2.50	6.00	12.00	8.79	2.23	6.00	12.00
	Mental health	44.22	8.81	33.00	62.00	48.07	8.77	32.00	64.00
	Child Quality of Life	3.70	0.38	2.80	4.00	3.86	0.28	2.90	4.30

Note. *f* = frequency, % = percentage, *M* = Mean, *SD* = Standard Deviation, *Min* = Minimum, *Max* = Maximum.

Regarding family characteristics, both C1 and C2 were composed of biparental families (C1 = 66.70%; C2 = 71.40%), nuclear families (C1 = 55.60%; C2 = 53.60%), with family stability (C1 = 55.60%; C2 = 71.40%). However, C1 families lived with fewer people than C2 families (M_{C1} = 3.89; SD_{C1} = 1.62; $Range_{C1}$ = 2–6; M_{C2} = 4.89; SD_{C2} = 1.20; $Range_{C2}$ = 3–8). The incomes of C1 families ranged between 1,000,000 and 50,000 escudos (*Range* = 11.20–22.20%), while in C2 families they were mostly between 10,000 and 30,000 escudos (25%). Regarding children, in both clusters the age ranged from 6 to 12 years (M_{C1} = 8.33; SD_{C1} = 2.50; M_{C2} = 8.79; SD_{C2} = 2.23), with C1 children being predominantly male (66.70%), while the C2 children were equally of both genders (50%).

Regarding past psychosocial risk, participants in C1 reported between 0 and 2 events (M = 0.67; SD = 0.87), and those in C2 experienced between 0 and 3 events (M = 0.71; SD = 0.90). At the level of current risk, the C1 participants reported a number of stressful life events (M = 1.00; SD = 1.00; *Range* = 0–3) consistent with low risk (100%), while C2 participants reported a slightly higher number (M = 0.71; SD = 1.18; *Range* = 0–4), distributed between low (96.40%) and medium risk levels (3.60%).

Regarding the mental health level of the participants, in C1 the scores ranged from 33.00 to 62.00 points (M = 44.22; SD = 8.81), and in C2 the scores ranged from 32.00 to 64.00 (M = 48.07; SD = 8.77). The results also revealed that, in terms of the evaluation of children's quality of life, C1 participants (M = 3.70; SD = 0.38) reported slightly lower levels than those in C2 (M = 3.86; SD = 0.28). Finally, as shown in Figure 2 and Table 3, there were differences in the characteristics of family functioning between the two clusters.

Regarding perceived parental competence, there were significant differences of moderate magnitude, with C1 participants showing higher gains in both efficacy ($Z = -3.98$; $p < 0.001$; $r = 0.65$) and satisfaction ($Z = -4.32$; $p < 0.001$; $r = 0.71$; $M_{Efficacy}$ = 1.02; $SD_{Efficacy}$ = 0.37; $M_{Satisfaction}$ = 1.35; $SD_{Satisfaction}$ = 0.62), compared to C2 ($M_{Efficacy}$ = 0.23; $SD_{Efficacy}$ = 0.33; $M_{Satisfaction}$ = 0.06; $SD_{Satisfaction}$ = 0.17). Regarding inappropriate expectations, both groups showed a statistically significant increase of moderate magnitude ($Z = -3.18$; $p < 0.001$; $r = 0.52$), but the increase was greater in C1 (M = 1.30; SD = 1.11) compared to C2 (M = 0.13; SD = 0.34). In terms of physical punishment, although the difference was marginally significant with low magnitude ($Z = -1.70$; $p = 0.088$; $r = 0.28$), the C1 participants showed a slight decrease in their average values ($M = -0.56$; SD = 1.01), while the C2 participants maintained their results (M = 0.02; SD = 0.29).

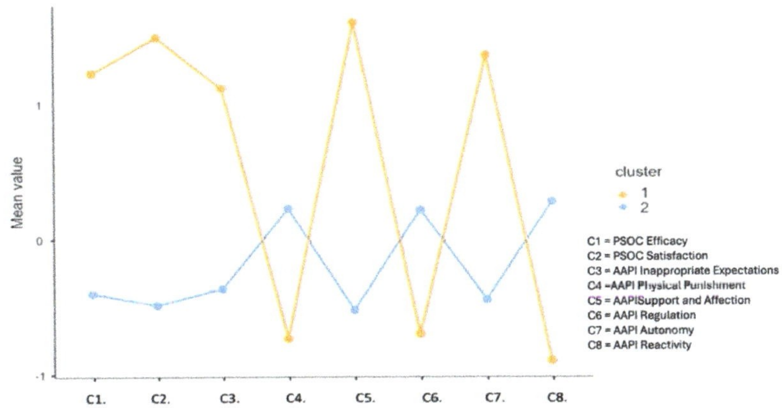

Figure 2. Average levels of variables characterizing parental behaviors by cluster.

Table 3. Effect of the intervention on parental behaviors and practices (difference between the average values of M1 and M2) by cluster.

Domains	Cluster 1 (n = 9)				Cluster 2 (n = 28)				Z	p	r
	M	SD	Min	Max	M	SD	Min	Max			
Efficacy	1.02	0.37	0.43	1.57	0.23	0.33	−0.57	1.14	−3.98	<0.001	0.65
Satisfaction	1.35	0.62	0.22	2.22	0.06	0.17	−0.22	0.44	−4.32	<0.001	0.71
Inap. Exp.	1.30	1.11	−0.14	2.86	0.13	0.34	−0.29	1.29	−3.18	0.001	0.52
Physical Punishment	−0.56	1.01	−2.00	1.09	0.02	0.29	−0.64	0.91	−1.70	0.088	0.28
Affection and Support	1.18	0.35	0.80	2.00	0.06	0.12	−0.20	0.40	−4.77	<0.001	0.78
Regulation	−2.04	0.51	−2.80	−1.20	−1.29	0.83	−3.00	0.20	−2.51	0.012	0.41
Autonomy	0.93	0.52	0.20	1.80	0.04	0.21	−0.80	0.40	−4.59	<0.001	0.75
Reactivity	−0.62	0.83	−2.40	0.00	−0.06	0.13	−0.40	0.20	−2.51	0.012	0.41

Note. Inap. Exp. = Inappropriate Expectations; M = Mean; SD = Standard Deviation; Min = Minimum; Max = Maximum; Z = test statistic; p = significance; r = effect size.

Regarding support and affection, there was a statistically significant difference of high magnitude ($Z = -4.77$; $p < 0.001$; $r = 0.78$), with C1 showing a higher result than C2 ($M_{C1} = 1.18$; $SD_{C1} = 0.35$; $M_{C2} = 0.06$; $SD_{C2} = 0.12$). In terms of regulation ($Z = -2.51$; $p = 0.012$; $r = 0.41$), C2 showed a smaller decrease ($M_{C1} = -2.04$; $SD_{C1} = 0.51$; $M_{C2} = -1.29$; $SD_{C2} = 0.83$), while C1 reported greater gains in autonomy ($Z = -4.59$; $p < 0.001$; $r = 0.75$; $M_{C1} = 0.93$; $SD_{C1} = 0.52$; $M_{C2} = 0.04$; $SD_{C2} = 0.21$) and a greater decrease in reactivity ($Z = -2.51$; $p = 0.012$; $r = 0.41$; $M_{C1} = -0.62$; $SD_{C1} = 0.83$; $M_{C2} = -0.06$; $SD_{C2} = 0.13$). All the differences were statistically significant, with moderate to high magnitudes.

In summary, the C1 participants overall reported higher gains on most of the evaluated dimensions (i.e., efficacy, satisfaction, inappropriate expectations, affection and support, and reactivity), while the C2 participants revealed changes only per the dimensions of physical punishment, regulation, and reactivity. To better interpret these results, a more detailed analysis of the values obtained by each cluster before the intervention was necessary (Table 4).

Table 4. Comparison between clusters in the pre-test.

Dimensions	C1		C2		*Z*	*p*	*r*
	M	*SD*	*M*	*SD*			
Efficacy	4.32	0.25	4.31	0.49	−0.27	0.789	0.04
Satisfaction	3.57	0.48	3.50	0.50	−0.28	0.776	0.05
Quality of Life	3.70	0.38	3.86	0.28	−1.33	0.183	0.22
Parental Mental Health	44.22	8.81	48.07	8.77	−1.45	0.146	0.24
Inappropriate Expectations	2.40	0.71	2.15	0.66	−1.14	0.255	0.19
Physical Punishment	2.77	0.63	2.71	0.68	−0.21	0.831	0.04
Affection and Support	3.76	0.36	3.95	0.43	−1.13	0.259	−0.19
Regulation	3.84	0.51	3.96	0.30	−0.72	0.475	−0.12
Autonomy	3.58	0.42	3.50	0.47	−0.41	0.680	−0.07
Reactivity	2.42	0.83	2.74	0.79	−1.16	0.248	−0.19

Note. *M* = Mean; *SD* = Standard deviation; *Z* = Test statistic; *p* = Significance; *r* = Effect size.

The comparison between C1 and C2 at the level of results obtained in the pre-test did not reveal significant differences or effects in any dimension. As Table 5 shows, the C2 participants attended slightly more program sessions (M_{C2} = 7.96; SD_{C2} = 2.56; $Range_{C2}$ = 3–12) than those in C1 (M_{C1} = 7.78; SD_{C1} = 2.44; $Range_{C1}$ = 3–10).

Table 5. Comparison between pre-test and post-test in both clusters.

Domains	Cluster 1 (*n* = 9)								*Z*	*p*	*r*	Cluster 2 (*n* = 28)								*Z*	*p*	*r*
	Pre				*Post*							*Pre*				*Post*						
	M	*SD*	*Min*	*Max*	*M*	*SD*	*Min*	*Max*				*M*	*SD*	*Min*	*Max*	*M*	*SD*	*Min*	*Max*			
No. of sessions	-	-	-	-	7.78	2.44	3.00	10.00	-	-	-	-	-	-	-	7.96	2.56	3.00	12.00	-	-	-
Efficacy	4.32	0.25	4.00	4.71	5.33	0.29	4.86	5.71	−2.67	0.008	0.47	4.31	0.49	3.14	5.43	4.55	0.41	3.57	5.29	−3.17	0.002	0.56
Satisfaction	3.57	0.48	3.00	4.44	4.91	0.47	4.11	5.56	−2.67	0.008	0.47	3.50	0.50	2.67	4.67	3.56	0.46	2.67	4.78	−1.66	0.097	0.29
Quality of Life	3.70	0.38	2.80	4.00	4.52	0.28	4.20	5.00	2.67	0.008	0.47	3.86	0.28	2.90	4.30	3.96	0.32	2.80	4.50	−3.03	0.002	0.54
Parental Mental Health	44.22	8.81	33.00	62.00	47.78	2.82	44.00	53.00	−1.87	0.236	0.33	48.07	8.77	32.00	64.00	48.04	8.29	33.00	64.00	−0.87	0.385	0.15
Inappropriate Expectations	2.40	0.71	1.43	3.29	3.70	0.49	3.00	4.43	−2.94	0.013	0.52	2.15	0.66	1.14	3.29	2.29	0.71	1.14	3.57	−2.20	0.028	0.39
Physical Punishment	2.77	0.63	2.00	3.55	2.21	0.67	1.18	3.18	−1.60	0.109	0.28	2.71	0.68	1.73	4.09	2.73	0.58	1.73	4.00	−0.51	0.609	0.09
Affection and Support	3.76	0.36	3.00	4.20	4.93	0.14	4.60	5.00	−2.69	0.007	0.48	3.95	0.43	3.00	5.00	4.01	0.38	3.00	4.80	−2.50	0.013	0.44
Regulation	3.84	0.51	3.00	4.60	4.87	0.22	4.40	5.00	−2.68	0.007	0.47	3.96	0.30	3.20	4.80	4.01	0.30	3.40	4.80	−2.83	0.005	0.50
Autonomy	3.58	0.42	2.80	4.00	4.51	0.39	4.00	5.00	−2.67	0.008	0.47	3.50	0.47	2.40	4.20	3.54	0.47	2.40	4.20	−1.65	0.098	0.29
Reactivity	2.42	0.83	1.40	3.60	1.80	0.46	1.20	2.40	−2.21	0.027	0.39	2.74	0.79	1.00	3.80	2.67	0.78	1.00	3.80	−2.31	0.021	0.41

Note. *M* = Mean; *SD* = Standard deviation; *Z* = Test statistic; *p* = Significance; *r* = Effect size.

The comparison between pre-test and post-test revealed statistically significant results in almost all dimensions in both clusters. However, values from C1 reflected greater gains than those from C2. Notable were satisfaction (Z_{C1} = −2.67; p_{C1} = 0.008; r_{C1} = 0.47; Z_{C2} = −1.66; p_{C2} = 0.097; r_{C2} = 0.29; pre-test: M_{C1} = 3.57; SD_{C1} = 0.48; M_{C2} = 3.50; SD_{C2} = 0.50; post-test: M_{C1} = 4.91; SD_{C1} = 0.47; M_{C2} = 3.56; SD_{C2} = 0.46) and autonomy (Z_{C1} = −2.67; p_{C1} = 0.008; r_{C1} = 0.47; Z_{C2} = −1.65; p_{C2} = 0.098; r_{C2} = 0.29; pre-test: M_{C1} = 3.58; SD_{C1} = 0.42; M_{C2} = 3.50; SD_{C2} = 0.47; post-test: M_{C1} = 4.51; SD_{C1} = 0.39; M_{C2} = 3.54; SD_{C2} = 0.47), where the difference in C2 was nearly significant. Regarding reactivity, it was also in C1 where a greater decrease was observed (Z_{C1} = 2.40; p_{C1} = 0.027; r_{C1} = 0.39; Z_{C2} = −2.31; p_{C2} = 0.021; r_{C2} = 0.41; pre-test: M_{C1} = 2.42; SD_{C1} = 0.83; M_{C2} = 2.74; SD_{C2} = 0.79; post-test: M_{C1} = 1.80; SD_{C1} = 0.46; M_{C2} = 2.67; SD_{C2} = 0.78).

Although the difference was not significant in both clusters, C1 reported a greater increase in parental mental health (Z_{C1} = −1.87; p_{C1} = 0.236; r_{C1} = 0.33; Z_{C2} = −0.87; p_{C2} = 0.385; r_{C2} = 0.15; pre-test: M_{C1} = 44.22; SD_{C1} = 8.81; M_{C2} = 48.07; SD_{C2} = 8.77; post-test: M_{C1} = 47.78; SD_{C1} = 2.82; M_{C2} = 48.04; SD_{C2} = 8.29), while C2 participants presented higher average levels, with stability between assessed moments. Also noteworthy in terms of physical punishment was that, although not statistically significant, the average value was higher in C1, and it was also in this group where the decrease between moments was highest (Z_{C1} = −1.60; p_{C1} = 0.109; r_{C1} = 0.28; Z_{C2} = −0.57; p_{C2} = 0.609; r_{C2} = 0.09; pre-test:

M_{C1} = 2.77; SD_{C1} = 0.63; M_{C2} = 2.71; SD_{C2} = 0.68; post-test: M_{C1} = 2.21; SD_{C1} = 0.67; M_{C2} = 2.73; SD_{C2} = 0.58).

4. Discussion

Considering the importance of positive parenting promotion programs in the development of parenting skills and the quality of life of children (e.g., Davies et al. [94]; Hidalgo et al. [95]), the present research aimed to study the changes promoted by the FAF intervention on parenting practices, perceived parental efficacy, and parents' attitudes and beliefs. Therefore, a cluster analysis was conducted to identify groups of participants with similar gains, resulting in the definition of two groups/clusters (i.e., C1 and C2).

A preliminary analysis of the clusters (Figure 2), showing the differences between the assessment moments, indicated that both groups benefited from the program, with neither group experiencing deterioration due to the intervention. These results are similar to those of previous applications of the FAF, both in the European context [63,65,66] and in Peru [67].

It was also found that there was a greater difference in the evaluated dimensions in C1 compared to C2. To rule out the possibility that these differences already existed beforehand, a comparison of the two clusters before the intervention was conducted (Table 4), which revealed no pre-existing differences. Thus, the analysis of the characteristics of the participants in each cluster proceeded.

Regarding the sociodemographic characteristics and functional profile of the parents, the results did not highlight any differences in their profiles that would justify the different changes observed in the clusters. In terms of session attendance, considering that 14 sessions were held, no participants in either cluster attended all sessions, although the maximum attendance in C2 was slightly higher (12 sessions; C1 = 10 sessions). Past research on the implementation of parenting promotion programs in African contexts had shown that parents' level of participation is quite high (e.g., Lachman et al. [70]), with low dropout rates, compared to developed countries [70,96]. However, it should be noted that parents' levels of participation are an important predictor of the changes promoted by the intervention analyzed [3,7,10,97].

Concerning the dimensions associated with parenting, in C1, the results showed significant differences, and in most cases, of greater magnitude before and after the implementation of the FAF, per the dimensions of parental efficacy and satisfaction, inappropriate expectations, affection and support, and reactivity. In this sense, it appears that this group of participants, who started with lower pre-test values compared to C2, gained more benefits in terms of improved attitudes, regulation, and interaction with their children, feeling more effective and satisfied in this process.

According to the literature, when parents feel competent in their parenting tasks, using effective educational practices, and feeling satisfied with their parenting performance [9,49], they tend to use more parenting practices that include support and affection, trust in, and enhance children's autonomy. As a result, they have less need to resort to regulation, use physical punishment, or find themselves in situations where they naturally feel more reactive. In summary, they are more inclined to engage in positive parenting practices rather than negative ones [6,16,17,98].

In turn, C2 showed a greater difference in regulation and reactivity, which appears to be a change largely focused on parenting practices and their implementation. Thus, the same activities can impact different parents differently [18]; however, the program resulted in changes across the various evaluated dimensions.

According to the standards of evidence developed by the Society for Prevention Research (SPR) for prevention programs and policies [99], the FAF can be considered an effective intervention because it was tested in at least two rigorous trials with defined samples from a specific population, using psychometrically sound measures and objective data collection procedures, and employing rigorous statistical approaches appropriate to the study's objective. The findings have demonstrated that the effects obtained were consistent and maintained at follow-up. Furthermore, this intervention was based on a manualized program, which included both an intervention group and a control group, and the results of the intervention emphasize the importance of parental programs in parenting skills [100].

Overall, the FAF, like other programs implemented in African contexts, helped to increase positive parenting practices (e.g., Lachman et al. [70,101]; Rose et al. [71]), particularly in terms of parent-child relationships, positive parenting practices, perceived parental efficacy and satisfaction [12], and child maltreatment [70,97,101]. However, past studies had also highlighted the importance of various stressors on parents' and groups' responses to the intervention (e.g., Shenderovich et al. [98]; Littell and Schuerman [99]; Farrelly and McLennan [102]), including economic, educational, social, and health barriers, among others [69,71,97,101], which can negatively affect parents' parenting skills and the development and well-being of their children [103].

In the present research, neither group showed a significant change in reducing physical punishment. It is important to emphasize that sociodemographic (e.g., family income and education level) and cultural characteristics can be important predictors of such practices [69,71,101]. Maya et al. [67] found similar results in Peru. These authors suggest that the practice of physical punishment as a form of behavioral control is more accepted in Latin American culture and, therefore, a more difficult dimension to change.

Some prior studies conducted in African contexts had indicated that families at psychosocial risk tend to exhibit higher levels of physical punishment. Other studies conducted among African cultural groups (e.g., Breen et al. [104]; Lachman et al. [70]) had suggested that physical punishment is a normative and culturally accepted disciplinary strategy. Therefore, programs and initiatives in this area have tended to show more modest results (e.g., Cluver et al. [105]; Lachman et al. [69,70,101]).

Limitations and Future Studies

While this study makes important contributions to the field, it also had several limitations, such as the small number of participants and the limited number of evaluated domains; the reliability of some measures used; and the focus solely on quantitative data, which restricted interpretation of the changes promoted by the FAF intervention. We recommend that future studies use previously adapted instruments to the context and employ mixed methods approaches. These approaches could involve returning the results to the parents and discussing them together, as well as including an assessment of the children's behavior and other evaluation sources. It is always important to consider that interventions in such programs should be evidence-based and meet the quality criteria for these types of actions [95,106]. Furthermore, it is crucial to exhaustively examine the various predictors and differentiators (e.g., mediators, moderators) of the changes achieved (or not) promoted (e.g., Decker et al. [73]). Future studies might also utilize qualitative methodologies and include an evaluation of the children's behavior, along with other assessment sources.

5. Conclusions

This study is an important contribution to promoting positive parenting programs, particularly in the African context. Past research had shown that such programs can have a positive impact on families, although their implementation must be subject to cultural adaptations. Our study, by analyzing the underlying profiles of these change processes, highlighted that some participants benefit more from the intervention than others, which is valuable information for professionals and researchers.

Author Contributions: Conceptualization, A.C., V.H. and C.N.; Data curation, A.C. and C.N.; Formal analysis, A.C., C.M. and C.N.; Funding acquisition, C.M. and C.N.; Investigation, A.C.; Methodology, A.C., V.H. and C.N.; Supervision, V.H., S.N.d.J. and C.N.; Writing—original draft, A.C., C.M., R.d.S., V.H., S.N.d.J. and C.N.; Writing—review & editing, A.C., C.M., R.d.S., V.H., S.N.d.J. and C.N. All authors have read and agreed to the published version of the manuscript.

Funding: This work was funded by national funds through FCT—Fundação para a Ciência e a Tecnologia—as part of the project CIP; Refª UIDB/PSI/04345/2020.

Institutional Review Board Statement: The study was conducted according to the guidelines of the Declaration of Helsinki and approved by the Scientific Commission of the Psychology and Sciences Education Department, University of Algarve, Reference No. 60_10/09/2018, on 10 September 2018.

Informed Consent Statement: Written informed consent was obtained from all subjects involved in the study.

Data Availability Statement: The data can be made available for consultation from the corresponding author upon request. The data are not publicly available due to privacy and ethical restrictions.

Conflicts of Interest: The authors declare no conflicts of interest.

References

1. Ayala-Nunes, L.; Jiménez, L.; Jesus, S.; Nunes, C.; Hidalgo, V. An Ecological Model of Well-Being in Child Welfare Referred Children. *Soc. Indic. Res.* **2018**, *140*, 811–836. [CrossRef]
2. United Nations Children's Fund [UNICEF]. *Fair Parent, Fair Child: Handbook on Positive Parenting*; UNICEF Office: Skopje, Macedonia, 2018. Available online: https://www.unicef.mk (accessed on 20 April 2024).
3. García-Poole, C.; Byrne, S.; Rodrigo, M.J. Implementation Factors that Predict Positive Outcomes in a Community-based Intervention Program for at-Risk Adolescents. *Psychosoc. Interv.* **2019**, *28*, 57–65. [CrossRef]
4. Hidalgo, M.V.; Ruiz, B.; Bacete, F.J.; González, R.A.; Verdugo, I.; Jiménez, L. The Evaluation of Family Support Programmes in Spain. An Analysis of their Quality Standards. *Psicol. Educ.* **2023**, *29*, 35–43. [CrossRef]
5. Nunes, C.; Martins, C.; Brás, M.; Carmo, C.; Gonçalves, A.; Pina, A. Impact of an online parenting support programme on children's quality of life. *Children* **2022**, *9*, 173. [CrossRef] [PubMed]
6. United Nations Children's Fund [UNICEF]. *O Cuidado Integral e a Parentalidade Positiva na Primeira Infância. Brasília: Fundo das Nações Unidas para a Infância*; Fundo das Nações Unidas para a Infância (UNICEF): Brasília, Brazil, 2023. Available online: https://www.unicef.org/brazil/biblioteca (accessed on 20 April 2024).
7. Hidalgo, V.; Jiménez, L. Os Programas de Educação e Apoio Parental Como Recurso para a Promoção da Parentalidade Positiva com Famílias em Situação de Risco Psicossocial. In *Famílias em Risco: Avaliação e Intervenção Psicoeducativa*; Nunes, C., Ayala, L., Eds.; Silabas & Desafios: Faro, Portugal, 2019; pp. 173–203.
8. Jiménez, L.; Hidalgo, M. La Incorporación de Prácticas Basadas en Evidencias en el Trabajo con Familias: Los Programas de Promoción de Parentalidad Positiva. *Apunt. Psicol.* **2017**, *34*, 91–100. [CrossRef]
9. Nunes, C.; Ayala-Nunes, L. Parenting sense of competence in at psychosocial risk families and child well-being. *Bordón* **2017**, *69*, 155–168. [CrossRef]
10. Rodrigo, M.J.; Almeida, A.; Reichle, B. Evidence-Based Parent Education Programs: A European Perspective. In *Evidence-Based Parenting Education: A Global Perspective*; Ponzetti, J., Ed.; Routledge: New York, NY, USA, 2016; pp. 85–104.
11. Altafim, E.; Linhares, M. Universal violence and child maltreatment prevention programs for parents: A systematic review. *Psychosoc. Interv.* **2016**, *25*, 27–38. [CrossRef]
12. Correia, A.; Matavelli, R.; Cunha, F.F.; Hidalgo, V.; Jesus, S.N.; Nunes, C. Family Education and support programme: Implementation and cultural adaptation in Cape Verde. *Soc. Sci.* **2022**, *11*, 1–14. [CrossRef]
13. Mikton, C.; Butchart, A. Child maltreatment prevention: A systematic review of reviews. *Bull. World Health Organ.* **2009**, *87*, 353–361. [CrossRef]
14. Sanders, M.R.; Higgins, D.; Prinz, R. A population approach to the prevention of child maltreatment: Rationale and implications for research, policy and practice. *Fam. Matters* **2018**, *100*, 62–70.
15. Council of Europe. Recommendation Rec(2006)7 of the Committee of Ministers to Member States on Management of Patient Safety and Prevention of Adverse Events in Health Care 2006. Available online: https://www.coe.int/en/web/portal/home (accessed on 20 April 2024).
16. Avezum, M.; Altafim, E.; Linhares, M. Spanking and corporal punishment parenting practices and child development: A systematic review. *Trauma Violence Abus.* **2023**, *24*, 3094–3111. [CrossRef] [PubMed]
17. Cuartas, J.; Weissman, D.; Sheridan, M.; Lengua, L.; McLaughlin, K. Corporal Punishment and Elevated Neural Response to Threat in Children. *Child Dev.* **2021**, *92*, 821–832. [CrossRef] [PubMed]
18. Lotto, C.; Altafim, E.; Linhares, M. Maternal history of childhood adversities and later negative parenting: A systematic review. *Trauma Violence Abus.* **2023**, *24*, 662–683. [CrossRef] [PubMed]
19. Martins, C.; Ayala-Nunes, L.; Nunes, C.; Pechorro, P.; Costa, E.; Matos, F. Confirmatory analysis of the Parenting Styles and Dimensions Questionnaire (PSDQ) short form in a portuguese sample. *Eur. J. Psychol. Educ.* **2018**, *11*, 77–91. [CrossRef]
20. Nunes, C.; Bodden, D.; Lemos, I.; Lorence, B.; Jiménez, L. Parenting practices and quality of life in Dutch and Portuguese adolescents: A cross-cultural study. *Rev. Psicodidact.* **2014**, *19*, 327–346. [CrossRef]

21. Macana, E.; Comim, F. O papel das práticas e estilos parentais no desenvolvimento da primeira infância. In *Fundamentos da Família como Promotora do Desenvolvimento Infantil: Parentalidade em Foco;* Pluciennik, G., Lazzari, M., Chicaro, M., Eds.; Fundação Maria Cecilia Souto Vidigal: São Paulo, Brazil, 2015; pp. 34–47.
22. Goagoses, N.; Bolz, T.; Eilts, J.; Schipper, N.; Schütz, J.; Rademacher, A.; Vesterling, C.; Koglin, U. Parenting dimensions/styles and emotion dysregulation in childhood and adolescence: A systematic review and meta-analysis. *Curr. Psychol.* **2023**, *42*, 18798–18822. [CrossRef]
23. Bornstein, M.H. Determinants of parenting. In *Developmental Psychopathology: Risk, Resilience, and Intervention*, 3rd ed.; Cicchetti, D., Ed.; Wiley: New York, NY, USA, 2016; Volume 4, pp. 180–270.
24. Nunes, C.; Martins, C.; Ayala-Nunes, L.; Matos, F.; Costa, E.; Gonçalves, A. Parents' perceived social support and children's psychological adjustment. *J. Soc. Work.* **2021**, *21*, 497–512. [CrossRef]
25. Belsky, J.; Jaffee, S.R. The multiple determinants of parenting. In *Developmental Psychopathology*, 2nd ed.; Cicchetti, D., Cohen, D., Eds.; Wiley: New York, NY, USA, 2006; pp. 38–77.
26. Belsky, J. The determinants of parenting: A process model. *Child Dev.* **1984**, *55*, 83–96. [CrossRef]
27. Gershoff, E.T.; Lee, S.J.; Durrant, J.E. Promising intervention strategies to reduce parents' use of physical punishment. *Child Abus. Negl.* **2017**, *71*, 9–23. [CrossRef]
28. Heilmann, A.; Mehay, A.; Watt, R.G.; Kelly, Y.; Durrant, J.E.; van Turnhout, J.; Gershoff, E.T. Physical punishment and child outcomes: A narrative review of prospective studies. *Lancet* **2021**, *398*, 355–364. [CrossRef]
29. Palacios, I.; Garcia, O.F.; Alcaide, M.; Garcia, F. Positive parenting style and positive health beyond the authoritative: Self, universalism values, and protection against emotional vulnerability from Spanish adolescents and adult children. *Front. Psychol.* **2022**, *13*, 1066282. [CrossRef] [PubMed]
30. Reyes, M.; Garcia, O.F.; Perez-Gramaje, A.F.; Serra, E.; Melendez, J.C.; Alcaide, M.; Garcia, F. Which is the optimum parenting for adolescents with low vs. high self-efficacy? Self-concept, psychological maladjustment and academic performance of adolescents in the Spanish context. *An. Psicol./Ann. Psychol.* **2023**, *39*, 446–457. [CrossRef]
31. Rodrigues, Y.; Veiga, F.; Fuentes, M.C.; García, F. Parenting and adolescents' self-esteem: The Portuguese context. *Rev. Psicodidact.* **2013**, *18*, 395–416. [CrossRef]
32. Bølstad, E.; Havighurst, S.S.; Tamnes, C.K.; Nygaard, E.; Bjørk, R.F.; Stavrinou, M.; Espeseth, T. A pilot study of a parent emotion socialization intervention: Impact on parent behavior, child self-regulation, and adjustment. *Front. Psychol.* **2021**, *12*, 730278. [CrossRef]
33. Dwairy, M.; Achoui, M. Adolescents-family connectedness: A first cross-cultural research on parenting and psychological adjustment of children. *J. Child Fam. Stud.* **2010**, *19*, 8–15. [CrossRef]
34. Gaspar, T.; Cerqueira, A.; Guedes, F.B.; de Matos, M.G. Parental Emotional Support, Family Functioning and Children's Quality of Life. *Psychol. Stud.* **2022**, *67*, 189–199. [CrossRef]
35. Pinquart, M. Associations of parenting dimensions and styles with externalizing problems of children and adolescents: An updated meta-analysis. *Dev. Psychol.* **2017**, *53*, 873. [CrossRef]
36. Roche, K.; Sharon, R.; Ghazarian, S.; Little, T.; Leventhal, T. Understanding links between punitive parenting and adolescent adjustment: The relevance of context and reciprocal associations. *J. Adolesc. Res.* **2010**, *21*, 448–460. [CrossRef]
37. Baker-Henningham, H.; Francis, T. Parents' use of harsh punishment and young children's behaviour and achievement: A longitudinal study of Jamaican children with conduct problems. *Glob. Ment. Health* **2018**, *5*, e32. [CrossRef]
38. Beckmann, L.; Bergmann, M.C.; Fischer, F.; Mößle, T. Risk and protective factors of child-to-parent violence: A comparison between physical and verbal aggression. *J. Interpers. Violence* **2021**, *36*, NP1309–NP1334. [CrossRef]
39. Davis, R.C.; Palumbo, I.M.; Tobin, K.E.; Latzman, R.D. Exploring the effects of parental involvement on broad and specific dimensions of behavioral problems in adolescence. *Child Psychiatry Hum. Dev.* **2022**, *53*, 1–13. [CrossRef] [PubMed]
40. Rodríguez Ruíz, M.M.; Carrasco, M.Á.; Holgado-Tello, F.P. Father involvement and children's psychological adjustment: Maternal and paternal acceptance as mediators. *J. Fam. Stud.* **2019**, *25*, 151–169. [CrossRef]
41. Sitnick, S.; Shaw, D.; Gill, A.; Dishion, T.; Winter, C.; Waller, R.; Gardner, F.; Wilson, M. Parenting and the Family Check-Up: Changes in observed parent-child interaction following early childhood intervention. *J. Clin. Child Adolesc. Psychol.* **2015**, *44*, 970–984. [CrossRef] [PubMed]
42. Ang, R.; Goh, D. Authoritarian parenting style in Asian societies. A cluster-analytic investigation. *Contemp. Fam. Ther.* **2006**, *28*, 131–151. [CrossRef]
43. Lamborn, S.; Dornbusch, S.; Stein-berg, L. Ethnicity and com-munity context as moderators of the relations between family decision making and adolescent adjustment. *Child Dev.* **1996**, *67*, 283–301. [CrossRef]
44. Costa, S.; Cruz, O. Atitudes e estilos parentais em mãe de crianças com processo de promoção e proteção. *Rev. Amaz.* **2012**, *8*, 310–337.
45. Black, D.; Heyman, R.; Smith Slep, A. Risk factors for child physical abuse. *Aggress. Violent Behav.* **2001**, *6*, 121–188. [CrossRef]
46. Perez-Albeniz, A.; de Paul, J. Gender diferences in empathy in parents at high- and low-risk of child physical abuse. *Child Abus. Negl.* **2004**, *28*, 289–300. [CrossRef] [PubMed]
47. Bavolek, S.; Keene, R. *Adult-Adolescent Parenting Inventory. AAPI—2: Assessing High-Risk Parenting Attitudes and Behaviors;* Family Development Resources, Inc.: Park City, UT, USA, 2001.

48. Aparício, G.; Cunha, M.; Duarte, J. Self-perception of parental competence in parents of pre-school children. *Aten. Prim.* **2016**, *48*, 247–252.
49. Jones, T.; Prinz, R. Potential roles of parental self-efficacy in parent and child adjustment: A review. *Clin. Psychol. Rev.* **2005**, *25*, 341–363. [CrossRef]
50. Ayala-Nunes, L.; Nunes, C.; Lemos, I. Social support and parenting stress in at-risk Portuguese families. *J. Soc. Work.* **2017**, *17*, 207–225. [CrossRef]
51. Nunes, C.; Ayala-Nunes, L.; Ferreira, L.; Pechorro, P.; Freitas, D.; Martins, C.; Santos, R. Parenting sense of competence: Psychometrics and invariance among community and at-risk sample of Portuguese parents. *Healthcare* **2023**, *11*, 15. [CrossRef] [PubMed]
52. Bauch, J.; Hefti, S.; Oeltjen, L.; Pérez, T.; Swenson, C.C.; Fürstenau, U.; Rhiner, B.; Schmid, M. Multisystemic therapy for child abuse and neglect: Parental stress and parental mental health as predictors of change in child neglect. *Child Abus. Negl.* **2022**, *126*, 105489. [CrossRef] [PubMed]
53. Ayala-Nunes, L.; Lemos, I.; Nunes, C. Predictores del estrés parental en madres de familias en riesgo psicosocial. *Univ. Psychol.* **2014**, *13*, 529–539. [CrossRef]
54. Pérez, J.; Nunes, L.; Victoria, M.V.; Nunes, C.; Lemos, I.; Menéndez, S. Parenting and stress: A study with Spanish and Portuguese at-risk families. *Int. Soc. Work.* **2017**, *60*, 1001–1014. [CrossRef]
55. Santos, A.M. Parentalidade na infância: Relação com a parentalidade e qualidade de vida atual [Childhood Parenting: Relationship with Parenting and Current Quality of Life]. Master's Thesis, Universidade Lusófona de Humanidades e Tecnologias, Lisboa, Portugal, 2022.
56. Feniger-Schaal, R.; Joels, T. Attachment quality of children with ID and its link to maternal sensitivity and structuring. *Res. Dev. Disabil.* **2018**, *76*, 56–64. [CrossRef] [PubMed]
57. Sanders, M. Harnessing the power of positive parenting to promote wellbeing of children, parents and communities over a lifetime. *Behav. Change* **2019**, *36*, 56–74. [CrossRef]
58. Correia, A.; Nunes, C.; Marotta, G.; Lopes, M.; Martins, C.; Hidalgo, V.; Jesus, S. Impacto do programa de formação e apoio familiar nas competências parentais e na qualidade de vida infantil percebida em Cabo-Verde. *Psychologica* **2024**, *67*, 1–20. [CrossRef]
59. Sanders, M.R. Triple P-Positive Parenting Program: Towards an empirically validated multilevel parenting and family support strategy for the prevention of behavior and emotional problems in children. *Clin. Child Fam. Psychol. Rev.* **1999**, *2*, 71–90. [CrossRef]
60. Gardner, F.; Burton, J.; Klimes, I. Randomised controlled trial of a parenting intervention in the voluntary sector for reducing child conduct problems: Outcomes and mechanisms of change. *J. Child Psychol. Psychiatry* **2006**, *47*, 1123–1132. [CrossRef]
61. Amorós-Martí, P.; Byrne, S.; Mateos-Inchaurrondo, A.; Vaquero-Tió, E.; Mundet-Bolós, A. "Learning together, growing with family": The implementation and evaluation of a family support programme. *Psychosoc. Interv.* **2016**, *25*, 87–93. [CrossRef]
62. Knerr, W.; Gardner, F.; Cluver, L. Improving positive parenting skills and reducing harsh and abusive parenting in low-and middle-income countries: A systematic review. *Prev. Sci.* **2013**, *14*, 352–363. [CrossRef] [PubMed]
63. Hidalgo, M.V.; Menéndez Álvarez-Dardet, S.; Sánchez Hidalgo, J.; Lorence Lara, B.; Jiménez, L. La intervención con familias en situación de riesgo psicosocial: Aportaciones desde un enfoque psicoeducativo. *Apunt. Psicol.* **2009**, *27*, 413–426.
64. Hidalgo, M.V.; Menéndez, S.; López, I.; Sánchez, J.; Lorence, B.; Jiménez, L. *Programa de Formación y Apoyo Familiar*; Ayuntamiento de Sevilla: Sevilla, Spain, 2011.
65. Hidalgo, M.V.; Jiménez, L.; López-Verdugo, I.; Lorence, B.; Sánchez, J. "Family education and support" program for families at psychosocial risk: The role of implementation process. *Psychosoc. Interv.* **2016**, *25*, 79–85. [CrossRef]
66. Hidalgo, V.; Sanchez, J.; Lorence, B.; Menendez, S.; Jiménez, L. Evaluación de la implementación del programa de formación y apoyo familiar en servicios sociales. *Escr. Psicol.* **2014**, *7*, 33–41. [CrossRef]
67. Maya, J.; Hidalgo, M.V. Evaluación de la implementación del Programa de Formación y Apoyo Familiar con familias peruanas. *Apunt. Psicol.* **2016**, *34*, 119–128. [CrossRef]
68. Hidalgo, M.V.; Menéndez, S.; López, I.; Sánchez, J.; Lorence, B.; Jiménez, L. *Programa de Formação e Apoio Familiar*; Nunes, C., Martins, C., Ayala Nunes, L., Gonçalves, A., Eds., Universidade do Algarve: Faro, Portugal, 2019.
69. Lachman, J.M.; Cluver, L.; Ward, C.L.; Hutchings, J.; Mlotshwa, S.; Wessels, I.; Gardner, F. Randomized controlled trial of a parenting program to reduce the risk of child maltreatment in South Africa. *Child Abus. Negl.* **2017**, *72*, 338–351. [CrossRef] [PubMed]
70. Lachman, J.M.; Kelly, J.; Cluver, L.; Ward, C.L.; Hutchings, J.; Gardner, F. Process evaluation of a parenting program for low-income families in South Africa. *Res. Social. Work. Prac.* **2018**, *28*, 188–202. [CrossRef]
71. Rose, J.; Roman, N.; Mwaba, K. Circle of Security parenting program efficacy for improving parental self-efficacy in a South African setting: Preliminary evidence. *J. Psychol. Afr.* **2018**, *28*, 518–521. [CrossRef]
72. Zand, D.H.; Bultas, M.W.; McMillin, S.E.; Halloran, D.; White, T.; McNamara, D.; Pierce, K.J. A pilot of a brief positive parenting program on children newly diagnosed with autism spectrum disorder. *Fam. Process* **2018**, *57*, 901–914. [CrossRef]
73. Decker, K.M.; Thurston, I.B.; Howell, K.H.; Hasselle, A.J.; Kamody, R.C. Associations between Profiles of Maternal Strengths and Positive Parenting Practices among Mothers Experiencing Adversity. *Parenting* **2021**, *21*, 1–23. [CrossRef]

74. McWayne, C.M.; Mattis, J.S.; Hyun, S. Profiles of culturally salient positive parenting practices among urban-residing Black Head Start families. *Cultur. Divers. Ethnic Minor. Psychol.* **2018**, *24*, 414–428. [CrossRef]
75. Hidalgo, M.V.; Menéndez, S.; Sánchez, J.; López, I.; Jiménez, L.; Lorence, B. *Inventario de Situaciones Estresantes y de Riesgo (ISER)*; University of Seville: Seville, Spain, 2005; Unpublished Document.
76. Nunes, C.; Lemos, I.; Ayala-Nunes, L.; Costa, D. Acontecimentos de vida stressantes e apoio social em famílias em risco psicossocial. *Psicol. Saúde Doenças* **2013**, *14*, 313–320. Available online: https://www.redalyc.org/pdf/362/36227023008.pdf (accessed on 20 April 2024).
77. Johnston, C.; Mash, E.J. A measure of parenting satisfaction and efficacy. *J. Clin. Child Psychol.* **1989**, *18*, 167–175. [CrossRef]
78. Goldberg, D.; Williams, P. *Cuestionario de Salud General GHQ (General Health Questionnaire): Guía para el Usuario de las Distintas Versiones*; Masson: Barcelona, Spain, 1996.
79. Pais-Ribeiro, J.L.; Antunes, S. Contribuição para o estudo de adaptação do questionário de saúde geral de 28 itens (General Health Questionnaire—GHQ28). *Rev. Port. Psicossomática* **2003**, *5*, 37–45.
80. The KIDSCREEN Group Europe. *The KIDSCREEN Questionnaires: Quality of Life Questionnaires for Children and Adolescents*; Pabst Science Publishers: Germany, 2006.
81. Gaspar, T.; Matos, M.G. *Qualidade de vida em Crianças e Adolescentes: Versão Portuguesa dos Instrumentos KIDSCREEN-52*; Aventura Social e Saúde: Cruz e Quebrada, Portugal, 2008.
82. Robinson, C.; Mandleco, B.; Olsen, S.; Hart, C.H. The Parenting Styles and Dimensions Questionnaire (PSDQ). In *Handbook of Family Measurement Techniques*; Perlmutter, B., Touliatos, J., Holden, G., Eds.; Sage: Thousand Oaks, CA, USA, 2001; Volume 3, pp. 319–321.
83. Arnold, D.; O'Leary, S.; Wolff, L.; Acker, M. The Parenting Scale: A measure of dysfunctional parenting in discipline situations. *Psychol. Assess.* **1993**, *5*, 137–144. [CrossRef]
84. Barber, B.K. Parental psychological control: Revisiting a neglected construct. *Child Dev.* **1996**, *67*, 3296–3319. [CrossRef] [PubMed]
85. Lopes, I.; Brandão, T. *AAPI—2, Versão de Investigação, Traduzida e Adaptada para Português Europeu*; Universidade Técnica de Lisboa: Lisbon, Portugal, 2005.
86. Brock, G.; Pihur, V.; Datta, S.; Datta, S. clValid: An R Package for Cluster Validation. *J. Stat. Softw.* **2008**, *25*, 1–22. [CrossRef]
87. Core Team, R. *R: A Language and Environment for Statistical Computing [Computer Software]*; R Foundation for Statistical Computing: Vienna, Austria, 2021.
88. Handl, J.; Knowles, J.; Kell, B.D. Computational cluster validation in post-genomic data analysis. *Bioinformatics* **2005**, *21*, 3201–3212. [CrossRef]
89. Dunn, J.C. Well separated clusters and fuzzy partitions. *J. Cybern.* **1974**, *4*, 95–104. [CrossRef]
90. Rousseeuw, P.J. Silhouettes: A graphical aid to the interpretation and validation of cluster analysis. *J. Comput. Appl. Math.* **1987**, *20*, 53–65. [CrossRef]
91. Datta, S.; Datta, S. Comparisons and validation of statistical clustering techniques for microarray gene expression data. *Bioinformatics* **2003**, *19*, 459–466. [CrossRef] [PubMed]
92. Freire, T.; S Almeida, L.S. *Metodologia da Investigação em Psicologia e Educação*; Psiquilibrios: Braga, Portugal, 2008.
93. Field, A. *Discovering Statistics Using SPSS*, 3rd ed.; Sage Publications Ltd.: London, UK, 2009.
94. Davies, L.M.; Janta, B.; Gardner, F. *Positive Parenting Interventions: Empowering Parents with Positive Parenting Techniques for Lifelong Health and Well-Being*; Publications Office of the European Union: Luxembourg, 2019.
95. Hidalgo, M.V. Procesos de innovación y mejora en el ámbito de la intervención familiar. El papel de las y los profesionales en la incorporación de buenas prácticas basadas en la evidencia. *Apunt. Psicol.* **2022**, *40*, 117–126. [CrossRef]
96. Axford, N.; Lehtonen, M.; Kaoukji, D.; Tobin, K.; Berry, V. Engaging parents in parenting programs: Lessons from research and practice. *Child. Youth Serv. Rev.* **2012**, *34*, 2061–2071. [CrossRef]
97. Shenderovich, Y.; Eisner, M.; Cluver, L.; Doubt, J.; Berezin, M.; Majokweni, S.; Murray, A.L. Delivering a parenting program in South Africa: The impact of implementation on outcomes. *J. Child Fam. Stud.* **2019**, *28*, 1005–1017. [CrossRef]
98. Batista, H.H.V.S.; Noronha, A.P.P.; Reppold, C.T. Associações entre forças de caráter e estilos parentais em adultos. *Rev. Psicol. Pesq.* **2022**, *16*, 1–24. [CrossRef]
99. Littell, J.; Schuerman, J. What works best for whom? A closer look at intensive family preservation services. *Child. Youth Serv. Rev.* **2002**, *24*, 673–699. [CrossRef]
100. Flay, B.; Biglan, A.; Boruch, R.F.; González, F.; Gottfredson, D.; Kellam, S.; Moscicki, E.; Schinke, S.; Valentine, J.C.; Ji, P. Standards of evidence: Criteria for efficacy, effectiveness and dissemination. *Prev. Sci.* **2005**, *6*, 151–175. [CrossRef] [PubMed]
101. Lachman, J.M.; Sherr, L.T.; Cluver, L.; Ward, C.L.; Hutchings, J.; Gardner, F. Integrating evidence and context to develop a parenting program for low-income families in South Africa. *J. Child Fam. Stud.* **2016**, *25*, 2337–2352. [CrossRef]
102. Farrelly, A.C.; McLennan, J.D. Participation in a parent education programme in the Dominican Republic: Utilization and barriers. *J. Trop. Pediatr.* **2010**, *56*, 149–158. [CrossRef]
103. Nunes, C.; Nunes, L.A. Famílias em risco psicossocial: Desafios para a avaliação e intervenção. *Child Adolesc. Psychol.* **2015**, *6*, 95–107. [CrossRef]
104. Breen, A.; Daniels, K.; Tomlinson, M. Children's experiences of corporal punishment: A qualitative study in an urban township of South Africa. *Child Abus. Negl.* **2015**, *48*, 131–139. [CrossRef] [PubMed]

105. Cluver, L.D.; Meinck, F.; I Steinert, J.; Shenderovich, Y.; Doubt, J.; Romero, R.H.; Lombard, C.J.; Redfern, A.; Ward, C.L.; Tsoanyane, S.; et al. Parenting for Lifelong Health: A pragmatic cluster randomised controlled trial of a non-commercialised parenting programme for adolescents and their families in South Africa. *BMJ Glob. Health* **2018**, *3*, e000539. [CrossRef] [PubMed]
106. Jiménez, L.; Antolín-Suárez, L.; Lorence, B.; Hidalgo, V. Family education and support for families at psychosocial risk in Europe: Evidence from a survey of international experts. *Health Soc. Care Community* **2019**, *27*, 449–458. [CrossRef] [PubMed]

children

MDPI

Article

Long-Term Mandatory Homeschooling during COVID-19 Had Compounding Mental Health Effects on Parents and Children

Lucretia V. M. Groff [1], Mariam M. Elgendi [1], Sherry H. Stewart [1,2,3] and Storm Hélène Deacon [1,*]

[1] Department of Psychology and Neuroscience, Dalhousie University, Halifax, NS B3H 4R2, Canada; lucretia.groff@dal.ca (L.V.M.G.); m.elgendi@dal.ca (M.M.E.); sherry.stewart@dal.ca (S.H.S.)
[2] Department of Psychiatry, Dalhousie University, Halifax, NS B3H 4R2, Canada
[3] Department of Community Health and Epidemiology, Dalhousie University, Halifax, NS B3H 4R2, Canada
* Correspondence: helene.deacon@dal.ca

Abstract: Background/Objectives: Most studies have linked mandatory homeschooling during COVID-19 to mental health harm in parents and children, while a minority have found non-significant or beneficial effects. Past studies have not measured mandatory homeschooling continuously over an extended period; consequently, they could not capture compounding mental health effects, which may explain conflicting results. We asked whether children's cumulative time spent homeschooled during COVID-19 school closure mandates caused compounding harm for parent and child mental health, and whether parent employment, child internet access and educational support from schools (live and pre-recorded online classes, home learning packs) impacted this relationship. We aimed to identify the families at greatest risk of mental health harm during mandatory homeschooling and the educational support that may have mitigated this risk. Methods: Couples completed retrospective, cross-sectional survey questionnaires assessing parent depression, anxiety and stress, child internalizing and externalizing symptoms, and the family's homeschooling experience. Data were analyzed using mediation analysis total effects, ordinary least squares regression and simple slopes analysis. Results: Both parents and children experienced compounding mental health harm during mandatory homeschooling. Live online classes protected parents and children, while home learning packs protected children. Unexpectedly, reliable internet access and the employment of both parents placed children at greater risk. Conclusions: Findings suggest that long-term mandatory homeschooling during COVID-19 placed families at greater risk of mental health harm. To protect family mental health during homeschooling mandates, schools should provide children with evidence-based educational support.

Keywords: COVID-19; homeschooling; parent mental health; child mental health

1. Introduction

On 11 March 2020, the World Health Organization declared the COVID-19 virus a pandemic [1]. To reduce transmission of the virus, over 90% of countries worldwide implemented school closures, forcing millions of children to continue their education through mandatory homeschooling [2]. Mandatory homeschooling refers to involuntary at-home learning resulting from mandated school closures, in which schooling responsibility is largely transferred onto parents and caregivers [3]. The COVID-19 pandemic has had negative impacts on parent and child mental health [4–7], which many studies have linked to mandatory homeschooling [3,8,9]. By contrast, a minority of studies have found that the effects of mandatory homeschooling on mental health were non-significant or beneficial [10,11].

Chronic (long-term) activation of stress response has been linked to greater adverse mental health impacts in adults and children than acute (short-lasting) stress [12–15]. These findings suggest that families engaged in long-term homeschooling may have been at greater risk of adverse mental health effects due to compounding (progressively worsening) effects over time [12,16]. However, existing research has not captured compounding mental health effects of mandatory homeschooling over an extended period, which may explain conflicting results across studies. Consequently, it is unknown whether mandatory homeschooling has compounding adverse mental health effects over time or if long-term mandatory homeschoolers are at greater risk.

Alongside the duration of mandatory homeschooling, several other factors may have influenced its effects on parent and child mental health. First, receiving inadequate educational support from schools during mandatary homeschooling may have placed additional academic strain on families, exacerbating mental health harm [17–19]. Second, since use of the internet was often necessary for mandatory homeschooling, families with poor internet access may have experienced greater mental health harm [20,21]. Finally, pre- and peri-pandemic research has linked parental unemployment to adverse mental health effects in families, which may point to parent unemployment as another risk factor during mandatory homeschooling [4,22–24].

The present study investigates whether children's cumulative time engaged in mandatory homeschooling has compounding adverse effects on family mental health, looking specifically at parent depression, anxiety, and stress, and child internalizing symptoms (emotional and peer problems) and externalizing symptoms (behavioral and hyperactivity problems). It also explores whether educational supports from schools, child internet access or parent employment status moderate this relationship. Our first aim was to identify which families are at greatest risk of adverse mental health effects during mandatory homeschooling, so they can be given access to the supports they need to recover. Our second aim was to identify educational supports that may mitigate these adverse effects, to assist schools in minimizing mental health harm for families during future mandates.

1.1. Mandatory Homeschooling during COVID-19

During mandatory homeschooling, educational and childcare responsibilities usually fulfilled by schools were shifted onto parents, who often lacked adequate training and resources [25]. One study of mandated homeschooling during COVID-19 found that children spent 30% of their learning time in contact with their parents, while just under 14% was spent in contact with teachers [18]. In-person school provides children with academic support, structured routines, and access to mental health and peer supports, which are beneficial to children's mental health [26,27]. However, during the COVID-19 school closures, children were cut off from many of these mental health protections [19,27]. Meanwhile, many parents were forced to navigate their newfound schooling responsibilities alongside other stressors, including employment insecurity, financial strain, and social inequities [4,7].

1.2. Mandatory Homeschooling and Parent and Child Mental Health

Most research examining mandatory homeschooling during the COVID-19 pandemic has linked it to declines in parent and child mental health. Kishida et al. [8] found that full school closures the previous week were linked to greater parent and child mental health harm compared to partial school closures, which in turn were linked to greater harm than full in-person learning. Schmidt et al. [9] found that parents and children experienced poorer affect on mandatory homeschooling days, while Deacon et al. [1] found that parents who spent more hours per week homeschooling their child due to COVID-19 mandates experienced higher anxiety, depression, and traumatic stress. Interestingly, a minority of studies did not support these findings. DesRoches [10] found that mandatory homeschooling had non-significant impacts on child mental health, while Monnier [11] found that more hours per day spent homeschooling were associated with lower externalizing symptoms in children. This lack of consensus on the effects of mandatory homeschooling on child mental health may be explained by how these studies conceptualized and measured mandatory homeschooling.

1.3. Homeschooling Time as a Continuous Measure

The duration of school closures during the COVID-19 pandemic varied by location and school board [28]. In Canada, school closure duration ranged from a minimum of 50 school days in British Columbia, to a minimum of 135 school days in Ontario [29]. Past research has studied mandatory homeschooling over short-term periods, often using non-continuous measures that do not capture variations in duration [3,8–11]. For example, some studies have measured mandatory homeschooling as a dichotomous yes/no variables [9,10], while others have measured it as the amount of time spent homeschooling per week [3,8] or day [11]. Consequently, these studies are unable to differentiate between families who experienced long-term versus short-term mandatory homeschooling.

Stressors are actual or perceived threats to an organism that provoke physiological, emotional and/or behavioral reactions from the body. These reactions, collectively called the stress response, prepare the body to cope with stressors [16]. Chronic (long-term) activation of the stress response has been linked to mental health problems in children and adults, including depression, anxiety and behavioral problems, which compound over time [12–15].

Based on findings that chronic stress causes compounding mental health harm over time, it is possible that families engaged in long-term mandatory homeschooling experienced greater mental health harm than those engaged in short-term homeschooling. Further, short-term homeschooling may have had positive mental health impacts on some families by providing increased opportunities for family support and removing children from potential school stressors such as bullying [30,31]. Because past research used non-continuous measures of mandatory homeschooling, the findings could not capture potential compounding mental health effects over time; this may account for the conflicting results on the effects of mandatory homeschooling. To our knowledge, the present study is the first to measure time spent engaging in mandated homeschooling continuously over an extended period. Consequently, it is unknown whether mandatory homeschooling has compounding negative mental health effects that place long-term homeschoolers at greater risk.

1.4. Educational Support from Schools

Throughout the COVID-19 pandemic, many countries provided minimal national guidance about which educational support should be provided by schools [32]. Consequently, there was wide variability in the support children received from their schools or governments [20,32]. Many families attributed mandatory homeschooling challenges during the COVID-19 pandemic to a lack of educational resources and support from schools [17,33], the latter of which was associated with greater parental distress [34]. Given these findings, it is possible that receiving educational support from school may have benefited mental health during mandatory homeschooling.

Many children received online classes from schools during mandated homeschooling [20]. Pre-recorded online classes may have provided students with scheduling flexibility and higher-quality presentations, while live online classes may have provided opportunities for live student–teacher interaction and questions [35,36]. Live online classes may have been especially beneficial for mental health, given findings that children who interacted more with their teacher found online learning more effective and were more satisfied with their experience [19]; however, not all students had access to online classes during mandated homeschooling [18,20]. It is possible that children struggled more when they did not receive online classes, especially live ones, resulting in greater mental health harm for families during mandatory homeschooling.

Many students also received other digital or physical resources such as assignments, worksheets or videos, which can be conceptualized as home learning packs [20,32,37,38]. Home learning packs may have likewise contributed to improved mental health during mandatory homeschooling by providing children with a flexible opportunity to supplement and apply knowledge they gained in class. Pre-pandemic research suggests that these opportunities may have improved children's academic experiences, suggesting that home learning packs may have decreased academic strain on families during mandatory homeschooling [39,40]. This study examines live and pre-recorded online classes, as well as home learning packs, as educational supports from schools that may have mitigated adverse mental health effects of mandatory homeschooling.

1.5. Child Internet Connection

While specific school supports varied during mandated homeschooling, most children had an online component to education during the pandemic [20], making reliable internet connectivity a crucial resource. Unreliable internet connection has been linked to distress and dissatisfaction during mandatory homeschooling [17,41], which may suggest that it contributed to families' mental health harm. Despite its importance, many children struggled to access reliable internet connection during the pandemic in Canada and the United States, with some children relying entirely on public Wi-Fi to complete homework [21,42]. Alternatively, it is possible that reliable internet access put children at greater risk of problematic internet use, which increased during the pandemic and has been linked to poor mental health in children [43,44]. Together, the prevalence of unreliable internet access and its potential to harm (or benefit) family mental health during mandatory homeschooling prompted us to investigate its effects in the present study.

1.6. Parent Employment

Many parents either lost their jobs during the COVID-19 pandemic or reduced their working hours to care for their children [45]. Findings are mixed regarding the effects of parent employment on family mental health during COVID-19. Pre-pandemic research has linked self- or spousal unemployment to stress, anxiety and depression in adults [23,46,47]. Some pre-pandemic studies have linked parental unemployment to poorer mental health outcomes for children due to family financial strain and reduced parental well-being [24], while others have found beneficial impacts on younger children due to increased availability of parent–child quality time [48]. In line with many pre-pandemic findings, parent unemployment during the pandemic has been associated with increased depression in parents [5] and increased negative affect in children [49]. Employed parents, however, reported that balancing the responsibility of their child's education with work was a major source of stress, and many felt unable to provide their child with adequate school support [4,7,22]. These findings prompted us to explore parent employment status as a factor that may have influenced family mental health during mandatory homeschooling.

1.7. Current Study

The goal of the present study is to assess the mental health impact of children's time spent engaged in mandated homeschooling during the COVID-19 pandemic for children and parents. We measure mandatory homeschooling continuously, as the percentage of time between September 2020 and 15 February 2021. In line with prior research, we conceptualize child mental health as internalizing symptoms and externalizing symptoms and parent mental health as depression, anxiety, and general stress [3,11,50]. The study further assesses whether this relationship is moderated by parent employment status, child internet access, or educational support from the child's school, including live online classes, pre-recorded classes, or home learning packs (e.g., worksheets, assignments, videos, etc.).

This study answers recent calls for research into the effects of COVID-19 restrictions on child and parent mental health [51]. By studying the compounding mental health effects of cumulative mandatory homeschooling over time, we aim to clarify contradictory findings in past research. By further exploring which factors may moderate this relationship, we aim to identify the families at greatest risk of adverse mental health effects during mandatory homeschooling and the educational support mitigating these effects. Our results may help governments and schools connect high-risk families with the support they need to recover from lingering mental health effects of the COVID-19 pandemic and may encourage schools to implement effective educational support in the future. Together, our results may shape how mandatory homeschooling is conceptualized in future research to capture compounding mental health effects. They may also guide policy aimed at minimizing mental health harm when implementing future homeschooling mandates, such as limiting duration. This study assesses the following hypotheses.

Hypothesis 1 (H1). *We predict that cumulative time spent homeschooling is positively associated with child internalizing and externalizing symptoms and parent anxiety, depression and stress, such that greater cumulative time spent homeschooling is associated with poorer mental health.*

Hypothesis 2a (H2a). *We predict that live online class moderate this relationship, such that receiving this educational support will predict decreased mental health harm of cumulative time spent homeschooling for parents and children.*

Hypothesis 2b (H2b). *We predict that pre-recorded online classes moderate this relationship, such that receiving this educational support will predict decreased mental health harm of cumulative time spent homeschooling for parents and children.*

Hypothesis 2c (H2c). *We predict that home learning packs moderate this relationship, such that receiving this educational support will predict decreased mental health harm of cumulative time spent homeschooling for parents and children.*

Hypothesis 3 (H3). *We predict that children's internet access moderates this relationship, such that unreliable internet access will predict increased mental health harm from cumulative time spent homeschooling for parents and children.*

Hypothesis 4 (H4). *We predict that parent employment moderates this relationship, such that unemployment of one or both parents will predict greater mental health harm from cumulative time spent homeschooling for parents and children.*

2. Materials and Methods

This study is based on an archival data set from the study COVID-19 Pandemic: Factors that Support and Impede Family Well-being During Mandatory Homeschooling conducted by the Language and Literacy Lab and the Mood, Anxiety and Co-Morbidity Lab at Dalhousie University.

2.1. Participants

Participants in this study were 718 romantic partners with at least one school-aged child in grades 1–5 (Table 1). Data were collected about each family's youngest school-aged child. Of these children, 332 were undergoing full- or part-time mandatory homeschooling due to COVID-19 mandates, while the remaining 338 were being schooled in person full time. Study eligibility required both parents to be at least 19 years old and living in Canada or the U.S. They had to have lived together during the COVID-19 pandemic and have been in a romantic relationship with each other for at least 3 months preceding the study. They also had to have at least one child in grades 1–5 involved in either mandatory homeschooling or full-time in-person learning between September 2020 and 15 February 2021.

Table 1. Demographic information for parents and children.

Variable	Families (n = 718)
Country	
Canada	647 (90%)
U.S.	71 (10%)
Parent Age—M (SD)	39 (6.4)

Table 1. *Cont.*

Variable	Families (n = 718)
Parent Gender	
Female	711 (<49.5%)
Male	722 (50.3%)
Non-binary/Unknown	3 (0.002%)
Parent Relationship Structure	
Mixed Sex	678 (94.4%)
Same Sex	27 (3.8%)
Other/Prefer Not to Answer	3 (0.004%)
Family Income	
USD 25,000 or less per year	30 (4.2%)
Between USD 26,000 and USD 50,000	74 (10.3%)
Between USD 51,000 and USD 75,000	103 (14.3%)
Between USD 76,000 and USD 100,000	140 (19.5%)
Between USD 101,000 and USD 125,000	102 (14.2%)
Between USD 126,000 and USD 150,000	109 (15.2%)
USD 151,000 or more per year	132 (18.4%)
Prefer not to answer	28 (3.9%)
Parent Highest Level of Education	
Some High School	32 (2.2%)
High School Graduate	155 (10.8%)
Some College/University	155 (10.8%)
College/University Graduate	715 (49.8%)
Some Post-Graduate	75 (5.2)
Post-Graduate Degree	304 (21.2%)
Parent Employment Status	
Employed	1170 (81.5%)
Employed Full Time	971 (67.6%)
Employed Part Time	199 (13.9%)
Unemployed	253 (17.6%)
Unemployed	115 (8%)
Not in Labor Force	138 (9.6%)
Parent Ethnicity	
White	992 (69.1%)
Asian	261 (18.2%)
Latin American	45 (3.1%)
Black	47 (3.3%)
Indigenous/First Nations	21 (1.5%)
Multiracial/Other	59 (4.1%)
Child Age—M (SD)	7.9 (1.7)
Child Gender	
Female	333 (46.4%)
Male	383 (53.3%)
Non-Binary/Unknown	0
Child Ethnicity	
White	481 (67%)
Asian	115 (16%)
Latin American	14 (1.9%)
Black	23 (3.2%)
Indigenous/First Nations	9 (1.3%)
Multiracial/Other	66 (9.2%)
Child Disability Status	
Diagnosed with Disability	88 (12.3%)
Not Diagnosed with Disability	628 (87.5%)

Notes. The numbers provided do not add up to the total of 718 (100%) due to missing data.

2.2. Procedure

After receiving approval from the Dalhousie University Research Ethics Board (#2020-5166), data collection for this study took place between 18 March and 18 May 2021. Couples were recruited via Qualtrics Survey Panels and provided data at a single time-point. After eligibility screenings, both members of eligible couples provided informed consent to participate. Via Qualtrics, each parent retrospectively reported on their own demographic information and mental health in the 30-day period between 15 January and 15 February (symptoms of depression, anxiety, and stress). One parent (called Parent A) reported on their youngest school-aged child, including the child's demographic information, mental health (internalizing and externalizing symptoms), the homeschooling support they received from school, and the percentage of time the child was engaged in mandated homeschooling between September 2020 and February 2021. The surveys also included attention-check questions and response-speed verifications to ensure that participants were considering their responses, and those who failed either verification were excluded. The 718 couples in the sample all passed verification. Participants were each compensated with one USD 10 Amazon gift card.

2.3. Measures

2.3.1. Demographics Questionnaire

Parents reported their age, gender, sex, race/ethnicity, relationship, income, education level, and employment status. Parent A reported their youngest school-aged child's age, gender, and race/ethnicity (Table 1).

2.3.2. Cumulative Time Spent Homeschooling

Cumulative time spent homeschooling was measured as the parent-reported percentage of time children were engaged in mandatory homeschooling between September 2020 and 15 February 2021. This period was chosen because it captures a significant wave of the COVID-19 pandemic, during which mandatory homeschooling and in-person learning were co-occurring across the U.S. and Canada [52].

2.3.3. Child Internalizing and Externalizing Symptoms

Child mental health symptoms were measured using the internalizing and externalizing subscales of the Strengths and Difficulties Questionnaire (SDQ), which can be completed by parents of 4–16-year-olds [50]. The SDQ consists of five subscales: emotional problems, peer problems, behavioral problems, hyperactivity, and prosocial behavior. The 10-item Child Internalizing Subscale (Cronbach's $\alpha = 0.83$) combines the emotional problems (e.g., "Many worries or often seems worried") and the peer-related problems (e.g., "Picked on or bullied") subscales, while the 10-item Child Externalizing Subscale (Cronbach's $\alpha = 0.79$) combines the behavioral problems (e.g., "Often loses temper") and hyperactive problems, (e.g., "Easily distracted") subscales [50]. Items from the SDQ are measured on a 3-point response scale ("Not true" = 0, "Somewhat true" = 1, "Certainly true" = 2), and scores for each subscale can range from 1 to 20, with higher scores representing greater presence of symptoms. In this version of the SDQ, parents were asked to what extent statements were true of their child within the 30-day period between 15 January and 15 February 2021. The SDQ has good internal consistency (Cronbach's $\alpha = 0.73$) [53] and good convergent and discriminant validity [50].

2.3.4. Parent Depression

Parent depression was measured using the 9-item Patient Health Questionnaire (PHQ-9; Parent A Cronbach's $\alpha = 0.92$; Parent B Cronbach's $\alpha = 0.91$), a self-report survey which assesses the DSM criteria for depression on a 4-point scale (0 = "not at all", 3 = "everyday") [54]. Scores on the PHQ-9 range from 0 to 27, with greater scores representing greater depressive symptoms. Scores from both parents were summed into a single couple score to capture collective parent depression. This creation of a composite score across parents is similar to the approach we used in past studies with couples to capture a dyadic level variable [55,56]. Depression scores between Parent A and Parent B were highly correlated ($r = 0.49$, $p \leq 0.001$), providing psychometric support for this approach. The PHQ-9 asks how frequently the respondent has been bothered by a symptom in the past two weeks (e.g., "Feeling down, depressed or hopeless"). In the current study, this time frame was modified to include the 30-day period between 15 January and 15 February

2021 to better capture the period of ongoing homeschooling. The PHQ-9 has shown good internal reliability (Cronbach's α = 0.89), criterion validity, and construct validity in adult patients [54].

2.3.5. Parent Anxiety

Parent anxiety was measured using the 7-item General Anxiety Disorder scale (GAD-7; Parent A Cronbach's α = 0.92; Parent B Cronbach's α = 0.92), a self-report survey which assesses anxiety symptoms (e.g., "Worrying too much about different things") on a 4-point scale (0 = "not at all", 3 = "nearly every day") [57]. Possible scores ranged from 1 to 27, with greater scores indicating higher levels of anxiety. Parent scores were summed into one collective anxiety score, which is similar to the approach we used in past studies with couples to capture a dyadic level variable [55,56]. The high correlation (r = 0.45, p = <0.001) between Parent A and Parent B provides psychometric support for this approach. The GAD-7 asks how frequently the respondent has been bothered by a symptom in the past two weeks, which was modified in the current study to capture the 30-day period between 15 January and 15 February 2021, a longer period of ongoing homeschooling. The GAD-7 has good internal consistency (Cronbach's α = 0.92) and good criterion and construct validity in adult patients [57].

2.3.6. Parent Stress

Parent stress was measured using the 4-item Perceived Stress Scale (PSS-4; Parent A Cronbach's α = 0.64; Parent B Cronbach's α = 0.59), a self-report survey which assesses stress symptoms on a 5-point scale (0 = "Never", 4 = "Very Often") [58]. The PSS-4 asks how frequently the respondent has experienced a symptom in the last month, which we modified to capture the 30-day between 15 January and 15 February 2021 (e.g., "Feeling unable to control the important things in life"). Possible scores on the PSS range from 0 to 28, with greater scores indicating greater levels of stress. Both parents' scores were summed into a single couple score, representing their collective stress. In past studies with couples, we used a similar approach to capture a dyadic level variable [55,56]. Parent A and Parent B stress scores were highly correlated (r = 0.5, $p \leq 0.001$), which provides psychometric support for this approach. The PSS-4 has good internal consistency (Cronbach's α = 0.77) [58] and good validity in adult populations [59].

2.3.7. Educational Support from Schools

Online live class. Parent A reported whether their child's school provided live online classes (e.g., yes or no).

Online pre-recorded class. Parent A reported whether their child's school provided pre-recorded online classes (e.g., yes or no).

Home learning packs. Parent A reported whether their child's school provided home learning packs (e.g., yes or no). Examples of home learning packs given to participants included "worksheets, assignments, videos, etc.".

2.3.8. Child Internet Connection

Children's access to reliable internet connection was measured using a 7-point Likert scale (0 = "not at all", 6 = "very much"). Parent A responded to the following question: "Between 15 January and 15 February, to what extent did your child have access to a reliable internet connection?". Internet connection was then re-coded into a binary variable to account for inadequate sample sizes in some response categories, such that Reliable Internet included scores of 6 and Unreliable Internet included scores from 0 to 5.

2.3.9. Parent Employment

Parent employment status was coded as Unemployed vs. Employed. The employed category included those employed full and part time, while the unemployed category included those who were unemployed (e.g., looking for work) or not in the labor force (e.g., not performing or looking for paid work). We combined unemployed people with those not in the labor force due to low sample sizes in some categories and because distinctions between these groups were blurred during the pandemic due to the volatile state of the labor force [60] and increases in unpaid care-giving labor [61]. We combined both parents into a single variable, coded as Both Employed vs. One or Both Unemployed, to capture compounding effects of parental employment.

2.4. Analysis Plan

We conducted statistical analyses for this study using version 4.2.2 of R [62]. Assumption screening revealed violation of normality, which was unlikely to impact our results due to our large sample size (>10 observations per variable) [63,64]. There was further violation of homogeneity of variance, which we addressed by conducting heteroskedasticity-consistent standard errors using PROCESS macro for R version 4.3.1 [65,66]. PROCESS macro is a modeling tool used for path analysis with ordinary least squares and logistic regressions [67]. It can be used to test two-way moderation models, simple slopes, and mediation models while incorporating heteroskedasticity-consistent standard errors [65,67]. Significance was determined using an alpha level of $p < 0.05$. Continuous variables were grand-mean-centered, and categorical variables were effect-coded.

We used mediation models to assess the total effects of cumulative time spent homeschooling on parent and child mental health (H1). This approach was used because PROCESS macro does not support basic linear regression. Using mediation models to extract the total effects of the predictor on the outcomes enabled us to use the same software for all our models, thus maintaining consistency across our analyses. Next, ordinary least squares regression and simple slopes analysis were used to test whether the relationships between cumulative time spent homeschooling and parent and child mental health are moderated by parent employment status, children's internet access, live online instructions, pre-recorded online instruction, or home learning packs (H2–H4). Ordinary least squares regressions tested for moderation by assessing whether interactions between cumulative time spent homeschooling and the moderators accounted for variation in the mental health outcomes, as indicated by significant ($p < 0.05$) changes in R^2 (Figure 1). For significant interactions, simple slopes analyses were used to assess the relationship between cumulative time spent homeschooling and mental health outcomes at different levels of the moderator to determine whether they supported our hypotheses. We ran one mediation model and four ordinary least squares regressions for each of our mental health outcomes (25 total).

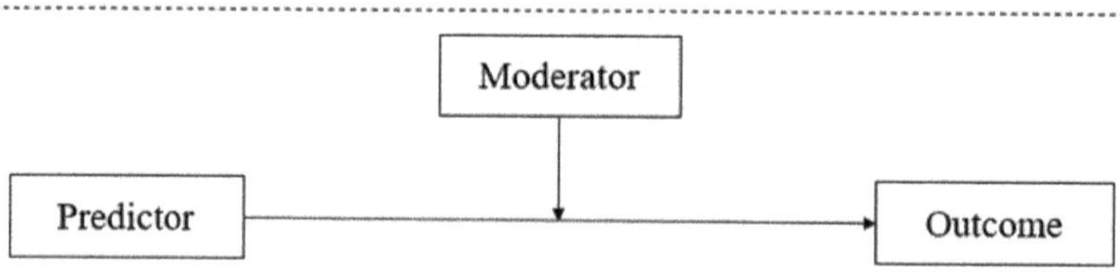

Predictor = Cumulative time spent homeschooling
Outcome = Parent anxiety, depression or stress, or child internalizing or externalizing symptoms
Moderator = Live online classes, pre-recorded online classes, home learning packs, parent employment or child internet access

Figure 1. Conceptual Model for Ordinary Least Squares Regression. Note. This conceptual model demonstrates the intention of the ordinary least squares regressions to determine whether the relationship between cumulative time spent homeschooling and the mental health outcome is changed by the moderator. This image is based on models from Moon [68] and Hayes [66].

3. Results

Demographic information and means for study variables are presented in Tables 1 and 2, respectively.

Table 2. Study variable means and counts.

Variable	*M (SD)*
% Time Spent Homeschooling	45.5 (36.3)
Child Externalizing Symptoms	6.8 (4)
Child Internalizing Symptoms	5.3 (4.2)
Parent Anxiety	10.3 (8.5)
Parent Depression	12.5 (10.1)
Parent Stress	12.7 (5.1)
	n
Live Online Class	
Yes	357
No	361
Pre-recorded Online Class	
Yes	89
No	629
Home Learning Pack	
Yes	178
No	540
Parent Employment	
Both Employed	489
One or Both Unemployed	207
Child Internet	
Reliable	460
Unreliable	257

Note. The numbers provided do not add up to the total of 718 due to missing data.

3.1. *Cumulative Time Spent Homeschooling and Parent and Child Mental Health (H1)*

Shown in Table 3, total effects from mediation models revealed that child internalizing symptoms, parent anxiety, and parent depression were all significantly and positively associated with time spent homeschooling. Child externalizing symptoms and parent stress were not significantly associated with cumulative time spent homeschooling.

Table 3. Total effects of cumulative time spent homeschooling on mental health outcomes.

	Cumulative Time Spent Homeschooling				
Predictors	**Est.**	*t*	**LLCI**	**ULCI**	*p*
Child Externalizing	0.01 (<0.01)	1.12	−0.003	0.013	0.26
Child Internalizing	*** 0.02 (<0.01)	4.39	0.01	0.026	<0.001
Parent Anxiety	* 0.02 (0.01)	2.12	0.001	0.036	0.03
Parent Depression	** 0.03 (0.01)	2.82	0.009	0.05	<0.01
Parent Stress	0.01 (0.01)	1.16	−0.005	0.018	0.246

Note. This table shows the total effects of cumulative time spent homeschooling (X) on parent and child mental health outcomes (Y) from the mediation analysis. There were positive, significant relationships for child internalizing symptoms and parent depression and anxiety. * $p < 0.05$, ** $p < 0.01$, *** $p < 0.001$.

3.2. *Live Online Classes as a Moderator (H2A)*

Ordinary least squares regressions revealed that live online classes significantly interacted with cumulative time spent homeschooling to predict child internalizing symptoms and parent anxiety and depression, but not parent stress or child externalizing symptoms (Table 4). Simple slopes probing revealed that cumulative time spent homeschooling was only significantly positively associated with child internalizing symptoms, parent anxiety (Figure 2), and parent depression when children did not receive live online classes. There was no significant association when children did receive live online classes (Table 5).

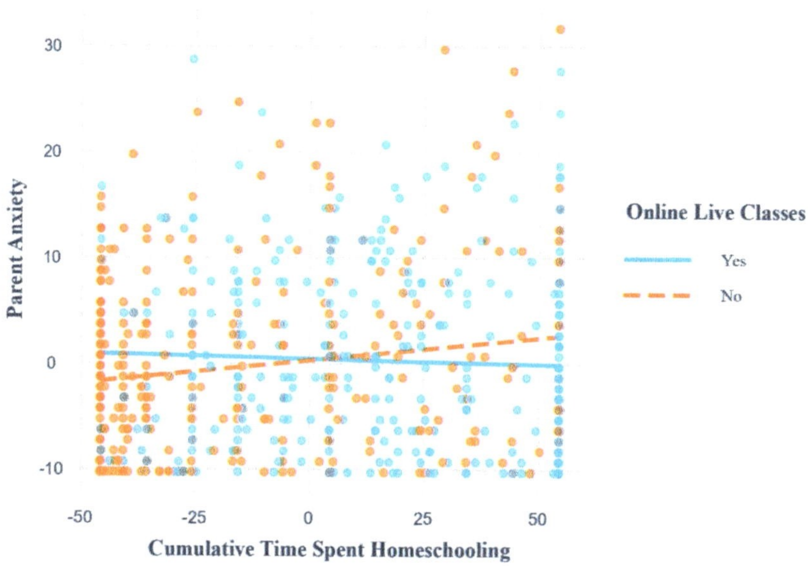

Figure 2. Simple slopes for parent anxiety outcome, online live classes moderator. Note. This plot shows the relationship between cumulative time spent homeschooling and parent anxiety at different levels of the moderator, online live classes. The relationship was significant and positive when children did not receive online classes but was non-significant when they did. Axis numerical ranges reflect grand mean centering or effect coding of variables.

3.3. *Pre-Recorded Online Classes as a Moderator (H2B)*

Ordinary least squares regressions revealed that pre-recorded online classes did not significantly interact with cumulative time spent homeschooling for any of the mental health outcomes (Table 4).

3.4. *Home Learning Packs as a Moderator (H2C)*

Ordinary least squares regressions revealed that home learning packs significantly interacted with cumulative time spent homeschooling to predict child internalizing symptoms and parent depression (Table 4). Simple slopes probing revealed that these relationships were significant and positive only when children did not receive home learning packs (Table 5; Figure 3).

Table 4. Ordinary least squares regressions with educational resources from school as moderators.

	Child Externalizing			Child Internalizing			Parent Anxiety			Parent Depression			Parent Stress		
Predictor	**Est (SE)**	**t**	**p**	**Est (SE)**	**t**	**p**	**Est (SE)**	**t**	**p**	**Est (SE)**	**t**	**p**	**Est (SE)**	**tl**	**p**
Live Class															
Intercept	0.12 (0.17)	0.71	0.477	0.18 (0.18)	0.98	0.326	0.39 (0.37)	1.04	0.298	0.46 (0.44)	1.05	0.294	0.36 (0.22)	0.287	0.774
CTSH	<0.01 (0.01)	0.23	0.82	** 0.02 (0.01)	3.2	0.001	0.02 (0.01)	1.58	0.115	* 0.03 (0.01)	2.26	0.024	<0.01 (0.01)	0.392	0.695
Live Class	0.56 (0.33)	1.7	0.092	0.34 (0.36)	0.94	0.35	0.18 (0.74)	0.24	0.808	0.01 (0.88)	0.007	0.994	0.68 (0.43)	1.577	0.115
Interaction	−0.02 (0.01)	−1.74	0.083	* −0.02 (0.01)	−2.46	0.014	* −0.05 (0.02)	−2.58	0.01	** −0.06 (0.02)	−2.62	0.009	−0.01 (0.01)	−0.665	0.506
Pre-recorded Class															
Intercept	0.06 (0.26)	0.23	0.82	0.45 (0.31)	1.45	0.147	0.06 (0.57)	0.11	0.914	0.39 (0.71)	0.55	0.586	−0.04 (0.37)	−0.116	0.908
CTSH	<0.01 (0.01)	0.03	0.979	0.01 (0.01)	1.24	0.215	0.02 (0.02)	1.11	0.267	0.03 (0.02)	1.2	0.247	0.01 (0.01)	0.536	0.592
Pre-recorded Class	0.1 (0.52)	0.19	0.849	1.15 (0.63)	1.83	0.068	0.25 (1.14)	0.22	0.827	1.04 (1.42)	0.73	0.465	−0.1 (0.74)	−0.131	0.896
Interaction	−0.01 (0.02)	−0.63	0.527	−0.01 (0.02)	−0.52	0.604	0.01 (0.04)	0.23	0.821	−<0.01 (0.05)	−0.05	0.963	<0.01 (0.03)	0.068	0.946
Learning Packs															
Intercept	0.12 (0.18)	0.1	0.55	0.21 (0.2)	1.05	0.296	0.49 (0.38)	1.28	0.201	0.46 (0.46)	0.99	0.322	0.25 (0.24)	1.0146	0.311
CTSH	<0.01 (0.01)	0.08	0.936	0.01 (0.01)	1.66	0.098	0.01 (0.01)	0.54	0.593	0.01 (0.01)	1	0.316	<0.01 (0.01)	0.072	0.943
Learning Packs	0.23 (0.36)	0.65	0.517	0.35 (0.4)	0.89	0.377	* 1.54 (0.77)	2	0.046	1.09 (0.92)	1.18	0.238	0.77 (0.48)	1.591	0.112
Interaction	−0.01 (0.01)	−1.3	0.196	** −0.03 (0.01)	−2.95	0.003	−0.03 (0.02)	−1.26	0.209	−0.05 (0.03)	−1.92	0.055	−0.01 (0.02)	−0.885	0.377

Note. These results from the ordinary least squares regressions show that Cumulative Time Spent Homeschooling (CTSH) interacted significantly with live online classes to predict child internalizing symptoms and parent anxiety and depression and interacted significantly with home learning packs to predict child internalizing symptoms. * $p < 0.05$, ** $p < 0.01$, *** $p < 0.001$.

Table 5. Simple slopes analysis.

	Child Externalizing			Child Internalizing			Parent Anxiety			Parent Stress		
Moderator	**Est (SE)**	**t**	**p**	**Est (SE)**	**t**	**p**	**Est (SE)**	**t**	**p**	**Est (SE)**	**t**	**p**
Live Classes												
No	—	—	—	0.03 *** (0.01)	3.98	<0.001	0.04 ** (0.02)	2.88	0.004	0.06 *** (0.02)	3.34	<0.001
Yes	—	—	—	<0.01 (0.01)	0.53	0.599	−0.01 (0.01)	−0.73	0.469	<−0.01 (0.02)	−0.27	0.792
No	—	—	—	0.02 *** (0.01)	4.86	<0.001	—	—	—	—	—	—
Yes	—	—	—	−0.01 (0.01)	−0.74	0.462	—	—	—	—	—	—
Employment												
Unemployed	−0.01 (0.01)	−1.47	0.141	0.01 (0.01)	1.09	0.276	—	—	—	—	—	—
Employed	0.01 * (0.01)	2.44	0.015	0.02 *** (0.01)	4.46	<0.001	—	—	—	—	—	—
Internet Access												
Unreliable	—	—	—	<0.01 (0.01)	0.32	0.748	—	—	—	—	—	—
Reliable	—	—	—	0.02 *** (0.01)	4.2	<0.001	—	—	—	—	—	—

Note. These results from the simple reveal the relationship between cumulative time spent homeschooling and parent and child mental health outcomes at each level of the moderator. * $p < 0.05$, ** $p < 0.01$, *** $p < 0.001$.

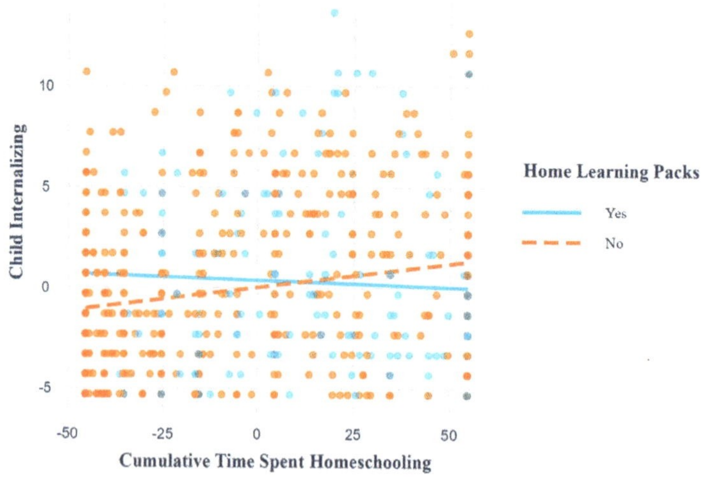

Figure 3. Simple slopes for child internalizing outcome, home learning pack moderator. Note. This plot shows the relationship between cumulative time spent homeschooling and child internalizing symptoms at different levels of the moderator, home learning packs. The relationship was significant and positive when children did not receive online classes but was non-significant when they did. Axis numerical ranges reflect grand mean centering or effect coding of variables.

3.5. *Internet Connection as a Moderator (H3)*

Ordinary least squares regressions revealed that internet connection interacted with cumulative time spent homeschooling to predict child internalizing symptoms (Table 6). Simple slopes revealed that cumulative time spent homeschooling was significantly positively associated with child internalizing symptoms when children had access to reliable internet connection, but not when they had unreliable internet connection (Table 5; Figure 4).

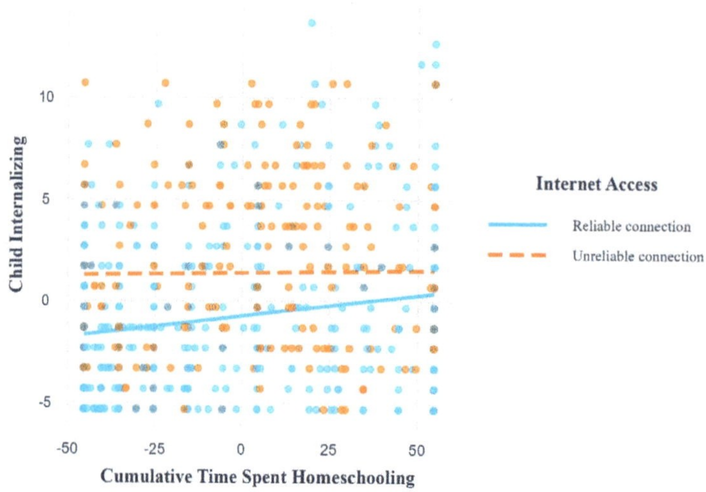

Figure 4. Simple slopes for child internalizing outcome, internet access moderator. Note. This plot shows the relationship between cumulative time spent homeschooling and child internalizing symptoms at different levels of the moderator, internet access. The relationship was significant and positive when they had reliable internet access but was non-significant when they had unreliable internet access. Axis numerical ranges reflect grand mean centering or effect coding of variables.

Table 6. Ordinary least squares regressions with parent employment and child internet access as moderators.

Predictor	Child Externalizing			Child Internalizing			Parent Anxiety			Parent Depression			Parent Stress		
	Est (*SE*)	*t*	*p*	Est (*SE*)	*t*	*p*	Est (*SE*)	*t*	*p*	Est (*SE*)	*t*	*p*	Est (*SE*)	*t*	*p*
Employment															
Intercept	−0.04 (0.17)	−0.21	0.837	−0.11 (0.16)	−0.69	0.493	−0.19 (0.35)	−0.53	0.595	−0.13 (0.42)	−0.316	0.752	−0.13 (0.23)	−0.57	0.57
CTSH	<0.01 (<0.01)	0.21	0.833	*** 0.02 (<0.01)	3.76	<0.001	0.02 (0.01)	1.88	0.061	* 0.03 (0.01)	2.36	0.018	0.02 (0.01)	0.85	0.395
Employment	0.26 (0.34)	0.75	0.455	* 0.64 (0.33)	1.95	0.052	0.78 (0.71)	1.1	0.271	0.76 (0.85)	0.9	0.368	0.42 (0.46)	0.92	0.36
Interaction	** 0.02 (0.01)	2.61	0.009	* 0.02 (0.01)	2.12	0.035	0.02 (0.02)	0.81	0.416	0.03 (0.02)	1.45	0.147	0.02 (0.01)	1.88	0.061
Internet Access															
Intercept	0.24 (0.15)	1.55	0.121	0.33 (0.16)	2.03	0.042	0.23 (0.33)	0.7	0.486	0.48 (0.39)	1.24	0.217	0.29 (0.18)	1.56	0.119
CTSH	<0.01 (0.01)	0.07	0.941	* 0.01 (0.01)	2.54	0.011	0.02 (0.01)	1.48	0.139	0.02 (0.01)	1.68	0.094	<0.01 (0.01)	0.24	0.813
Internet Access	*** −1.56 (0.31)	−5.1	<0.001	*** −2.1 (0.32)	−6.49	<0.001	* −1.6 (0.67)	−2.39	0.017	*** −3.09 (0.78)	−3.94	<0.001	*** −1.88 (0.37)	−5.1	<0.001
Interaction	0.01 (0.01)	1.26	0.207	* 0.02 (0.01)	2	0.046	0.01 (0.02)	0.52	0.601	0.03 (0.02)	1.38	0.168	0.01 (0.01)	1.17	0.242

Note. These results from the ordinary least squares regressions show that cumulative time spent homeschooling (CTSH) interacted significantly with child internet access to predict child internalizing symptoms and interacted significantly with parent employment to predict child externalizing and internalizing symptoms. * $p < 0.05$, ** $p < 0.01$, *** $p < 0.001$.

3.6. Parent Employment as a Moderator (H4)

Ordinary least squares regressions revealed that parent employment interacted significantly with cumulative time spent homeschooling to predict child internalizing and externalizing symptoms (Table 6). Simple slopes analysis revealed that cumulative time spent homeschooling was significantly positively associated with child externalizing (Figure 5) and internalizing symptoms when parents were employed, but not when one or both parents were unemployed (Table 5).

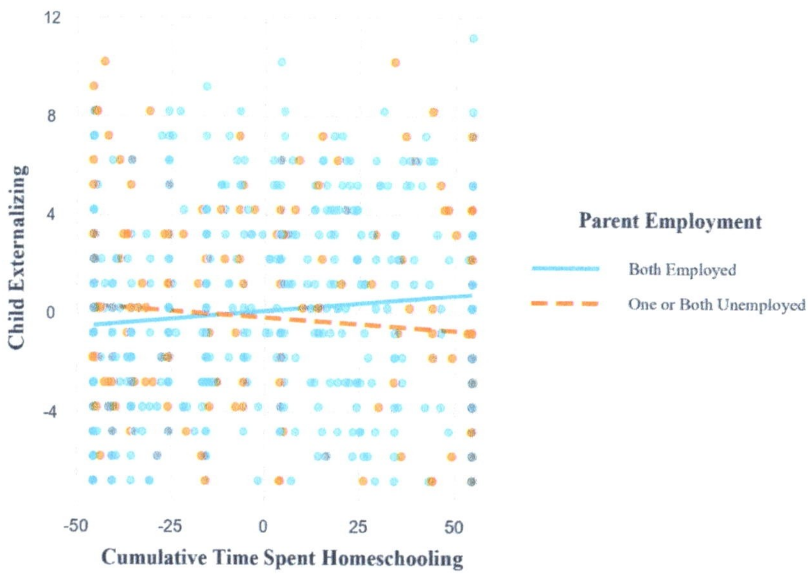

Figure 5. Simple slopes for child externalizing outcome, parent employment moderator. Note. This plot shows the relationship between cumulative time spent homeschooling and child internalizing symptoms at different levels of the moderator, parent employment. The relationship was significant and positive when both parents were employed but was non-significant when one or both were unemployed. Axis numerical ranges reflect grand mean centering or effect coding of variables.

4. Discussion

In the present study, we explored compounding adverse mental health effects of mandatory homeschooling for families during the COVID-19 pandemic by assessing parent and child mental health and children's cumulative time spent homeschooling over several months. We further explored the effects of potential risk and protective factors on this relationship, including educational support from schools, child internet access, and parent employment.

We found that greater cumulative time spent homeschooling was significantly associated with greater child internalizing symptoms and parent depression and anxiety, but not child externalizing symptoms or parent stress, showing partial support for H1. This supports findings from most past research linking mandatory homeschooling to adverse mental health effects for parents and children [3,8,9]. It also extends this research by suggesting that these effects compound over time, placing long-term homeschoolers at greater risk of mental health harm. These findings align with chronic stress research, which shows that long-term exposure to stressors (such as mandatory homeschooling) is harmful for adult and child mental health [12–15]. These findings also suggest that measuring mandatory homeschooling continuously over longer periods may be a more effective means of investigating its effects on mental health.

Our results also suggest that the effects of mandated homeschooling may be more salient for some mental health outcomes than others. The non-significant association between cumulative time spent homeschooling and child externalizing symptoms may relate to findings by Monnier et al. [11], which show that three or more hours spent homeschooling per day improved children's hyperactivity symptoms. Research has found that daily routines, which could be built around homeschooling tasks, may have had positive impacts on children's externalizing symptoms [10,69]. There may exist a "sweet spot" of time spent homeschooling during school closure mandates that is protective for children's externalizing symptoms, which would not be captured in the total effects of our mediation models. The non-significant relationship between cumulative time spent homeschooling and parent stress may be explained by our measure of stress, the PSS-4, which captures general stress [58]. During mandatory homeschooling, parents may have been experiencing forms of stress specific to the COVID-19 pandemic, which may not have been captured by this measure. A stress measure specific to COVID-19, such as the COVID-19 Stress Scale developed by Taylor et al. [70], may therefore be more appropriate. Deacon et al. [1] used this scale to find that greater time engaged in mandatory homeschooling was linked to increased COVID-19-related stress in parents, supporting this possibility.

Looking at educational support provided by schools (H2), we found that live online classes (H2a) and home learning packs (H2c) but not pre-recorded online classes (H2b) moderated the relationships between cumulative time spent homeschooling and some mental health outcomes. First, we found that cumulative time spent homeschooling was only positively associated with child internalizing symptoms and parent depression and anxiety when children did not receive live online classes. These findings may reflect the importance of live student–teacher interactions for academic success and satisfaction during mandatory homeschooling [19]. Live classes may have allowed children to depend more on teachers for ongoing academic support, easing the educational strain felt by families when tackling academic and technological challenges at home [25,33]. Live online classes also create routine in the child's day, which has been identified as a protective factor for children's mental health during COVID-19 [10,69]. This routine may have helped parents by offering them structured time to focus on other responsibilities while children are occupied by teachers. By contrast, pre-recorded online classes did not offer live academic support or routine, which may explain their non-significant interaction effects. Instead, children learning from pre-recorded classes may have sought support from parents, adding to the family's academic strain. The added responsibility of scheduling class time may have also fallen to parents.

We also found that home learning packs protected against the effects of cumulative time spent homeschooling on child internalizing symptoms and parent depression. The relationships between mandatory homeschooling and child internalizing symptoms or parent depression were only significant and positive when children did not receive home learning packs. This suggests that children and parents benefitted when children received educational support such as assignments, worksheets, or videos during mandated homeschooling. For parents, having additional resources to rely on may have helped them instruct their children more effectively while sparing them the additional effort of assembling materials on their own. This may have protected parents by reducing the burden of their newfound educator roles. These resources may also have provided children with opportunities to learn independently and apply their knowledge, which has been linked to improved academic performance [40]. If home learning packs helped students and parents engage with course content more effectively and overcome academic challenges, this may explain their protective effects on child mental health. Together, these results suggest that educational support for schools, especially live online class and home learning packs, protect families against the adverse mental health impact of mandatory homeschooling.

Our results suggest that reliable internet access is a risk factor for children's mental health during mandatory homeschooling, contrary to our hypothesis (H3). Cumulative time spent homeschooling was only significantly positively associated with child internalizing symptoms when children had reliable internet access. We hypothesized that reliable internet connection would protect mental health because of its crucial importance for school, work, social connection, entertainment, and health care during the pandemic [71,72]. However, excessive internet use before and during COVID-19 has been linked to adverse mental health and academic outcomes in children [25,44,73,74]. Further, problematic internet use among children, including elevated time online, increased throughout the COVID-19 pandemic [43,44]. Therefore, children with reliable internet may have been using the internet excessively or in otherwise problematic ways, which may in turn have interfered with their schooling and had adverse impacts on their mental health. By contrast, when children were distracted by the internet, parents' mental health may have benefitted from having time to themselves, explaining why adverse effects did not extend to parents.

Finally, our results suggest that having both parents employed is a risk factor for child mental health during mandatory homeschooling, contrary to our hypothesis (H4). There was only a significant positive relationship between cumulative time spent homeschooling and child internalizing and externalizing symptoms when both parents were employed. These findings suggest that cumulative time spent homeschooling only has adverse impacts on child mental health when both parents are employed. This finding may reflect reports that balancing work and homeschooling is a major source of stress for employed parents [4,7,22] and past findings that children show more internalizing and externalizing symptoms when parents experience greater work–family conflict [75]. It is possible that working parents had less time to support their children academically, which may have caused their children to struggle more with school and consequently experience mental health declines. By contrast, unemployed parents may have had more time and energy to support their children with school. For parents, the unique challenges of being unemployed during a pandemic may have negated the benefits experienced by their children, explaining the non-significant results for parent mental health [4,7,22]. These findings suggest that the effects of unemployment differed in the context of the COVID-19 pandemic, and that families with two working parents may have been at greater risk of mental health harm.

Limitations and Future Directions

Our study includes some limitations. First, our data were collected at a single time point and accounts were retrospective, preventing causal conclusions. Parents and children were mostly white (parent = 69%, children = 67%), parent relationships were mostly heterosexual (94%), and only 14% of families had incomes of USD 50,000 or less. It is important that future research include more diverse samples, given that racial, ethnic, and sexual minorities and people of lower socioeconomic status experienced disproportionate challenges during the COVID-19 pandemic due to inequities [4,76]. Given the disproportionate impacts experienced by people of lower socioeconomic status, we ran additional sensitivity tests using family income (adjusted for family size) as a covariate. Our results unchanged, suggesting that the effects of family income on mental health likely do not account for our results; however, future research should continue to include relevant sociodemographic variables as covariates in their models.

Another limitation is that we used binary yes/no measures for educational support from school and did not collect information on its quality or the training provided to families for this support. Families reported that poor-quality educational support and lack of training on how to use it contributed to adverse mandatory homeschooling experiences [25,37], suggesting that these factors should be explored in future research.

This study also ran multiple (30 total) tests, which can increase the risk of Type 1 error. A stringent method to protect against Type 1 error with multiplicity testing is the Bonferroni correction, which is calculated by dividing the standard significance threshold of $p < 0.05$ by the number of tests [77]—in our case, 30. With a stringent Bonferroni-corrected alpha of 0.0017 (0.05/30), only one of our findings remained significant, namely the positive relationship between time spent homeschooling and child internalizing symptoms ($p < 0.001$). Thus, we can have confidence in the observed positive link of time spent homeschooling with child internalizing symptoms. Other findings reported as statistically significant in the main analyses using traditional significance levels ($p < 0.05$) should be interpreted with caution and must be replicated in future studies. Our survey data were also collected at a single time point, which limits our ability to determine causality and temporality [78]. While our cross-sectional design is a useful first step, further studies using longitudinal designs are needed to replicate our findings and confirm causality [79]. Our findings therefore represent important early findings.

Our conceptualization of parent employment also presents limitations. We combined "Unemployed" parents with those "Not in the labor force" to account for low sample sizes, based on findings that these employment statuses resembled each other during the pandemic [60,61]. However, these categories are usually viewed as distinct from each other, and should also be explored separately in future research to determine whether their effects differ [80]. To further account for the small sample size of families in which both parents were unemployed ($n = 35$), the "Unemployed" category combined families with one and two unemployed parents. This may present a limitation, as experiences of families with two unemployed parents may have differed from those with one employed and one unemployed parent [81]. For example, the latter families may have benefited from having one parent with stable employment and one parent with extra time to support the child's homeschooling [82], which could have influenced our results. To address this limitation, we ran supplementary analyses that assessed the parent employment moderator at three levels: Both Employed, Both Unemployed and Mixed (One Employed, one Unemployed). Results were virtually unchanged, suggesting that combining these groups did not adversely affect our results. However, future studies should still consider exploring potential differences between families with one versus two unemployed parents.

Past research has also found that mothers took on a disproportionate share of child-care responsibilities during the pandemic compared to fathers and may have experienced more adverse mental health effects [83,84]. Further, paternal and maternal unemployment may impact child mental health differently [48]. Considering these findings, future studies should also assess differences in the effects of maternal versus paternal employment on family mental health during COVID-19. Future studies should also explore whether families with multiple school-aged children experienced mandatory homeschooling differently.

5. Conclusions

The present study investigated the compounding mental health impacts of cumulative time spent homeschooling for parents and children and sought to identify relevant risk and protective factors that may moderate these relationships. Our study extends past research on mental health during mandatory homeschooling by demonstrating that cumulative mandatory homeschooling had compounding adverse effects on mental health over time, which suggests that families engaged in long-term mandatory homeschooling were at greater risk. These findings may prompt policy makers to limit the duration of future homeschooling mandates or to explore alternatives instead. They also suggest that measuring mandatory homeschooling as a continuous variable over time may be a more effective strategy for studying its effects on mental health, which future researchers should consider adopting.

Our results also suggest that the cumulative mental health harm faced by families during mandatory homeschooling was exacerbated when both parents were employed. These families may require additional mental health and academic support to recover from the effects of mandatory homeschooling. Teachers and schools should work with affected students and their families to develop plans for recovery. Schools and governments should likewise consider subsidizing tutoring support programs for families that may be struggling with lingering impacts of mandatory homeschooling. Finally, our results highlight the crucial role schools and teachers play in maintaining family mental health during mandatory homeschooling. Effective support from schools, especially in the form of live online classes, appears hugely impactful in improving mental health outcomes for families.

Schools should provide live online classes and other evidence-based educational support as a required component of education during mandatory homeschooling. School boards must likewise ensure that teachers, parents, and students all receive access to the technologies and training needed for these educational approaches to be implemented effectively.

Author Contributions: Conceptualization, L.V.M.G., M.M.E., S.H.D. and S.H.S.; methodology, M.M.E., S.H.D. and S.H.S.; validation, M.M.E.; formal analysis, L.V.M.G. and M.M.E.; investigation, M.M.E., S.H.D. and S.H.S.; resources, S.H.D. and S.H.S.; data curation, M.M.E.; writing—original draft preparation, L.V.M.G.; writing—review and editing, L.V.M.G., M.M.E., S.H.D. and S.H.S.; visualization, L.V.M.G.; supervision, S.H.D. and S.H.S.; project administration, M.M.E. and S.H.D.; funding acquisition, S.H.D. and S.H.S. All authors have read and agreed to the published version of the manuscript.

Funding: This study was funded by a Social Science and Humanities Research Council of Canada Partnership Engagement Grant (#1008-2020-0220).

Institutional Review Board Statement: This study received ethics approval from the Social Science and Humanities Research Ethics Board of Dalhousie University (#2020-5166, date of approval 19 June 2020).

Informed Consent Statement: All participants involved in the study provided informed consent.

Data Availability Statement: The data presented in this study are available on request from the corresponding author due to ethical reasons.

Conflicts of Interest: The authors declare no conflicts of interest.

References

1. World Health Organization (WHO). WHO Director-General's Opening Remarks at the Media Briefing on COVID-19. 11 March 2020. Available online: https://www.who.int/director-general/speeches/detail/who-director-general-s-opening-remarks-at-the-media-briefing-on-covid-19---11-march-2020 (accessed on 23 October 2022).
2. UNICEF. Covid-19 and School Closures: Are Children Able to Continue Learning. UNICEF DATA. 22 September 2021. Available online: https://data.unicef.org/resources/remote-learning-reachability-factsheet/ (accessed on 23 October 2022).
3. Deacon, S.H.; Rodriguez, L.M.; Elgendi, M.; King, F.E.; Nogueira-Arjona, R.; Sherry, S.B.; Stewart, S.H. Parenting through a pandemic: Mental health and substance use consequences of mandated homeschooling. *Couple Fam. Psychol. Res. Pract.* **2021**, *10*, 281–293. [CrossRef]
4. American Psychological Association (APA). Stress in America™ 2020: Stress in the Time of COVID-19, Volume One. May 2020. Available online: https://www.apa.org/news/press/releases/stress/2020/report (accessed on 23 October 2022).
5. Crescentini, C.; Feruglio, S.; Matiz, A.; Paschetto, A.; Vidal, E.; Cogo, P.; Fabbro, F. Stuck Outside and Inside: An Exploratory Study on the Effects of the COVID-19 Outbreak on Italian Parents and Children's Internalizing Symptoms. *Front. Psychol.* **2020**, *11*, 586074. [CrossRef] [PubMed]
6. Di Giorgio, E.; Di Riso, D.; Mioni, G.; Cellini, N. The interplay between mothers' and childrens' behavioral and psychological factors during COVID-19: An Italian study. *Eur. Child Adolesc. Psychiatry* **2020**, *30*, 1401–1412. [CrossRef]
7. Gadermann, A.C.; Thomson, K.C.; Richardson, C.G.; Gagné, M.; McAuliffe, C.; Hirani, S.; Jenkins, E. Examining the impacts of the COVID-19 pandemic on family mental health in Canada: Findings from a national cross-sectional study. *BMJ Open* **2021**, *11*, e042871. [CrossRef] [PubMed]
8. Kishida, K.; Tsuda, M.; Waite, P.; Creswell, C.; Ishikawa, S.-I. Relationships between local school closures due to the COVID-19 and mental health problems of children, adolescents, and parents in Japan. *Psychiatry Res.* **2021**, *306*, 114276. [CrossRef] [PubMed]
9. Schmidt, A.; Kramer, A.C.; Brose, A.; Schmiedek, F.; Neubauer, A.B. Distance learning, parent–child interactions, and affective well-being of parents and children during the COVID-19 pandemic: A daily diary study. *Dev. Psychol.* **2020**, *57*, 1719–1734. [CrossRef]
10. DesRoches, D. Mental Health Outcomes for Children Engaging in Home-Based Learning During COVID-19: The Role of Routines and Household Chaos. Unpublished. Master's Thesis, Dalhousie University, Halifax, NS, Canada, 2021.
11. Monnier, M.; Moulin, F.; Thierry, X.; Vandentorren, S.; Côté, S.; Barbosa, S.; Falissard, B.; Plancoulaine, S.; Charles, M.-A.; Simeon, T.; et al. Children's mental and behavioral health, schooling, and socioeconomic characteristics during school closure in France due to COVID-19: The SAPRIS project. *Sci. Rep.* **2021**, *11*, 22373. [CrossRef]
12. American Psychological Association (APA). How Stress Affects Your Health. 31 October 2022. Available online: https://www.apa.org/topics/stress/health (accessed on 4 April 2023).
13. Dieleman, G.C.; Huizink, A.C.; Tulen, J.H.; Utens, E.M.; Creemers, H.E.; van der Ende, J.; Verhulst, F.C. Alterations in HPA-axis and autonomic nervous system functioning in childhood anxiety disorders point to a chronic stress hypothesis. *Psychoneuroendocrinology* **2015**, *51*, 135–150. [CrossRef]

14. Hammen, C.; Kim, E.Y.; Eberhart, N.K.; Brennan, P.A. Chronic and acute stress and the prediction of major depression in women. *Depress. Anxiety* **2009**, *26*, 718–723. [CrossRef]
15. Snyder, H.R.; Young, J.F.; Hankin, B.L. Chronic stress exposure and generation are related to the p-factor and externalizing specific psychopathology in youth. *J. Clin. Child Adolesc. Psychol.* **2017**, *48*, 306–315. [CrossRef]
16. Crum, A.J.; Jamieson, J.P.; Akinola, M. Optimizing stress: An integrated intervention for regulating stress responses. *Emotion* **2020**, *20*, 120–125. [CrossRef] [PubMed]
17. Layachi, A.; Schuelka, M.J. The impact of the COVID-19 related school closure on the mental health and well-being of children with SEN and their parents in Algeria. *Int. J. Disabil. Dev. Educ.* **2022**, *71*, 24–41. [CrossRef]
18. Thorell, L.B.; Skoglund, C.; De La Peña, A.G.; Baeyens, D.; Fuermaier, A.B.M.; Groom, M.J.; Mammarella, I.C.; Van Der Oord, S.; Hoofdakker, B.J.V.D.; Luman, M.; et al. Parental experiences of homeschooling during the COVID-19 pandemic: Differences between seven European countries and between children with and without mental health conditions. *Eur. Child Adolesc. Psychiatry* **2021**, *31*, 649–661. [CrossRef] [PubMed]
19. Zheng, X.; Zhang, D.; Lau, E.N.; Xu, Z.; Zhang, Z.; Mo, P.K.; Yang, X.; Mak, E.C.; Wong, S.Y. Primary school students' online learning during coronavirus disease 2019: Factors associated with satisfaction, perceived effectiveness, and preference. *Front. Psychol.* **2022**, *13*, 784826. [CrossRef]
20. Andrew, A.; Cattan, S.; Costa Dias, M.; Farquharson, C.; Kraftman, L.; Krutikova, S.; Phimister, A.; Sevilla, A. Inequalities in children's experiences of home learning during the COVID-19 lockdown in England. *Fisc. Stud.* **2020**, *41*, 653–683. [CrossRef]
21. McClain, C.; Vogels, E.A.; Perrin, A.; Sechopoulos, S.; Rainie, L. *The Internet and the Pandemic. Internet, Science & Technology*; Pew Research Center: Washington, DC, USA, 28 April 2022; Available online: https://www.pewresearch.org/internet/2021/09/01/the-internet-and-the-pandemic/ (accessed on 24 October 2022).
22. Catalyst. The Impact of COVID-19 on Working Parents (Report). 29 September 2020. Available online: https://www.catalyst.org/research/impact-covid-working-parents/ (accessed on 2 April 2023).
23. Marcus, J. The effect of unemployment on the mental health of spouses—Evidence from plant closures in Germany. *J. Health Econ.* **2013**, *32*, 546–558. [CrossRef]
24. Mooi-Reci, I.; Wooden, M. Jobless parents, unhealthy children? How past exposure to parental joblessness influences children's future health. *SSM—Popul. Health* **2022**, *19*, 101144. [CrossRef]
25. Dong, C.; Cao, S.; Li, H. Young children's online learning during COVID-19 pandemic: Chinese parents' beliefs and attitudes. *Child. Youth Serv. Rev.* **2020**, *118*, 105440. [CrossRef]
26. Fiese, B.H.; Tomcho, T.J.; Douglas, M.; Josephs, K.; Poltrock, S.; Baker, T. A review of 50 years of research on naturally occurring family routines and rituals: Cause for celebration? *J. Fam. Psychol.* **2002**, *16*, 381–390. [CrossRef]
27. Lee, J. Mental health effects of school closures during COVID-19. *Lancet Child Adolesc. Health* **2020**, *4*, 421. [CrossRef]
28. Gallagher-Mackay, K.; Srivastava, P.; Underwood, K.; Dhuey, E.; McCready, L.; Born, K.B.; Maltsev, A.; Perkhun, A.; Steiner, R.; Barrett, K.; et al. COVID-19 and education disruption in Ontario: Emerging evidence on impacts. In *Law and Society Faculty Publications*; Wilfrid Laurier University Press: Waterloo, ON, Canada, 2021.
29. Dawson, T. Some Canadian Schools Were Shut More than 135 Days for COVID, and Students Suffered: Study. *National Post*. 7 September 2023. Available online: https://nationalpost.com/news/canada/canadian-schools-covid-closures (accessed on 2 April 2023).
30. Evans, S.; Mikocka-Walus, A.; Klas, A.; Olive, L.; Sciberras, E.; Karantzas, G.; Westrupp, E.M. From "it has stopped our lives" to "spending more time together has strengthened bonds": The varied experiences of Australian families during COVID-19. *Front. Psychol.* **2020**, *11*, 588667. [CrossRef] [PubMed]
31. Vaillancourt, T.; Brittain, H.; Krygsman, A.; Farrell, A.H.; Landon, S.; Pepler, D. School bullying before and during COVID-19: Results from a population-based randomized design. *Aggress. Behav.* **2021**, *47*, 557–569. [CrossRef] [PubMed]
32. Teacher Tapp. What Does Distance Learning Look Like in England? (And Where Will Teachers' Kids Be Today?). 23 March 2020. Available online: https://teachertapp.co.uk/what-does-distance-learning-look-like-in-england-and-where-will-teachers-kids-be-today/ (accessed on 29 October 2022).
33. Fontenelle-Tereshchuk, D. 'Homeschooling' and the COVID-19 crisis: The insights of parents on curriculum and remote learning. *Interchange* **2021**, *52*, 167–191. [CrossRef] [PubMed]
34. Calear, A.L.; McCallum, S.; Morse, A.R.; Banfield, M.; Gulliver, A.; Cherbuin, N.; Farrer, L.M.; Murray, K.; Harris, R.M.R.; Batterham, P.J. Psychosocial impacts of home-schooling on parents and caregivers during the COVID-19 pandemic. *BMC Public Health* **2022**, *22*, 119. [CrossRef]
35. Islam, M.; Kim, D.-A.; Kwon, M. A comparison of two forms of instruction: Pre-recorded video lectures vs. live ZOOM lectures for education in the business management field. *Sustainability* **2020**, *12*, 8149. [CrossRef]
36. Le, K. Pre-recorded lectures, live online lectures, and student academic achievement. *Sustainability* **2022**, *14*, 2910. [CrossRef]
37. Onstad, K. The Miserable Truth about Online School. 19 February 2021. Available online: https://torontolife.com/city/the-miserable-truth-about-online-school/ (accessed on 4 April 2023).
38. New Zealand Government. 2022 Learning from Home Packs. 2022. Available online: https://learningfromhome.govt.nz/2022-learning-packs (accessed on 4 April 2023).
39. Rønning, M. Who benefits from homework assignments? *Econ. Educ. Rev.* **2011**, *30*, 55–64. [CrossRef]

40. Topping, K.; Samuels, J.; Paul, T. Does practice make perfect? Independent reading quantity, quality and student achievement. *Learn. Instr.* **2007**, *17*, 253–264. [CrossRef]
41. Saha, A.; Dutta, A.; Sifat, R.I. The mental impact of digital divide due to COVID-19 pandemic induced emergency online learning at undergraduate level: Evidence from undergraduate students from Dhaka City. *J. Affect. Disord.* **2021**, *294*, 170–179. [CrossRef]
42. Government of Canada. *Communications Monitoring Report*; CRTC: Ottawa, ON, Canada, 10 December 2020; Available online: https://crtc.gc.ca/eng/publications/reports/policyMonitoring/2020/cmr4.htm (accessed on 2 April 2023).
43. Kamaşak, T.; Topbaş, M.; Ozen, N.; Esenülkü, G.; Yıldız, N.; Şahin, S.; Arslan, E.A.; Çil, E.; Kart, P.; Cansu, A. An investigation of changing attitudes and behaviors and problematic internet use in children aged 8 to 17 years during the COVID-19 pandemic. *Clin. Pediatr.* **2021**, *61*, 194–205. [CrossRef]
44. Toombs, E.; Mushquash, C.J.; Mah, L.; Short, K.; Young, N.L.; Cheng, C.; Zhu, L.; Strudwick, G.; Birken, C.; Hopkins, J.; et al. Increased Screen Time for Children and Youth during the COVID-19 Pandemic. In *Science Brief of the Ontario COVID-19 Science Advisory Table*; 2022; Volume 3, The Ontario COVID-19 Science Advisory Table: Toronto, ON, Canada. [CrossRef]
45. Zeman, K.; McLeish, S. *School Closures and COVID-19: Interactive Tool*; Government of Canada, Statistics Canada: Ottawa, ON, Canada, 2021. Available online: https://www150.statcan.gc.ca/n1/pub/71-607-x/71-607-x2021009-eng.htm (accessed on 23 October 2022).
46. Murphy, G.C.; Athanasou, J.A. The effect of unemployment on Mental Health. *J. Occup. Organ. Psychol.* **1999**, *72*, 83–99. [CrossRef]
47. Institute for Work & Health. Unemployment and Mental Health. August 2009. Available online: https://www.iwh.on.ca/summaries/issue-briefing/unemployment-and-mental-health (accessed on 4 April 2023).
48. Powdthavee, N.; Vernoit, J. Parental unemployment and children's happiness: A longitudinal study of young people's well-being in unemployed households. *Labour Econ.* **2013**, *24*, 253–263. [CrossRef]
49. Wang, M.-T.; Henry, D.A.; Del Toro, J.; Scanlon, C.L.; Schall, J.D. Covid-19 employment status, Dyadic family relationships, and child psychological well-being. *J. Adolesc. Health* **2021**, *69*, 705–712. [CrossRef] [PubMed]
50. Goodman, A.; Lamping, D.L.; Ploubidis, G.B. When to use broader internalising and externalizing subscales instead of the hypothesised five subscales on the Strengths and Difficulties Questionnaire (SDQ): Data from British parents, teachers and children. *J. Abnorm. Child Psychol.* **2010**, *38*, 1179–1191. [CrossRef] [PubMed]
51. Racine, N.; Korczak, D.J.; Madigan, S. Evidence suggests children are being left behind in COVID-19 mental health research. *Eur. Child Adolesc. Psychiatry* **2020**, *31*, 1479–1480. [CrossRef] [PubMed]
52. UNESCO. UNESCO Web Archive. 14 January 2020. Available online: https://www.unesco.org/en/archives (accessed on 26 November 2022).
53. Goodman, R. Psychometric Properties of the Strengths and Difficulties Questionnaire. *J. Am. Acad. Child Adolesc. Psychiatry* **2001**, *40*, 1337–1345. [CrossRef]
54. Kroenke, K.; Spitzer, R.L.; Williams, J.B. The PHQ-9. *J. Gen. Intern. Med.* **2001**, *16*, 606–613. [CrossRef]
55. Hagen, A.E.F.; Rodriguez, L.M.; Neighbors, C.; Nogueira-Arjona, R.; Sherry, S.B.; Lambe, L.; Deacon, S.H.; Meier, S.; Abbass, A.; Stewart, S.H. Drinking to cope mediates the association between dyadic conflict and drinking behavior: A study of romantic couples during the COVID-19 pandemic. *Int. J. Environ. Res. Public Health* **2023**, *20*, 6332. [CrossRef]
56. Lambe, L.; Mackinnon, S.P.; Stewart, S.H. Dyadic conflict, drinking to cope, and alcohol-related problems: A psychometric study and longitudinal actor–partner interdependence model. *J. Fam. Psychol.* **2015**, *29*, 697–707. [CrossRef]
57. Spitzer, R.L.; Kroenke, K.; Williams, J.B.; Löwe, B. A brief measure for assessing generalized anxiety disorder. *Arch. Intern. Med.* **2006**, *166*, 1092–1097. [CrossRef]
58. Warttig, S.L.; Forshaw, M.J.; South, J.; White, A.K. New, normative, English-sample data for the short form perceived stress scale (PSS-4). *J. Health Psychol.* **2013**, *18*, 1617–1628. [CrossRef] [PubMed]
59. Karam, F.; Bérard, A.; Sheehy, O.; Huneau, M.-C.; Briggs, G.; Chambers, C.; Einarson, A.; Johnson, D.; Kao, K.; Koren, G.; et al. Reliability and validity of the 4-item perceived stress scale among pregnant women: Results from the Otis Antidepressants Study. *Res. Nurs. Health* **2012**, *35*, 363–375. [CrossRef]
60. Lemieux, T.; Milligan, K.; Schirle, T.; Skuterud, M. Initial Impacts of the COVID-19 Pandemic on the Canadian Labour Market. *Can. Public Policy* **2020**, *46* (Suppl. S1), S55–S65. [CrossRef]
61. Government of Canada, Statistics Canada. More than Half of Women Provide Care to Children and Care-Dependent Adults in Canada, 2022. *The Daily*. 8 November 2022. Available online: https://www150.statcan.gc.ca/n1/daily-quotidien/221108/dq221108b-eng.htm (accessed on 26 November 2022).
62. R Core Team. *R: A Language and Environment for Statistical Computing*; R Foundation for Statistical Computing: Vienna, Austria, 2022; Available online: https://www.R-project.org/ (accessed on 2 April 2023).
63. Kwak, S.G.; Kim, J.H. Central limit theorem: The cornerstone of modern statistics. *Korean J. Anesthesiol.* **2017**, *70*, 144–156. [CrossRef] [PubMed]
64. Schmidt, A.F.; Finan, C. Linear regression and the normality assumption. *J. Clin. Epidemiology* **2018**, *98*, 146–151. [CrossRef]
65. Hayes, A.F. *Introduction to Mediation, Moderation, and Conditional Process Analysis: A Regression-Based Approach*, 3rd ed.; The Guilford Press: New York, NY, USA, 2022.
66. Hayes, A.F.; Cai, L. Using heteroskedasticity-consistent standard error estimators in OLS regression: An introduction and software implementation. *Behav. Res. Methods* **2007**, *39*, 709–722. [CrossRef]

67. Hayes, A.F. The PROCESS Macro for SPSS, SAS, and R. Available online: https://www.processmacro.org/index.html (accessed on 2 April 2023).
68. Moon, K.-W. Welcome to Process R Shiny Apps. Available online: https://cardiomoon.shinyapps.io/processR/ (accessed on 14 November 2022).
69. Glynn, L.M.; Davis, E.P.; Luby, J.L.; Baram, T.Z.; Sandman, C.A. A predictable home environment may protect child mental health during the COVID-19 pandemic. *Neurobiol. Stress* **2021**, *14*, 100291. [CrossRef] [PubMed]
70. Taylor, S.; Landry, C.A.; Paluszek, M.M.; Fergus, T.A.; McKay, D.; Asmundson, G.J.G. COVID stress syndrome: Concept, structure, and correlates. *Depression Anxiety* **2020**, *37*, 706–714. [CrossRef] [PubMed]
71. Bilodeau, H.; Minnema, N.; Kehler, A. Internet Use and COVID-19: How the Pandemic Increased the Amount of Time Canadians Spend Online. 24 June 2021. Available online: https://www150.statcan.gc.ca/n1/pub/45-28-0001/2021001/article/00027-eng.htm (accessed on 4 April 2023).
72. McBain, R.K.; Cantor, J.; Pera, M.F.; Breslau, J.; Bravata, D.M.; Whaley, C.M. Mental health service utilization rates among commercially insured adults in the us during the first year of the COVID-19 pandemic. *JAMA Health Forum* **2023**, *4*, e224936. [CrossRef]
73. Chen, Y.-F.; Peng, S.S. University students' internet use and its relationships with academic performance, interpersonal relationships, psychosocial adjustment, and self-evaluation. *CyberPsychol. Behav.* **2008**, *11*, 467–469. [CrossRef]
74. El Asam, A.; Samara, M.; Terry, P. Problematic internet use and mental health among British children and adolescents. *Addict. Behav.* **2019**, *90*, 428–436. [CrossRef] [PubMed]
75. Vahedi, A.; Krug, I.; Westrupp, E.M. Crossover of parents' work-family conflict to family functioning and child mental health. *J. Appl. Dev. Psychol.* **2019**, *62*, 38–49. [CrossRef]
76. Hawrilenko, M.; Kroshus, E.; Tandon, P.; Christakis, D. The association between school closures and child mental health during COVID-19. *JAMA Netw. Open* **2021**, *4*, e2124092. [CrossRef] [PubMed]
77. Armstrong, R.A. When to use the Bonferroni correction. *Ophthalmic Physiol. Opt.* **2014**, *34*, 502–508. [CrossRef] [PubMed]
78. Chilcoat, H.D.; Breslau, N. Investigations of causal pathways between ptsd and drug use disorders. *Addict. Behav.* **1998**, *23*, 827–840. [CrossRef]
79. Hayes, A.F. *Introduction to Mediation, Moderation, and Conditional Process Analysis: A Regression-Based Approach*; Guilford: New York, NY, USA, 2017.
80. Statistics Canada. Guide to the Labour Force Survey. 7 September 2018. Available online: https://www150.statcan.gc.ca/n1/pub/71-543-g/71-543-g2018001-eng.htm (accessed on 4 April 2023).
81. Sleskova, M.; Salonna, F.; Geckova, A.M.; Nagyova, I.; Stewart, R.E.; van Dijk, J.P.; Groothoff, J.W. Does parental unemployment affect adolescents' health? *J. Adolesc. Health* **2006**, *38*, 527–535. [CrossRef]
82. Bettinger, E.; Hægeland, T.; Rege, M. Home with mom: The effects of stay-at-home parents on children's long-run educational outcomes. *J. Labor Econ.* **2014**, *32*, 443–467. [CrossRef]
83. Elgendi, M.M.; Stewart, S.H.; DesRoches, D.I.; Corkum, P.; Nogueira-Arjona, R.; Deacon, S.H. Division of labour and parental mental health and relationship well-being during COVID-19 pandemic-mandated homeschooling. *Int. J. Environ. Res. Public Health* **2022**, *19*, 17021. [CrossRef]
84. Lyttelton, T.; Zang, E.; Musick, K. Parents' work arrangements and gendered time use during the COVID-19 pandemic. *J. Marriage Fam.* **2022**, *85*, 657–673. [CrossRef]

MDPI AG
Grosspeteranlage 5
4052 Basel
Switzerland
Tel.: +41 61 683 77 34

Children Editorial Office
E-mail: children@mdpi.com
www.mdpi.com/journal/children

www.ingramcontent.com/pod-product-compliance
Lightning Source LLC
Chambersburg PA
CBHW061551210926
51850CB00009B/2073
9783725861613